Re e
A !

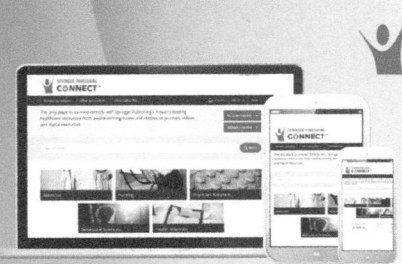

Your print purchase of *Evidence-Based Physical Examination Handbook, Second Edition,* **includes online access to the contents of your book**—increasing accessibility, portability, and searchability!

Access today at:
http://connect.springerpub.com/content/ book/978-0-8261-8852-6 or scan the QR code at the right with your smartphone. Log in or register, then click "Redeem a voucher" and use the code below.

7K64NRPF

Scan here for quick access.

Having trouble redeeming a voucher code?
Go to https://connect.springerpub.com/redeeming-voucher-code

If you are experiencing problems accessing the digital component of this product, please contact our customer service department at cs@springerpub.com

The online access with your print purchase is available at the publisher's discretion and may be removed at any time without notice.

Publisher's Note: New and used products purchased from third-party sellers are not guaranteed for quality, authenticity, or access to any included digital components.

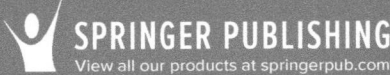

Evidence-Based Physical Examination
HANDBOOK

Kate Sustersic Gawlik, DNP, APRN-CNP, FAANP, FNAP, FAAN, is an associate professor of clinical nursing at The Ohio State University. She is certified by the American Nurses Credentialing Center as a family nurse practitioner. She has extensive background in primary care, with experience in family practice, college health, urgent care, and reproductive care. Her clinical interests are evidence-based practice, health professionals' education, population health, preventive care through lifestyle change, clinician well-being, wellness, parental burnout, and cardiovascular disease prevention. She currently serves as the director of Undergraduate Health and Wellness Academic Programming, codirector of the Health and Wellness in Healthcare program, and the project manager for the Million Hearts initiatives at Ohio State's College of Nursing. She has received multiple awards for her clinical practice and teaching, including the 2018 American Association of Nurse Practitioner State Award for Excellence. Dr. Gawlik is a Fellow of the American Academy of Nurse Practitioners and of the National Academies of Practice. She has taught undergraduate, RN-BSN, and graduate nursing students and has taught advanced health assessment for over 15 years.

Bernadette Mazurek Melnyk, PhD, APRN-CNP, EBP-C, FAANP, FNAP, FAAN, is the Vice President for Health Promotion and is University Chief Wellness Officer at The Ohio State University. She is the Helene Fuld Health Trust Professor of Evidence-Based Practice with the Fuld National Institute for Evidence-based Practice at the College of Nursing, where she just finished a 12-year term as dean. Dr. Melnyk is also a professor of pediatrics and psychiatry at Ohio State's College of Medicine. Dr. Melnyk is a nationally/internationally recognized expert in evidence-based practice, intervention research, child and adolescent mental health, health and wellness, and clinician well-being, and is a frequent keynote speaker at national and international conferences. She has consulted with hundreds of healthcare systems and colleges throughout the nation and globe on how to improve quality of care and patient outcomes through implementing and sustaining evidence-based practice. Her record includes over $35 million of sponsored funding from federal agencies and foundations as principal investigator and over 520 publications along with seven books. Dr. Melnyk is an elected fellow of the National Academy of Medicine, the American Academy of Nursing, the National Academies of Practice, and the American Association of Nurse Practitioners. She currently serves as editor in chief of *Worldviews on Evidence-Based Nursing*. She served a 4-year term with the U.S. Preventive Services Task Force and the National Institute for Nursing Research Advisory Council and is a member of the National Quality Forum's (NQF) Behavioral Health Standing Committee, along with serving as vice-chair of the National Forum for Heart Disease and Stroke Prevention. She is a current member of the National Academy of Medicine's Action Collaborative on Clinician Well-Being and Resilience and is the founder and current president of the National Consortium for Building Healthy Academic Communities.

Alice M. Teall, DNP, APRN-CNP, NC-BC, FAANP, FNAP, is an associate clinical professor at The Ohio State University. She was a founding member of the College of Nursing's team delivering online education, and currently serves as the Director of Graduate Health and Wellness Academic Programming. Dr. Teall has received leadership, teaching, and practice awards, including the University Provost's Award for Distinguished Teaching and the American Association of Colleges of Nursing Award for Innovations in Professional Nursing Education. As a certified nurse practitioner and integrative nurse coach, her areas of expertise include clinician well-being, college health, primary care of at-risk youth and families, recovery from substance use disorder, and delivery of care by telehealth. Dr. Teall is a Fellow of the American Academy of Nurse Practitioners and of the National Academies of Practice.

Evidence-Based Physical Examination
HANDBOOK

SECOND EDITION

Kate Sustersic Gawlik
DNP, APRN-CNP, FAANP, FNAP, FAAN

Bernadette Mazurek Melnyk
PhD, APRN-CNP, EBP-C, FAANP, FNAP, FAAN

Alice M. Teall
DNP, APRN-CNP, NC-BC, FAANP, FNAP

Editors

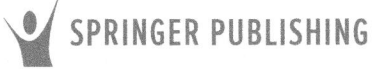

SPRINGER PUBLISHING

First Springer Publishing edition 978-0-8261-6465-0 (2022)

Springer Publishing Company, LLC
902 Carnegie Center/Suite 140, Princeton, NJ 08540
www.springerpub.com
connect.springerpub.com

Executive Acquisitions Editor: Joseph Morita
Director, Content Development: Taylor Ball
Production Manager: Kris Parrish
Compositor: S4Carlisle Publishing Services

ISBN: 978-0-8261-8851-9
ebook ISBN: 978-0-8261-8852-6
DOI: 10.1891/9780826188526

24 25 26 27 / 5 4 3 2 1

The author and the publisher of this Work have made every effort to use sources believed to be reliable to provide information that is accurate and compatible with the standards generally accepted at the time of publication. Because medical science is continually advancing, our knowledge base continues to expand. Therefore, as new information becomes available, changes in procedures become necessary. We recommend that the reader always consult current research and specific institutional policies before performing any clinical procedure or delivering any medication. The author and publisher shall not be liable for any special, consequential, or exemplary damages resulting, in whole or in part, from the readers' use of, or reliance on, the information contained in this book. The publisher has no responsibility for the persistence or accuracy of URLs for external or third-party Internet websites referred to in this publication and does not guarantee that any content on such websites is, or will remain, accurate or appropriate.

Library of Congress Cataloging-in-Publication Data

Names: Gawlik, Kate Sustersic, editor. | Melnyk, Bernadette Mazurek, editor. | Teall, Alice M., editor.
Title: Evidence-based physical examination handbook / Kate Sustersic Gawlik, DNP, APRN-CNP, FAANP, FNAP, FAAN, Bernadette Mazurek Melnyk, PhD, APRN-CNP, EBP-C, FAANP, FNAP, FAAN, Alice M. Teall, DNP, APRN-CNP, NC-BC, FAANP, FNAP, editors.
Description: Second edition. | New York, NY : Springer Publishing Company, LLC, [2025] | Includes bibliographical references and index.
Other titles: Handbook
Identifiers: LCCN 2023046048 (print) | LCCN 2023046049 (ebook) | ISBN 9780826188519 | ISBN 9780826188526 (ebook)
Subjects: LCSH: Physical diagnosis. | MESH: Physical Examination—methods | Evidence-Based Medicine | Handbook
Classification: LCC RC76 .E96 2024 (print) | LCC RC76 (ebook) | DDC 616.07/54—dc23/eng/20231213

LC record available at https://lccn.loc.gov/2023046048
LC ebook record available at https://lccn.loc.gov/2023046049

Contact sales@springerpub.com to receive discount rates on bulk purchases.

Publisher's Note: **New and used products purchased from third-party sellers are not guaranteed for quality, authenticity, or access to any included digital components.**

Printed in the United States of America.

To all of the health science students and practicing clinicians
who use this handbook to study, refresh, and renew their
skills, thank you for demonstrating a willingness to learn and
for your dedication to providing the best, evidence-based,
patient-centered care for individuals, families, communities,
and populations. You make us proud.

Contents

Abbreviations   Inside front and back covers
Contributors   xi
Preface   xv

1. Evidence-Based History Taking   1

2. Evidence-Based General Survey Including Vital Signs   11

3. Evidence-Based Assessment of the
   Heart and Vascular System   35

4. Evidence-Based Assessment of the Lungs
   and Respiratory System   66

5. Evidence-Based Assessment of the Skin, Hair, and Nails   87

6. Evidence-Based Assessment of the Lymphatic System   117

7. Evidence-Based Assessment of the Head and Neck   130

8. Evidence-Based Assessment of the Eyes   145

9. Evidence-Based Assessment of the
   Ears, Nose, and Throat   169

10. Evidence-Based Assessment of the Neurologic System   194

11. Evidence-Based Assessment of the Musculoskeletal
    System   222

12. Evidence-Based Assessment of the Abdomen and
    Gastrointestinal and Urological Systems   260

13. Evidence-Based Assessment of the Male
    Genitalia, Prostate, Rectum, and Anus   289

14. **Evidence-Based Assessment of the Breasts, Female Genitalia, and Reproductive System** 309

15. **Evidence-Based Obstetric Assessment** 343

16. **Evidence-Based Assessment of Mental Health Including Substance Use Disorders** 363

17. **Evidence-Based Considerations for Assessment Across the Life Span** 393

Index 421

Contributors

Barbara K. Bailes, EdD, RN, CS, NP-C
Associate Professor
Department of Graduate Studies
Cizik School of Nursing
University of Texas Health Science Center
Houston, Texas

Sherry Bumpus, PhD, FNP-BC
Special Associate to the Provost and Associate Professor of Nursing
Eastern Michigan University
Ypsilanti, Michigan

Amber Carriveau, DNP, FNP-BC, NCMP
DNP Program Director
College of Nursing and Health Sciences
United States University
San Diego, California

Kelly Casler, DNP, APRN, FNP-BC, EBP-C
Assistant Professor of Clinical Practice
College of Nursing
The Ohio State University
Columbus, Ohio

Maria Colandrea, DNP, NP-C, CORLN, CCRN, FAANP
Clinical Consulting Associate
Department of Otolaryngology
Duke School of Nursing
Durham VA Medical Center
Durham, North Carolina

Jennifer Dush, PhD, APRN-CNP
Assistant Clinical Professor
College of Nursing
The Ohio State University
Columbus, Ohio

Kristie L. Flamm, DNP, FNP-BC, ACNP-BC, FAANP
Clinical Assistant Professor
College of Nursing
University of Arizona
Tucson, Arizona

Kate Sustersic Gawlik, DNP, APRN-CNP, FAANP, FNAP, FAAN
Associate Professor of Clinical Nursing
College of Nursing
The Ohio State University
Columbus, Ohio

Retha D. Gentry, DNP, FNP-C
Assistant Professor
College of Nursing Graduate Programs
East Tennessee State University
Johnson City, Tennessee

Brenda M. Gilmore, DNP, CNM, FNP-BC, CNE, NCMP
Assistant Professor
College of Nursing
University of South Florida
Tampa, Florida

Matthew R. Granger, MS, FNP-BC
Adjunct Instructor of Clinical Practice
College of Nursing
The Ohio State University
Columbus, Ohio

Brittany B. Hay, DNP, APRN, ANP-BC, FNP-BC
Assistant Professor
College of Nursing
University of South Florida
Tampa, Florida

Shannon L. Linder, DNP, APRN-CNP, FNP-BC, PMHNP-BC
Clinical Assistant Professor of Practice
College of Nursing
The Ohio State University
Columbus, Ohio

Bernadette Mazurek Melnyk, PhD, APRN-CNP, EBP-C, FAANP, FNAP, FAAN
Vice President for Health Promotion
University Chief Wellness Officer
Dean and Helene Fuld Health Trust Professor of Evidence-Based Practice, College of Nursing Professor of Pediatrics and Psychiatry, College of Medicine
Executive Director, the Helene Fuld Health Trust Institute for Evidence-Based Practice in Nursing and Healthcare College of Nursing
The Ohio State University
Columbus, Ohio

Emily Neiman, MS, ARPN-CNM, C-EFM, FACNM
Instructor of Clinical Practice
College of Nursing
The Ohio State University
Columbus, Ohio

Lisa Ousley, DNP, FNP-C
Associate Professor
Department of Nursing
University of North Georgia
Dahlonega, Georgia
Faculty Emeritus
College of Nursing Graduate Programs
East Tennessee State University
Johnson City, Tennessee

Eileen M. Raynor, MD, FACS, FAAP
Associate Professor Pediatric Otolaryngology
Duke Head and Neck Surgery & Communication Sciences
Duke University School of Medicine
Durham, North Carolina

Katie Roll, APRN-CNP
Certified Nurse Practitioner
The Ohio State University Wexner Medical Center
Columbus, Ohio

Kathleen L. Siders, DNP, APRN, FNP-C
Associate Professor
Department of Graduate Studies
Cizik School of Nursing
University of Texas Health Science Center
Houston, Texas

Leigh Small, PhD, RN, CPNP-PC, FNAP, FAANP, FAAN
Dean and Professor
College of Nursing
Michigan State University
East Lansing, Michigan

Zach Stutzman, MS, PA-C, ATC
Department of Orthopaedic Surgery
Northwestern Medicine Regional Medical Group
Glen Ellyn, Illinois

Alice M. Teall, DNP, APRN-CNP, NC-BC, FAANP, FNAP
Associate Clinical Professor
College of Nursing
The Ohio State University
Columbus, Ohio

Kathryn Tierney, MSN, APRN, FNP-BC
Family Nurse Practitioner
Middlesex Health
Middletown, Connecticut

Rosie Zeno, DNP, APRN-CNP, CPNP-PC
Associate Professor of Clinical Practice
College of Nursing
The Ohio State University
Columbus, Ohio

Preface

> *I have no special talent. I am only passionately curious.*
> —Albert Einstein

Evidence-Based Physical Examination Handbook, Second Edition, was developed as a guide to the strategies and best practices needed by clinicians to assess an individual's health and well-being. This handbook is intended to be used by a broad audience of health science students and clinicians across disciplines who strive to exemplify excellence in evidence-based assessment and practice.

The overall goal of the handbook is to provide a practical, scientific, and holistic approach to assessment, in a summarized format that provides ease of access to students and clinicians while in lab and clinical settings. Additional goals of this text include the following:

- To promote evidence-based assessment to ensure that clinicians are using valid and reliable examination methods in which to base future decision-making
- To incorporate physical and mental dimensions of wellness, social determinants of health, prevention, and self-care needs into assessment in a manner that respects an individual's personal perspectives, family, and community
- To provide information on specific assessment skills that are often overlooked or misunderstood
- To summarize abnormal subjective (history) and objective (physical exam) findings for common disease states across the life span
- To ensure that clinicians are able to conduct a self-assessment of their own personal health and wellness

Learning to effectively assess the health and well-being of an individual involves integrating skills of history taking, physical examination, and diagnostic decision-making within the context of patient-centered, culturally sensitive, evidence-based clinical practice. Each chapter of *Evidence-Based Physical Examination Handbook* begins with priority clinical considerations. The first two chapters review evidence-based approaches to assessment—the importance of history taking and the approach to general survey. Chapters 3 to 12 review assessment priorities and common diagnoses relative to specific body systems. Chapters 13 to 15 focus on assessments related to sexual and reproductive health and obstetric assessment. Chapter 16 focuses on mental status and mental health. Chapter 17 outlines key considerations for assessment across the life span, with a focus on children, adolescents, and older adults.

The second edition of *Evidence-Based Physical Examination Handbook* incorporates a broad understanding of wellness, presents evidence-based recommendations for history taking, reviews the physical examination components required to inform clinical decision-making, and lists the findings that are generally associated with differential diagnoses. Only with evidence-based assessment can a clinician ensure patient safety and high-quality, cost-effective care. The valid, reliable assessment techniques and approaches in this text are intended to prepare clinicians to deliver evidence-based, safe, quality clinical care.

Kate Sustersic Gawlik
Bernadette Mazurek Melnyk
Alice M. Teall

1

Evidence-Based History Taking

CLINICAL CONSIDERATIONS

- Individuals seek visits with clinicians to address episodic concerns, manage chronic illnesses, maintain wellness, or follow up from previous visits. During these visits, clinicians assess a patient's history and obtain subjective information.
- A thorough patient history consists of the chief concern (CC) or reason for seeking care; history of present illness (HPI); past medical history, including medication and allergy history; family history; social history; and review of systems (ROS).
- Although objective assessments can be made during history taking, the data gathered are primarily subjective (i.e., information reported, experienced, or understood by the patient).
- One of the most important priorities for evidence-based care is establishment of therapeutic rapport, which begins with active listening. Listening and responding empathetically to an individual's history serves to establish trust. Active listening requires the clinician to eliminate distractions and focus on an individual's verbal and nonverbal communication.

HISTORY TAKING FOR AN EPISODIC VISIT

- The episodic visit, scheduled for a recent, bothersome, acute, urgent, or emergent health problem, accounts for the majority of clinician visits.
- Episodic visits focus on a specific concern of the patient. The patient can be either an established patient or a new patient.
- For an episodic visit, the extent of the history collected is variable, based on the clinician's judgment and the patient's presenting symptoms. For new patients, a comprehensive health history should be conducted. For established patients, a more limited health history is collected, tailored to the CC.
- The following sections provide the general framework for the elements of history taking during an episodic visit. To begin the visit, the clinician introduces themselves, confirms the patient's identity, and washes their hands.

CHIEF CONCERN OR REASON FOR SEEKING CARE

- History taking begins with clarifying the patient's main reason for the visit. Clarifying an individual's CC is a priority.
- The CC is the description of the symptom, problem, condition, diagnosis, or reason for seeking care. Often, documentation of the CC is in the patient's own words—for example, "my left elbow hurts."

HISTORY OF PRESENT ILLNESS

- The HPI provides key information required for developing differential diagnoses, determining a diagnosis, and guiding treatment. Often, a diagnosis can be made from the history alone, so this step is crucial.
- In the HPI, the patient provides detailed reasons for the visit and describes how the illness has progressed. Allow the patient to tell the story about their concerns in their own words, including their perception of the illness or health problem. The HPI contains eight core elements to assess, summarized with the mnemonic OLDCARTS:
  - ○ **Onset:** When did the symptoms start? Are the symptoms recent? How did the symptoms begin?
  - ○ **Location:** Specific location of the symptoms? Do the symptoms move or spread to other areas of the body?
  - ○ **Duration:** Are the symptoms persistent or transitory? Increasing or unchanged?
  - ○ **Characteristics:** How would you describe the symptoms? Is there itching, burning, drainage, pain, swelling, bruising, or redness? How does the symptom feel (e.g., sharp, dull, stabbing, burning, crushing, throbbing, nauseating, shooting, twisting, or stretching)?
  - ○ **Aggravating factors:** What actions or activities may have triggered the symptoms or caused them to worsen?
  - ○ **Relieving factors:** What actions or activities decrease the symptoms? What medications have been taken to help with the symptoms? (Note that treatment may be listed as a distinct component of the HPI.)
  - ○ **Temporal factors/timing:** How do the symptoms respond to treatment, relieving factors, situations, or conditions? Are the symptoms constant? How have the symptoms changed over time?
  - ○ **Severity:** How severe are the symptoms on a scale of 0 to 10? Do the symptoms limit participation in activities at school/work/home?

PAST MEDICAL HISTORY

- Also referred to as history of illness, health history, or past medical and surgical history, the assessment of past medical history is important to obtain and review during all visits; even when established patients follow up with clinicians, their health history should be updated.

- Assessment includes asking the patient about their experiences with illnesses, both acute and chronic (may include pertinent childhood illnesses), hospitalizations, surgeries, sexual/reproductive health issues, and hereditary conditions that could place the patient at risk.
- When asking health history questions, review all current medications, prescribed, over-the-counter (OTC), and/or herbal; when an individual shares history of allergies, ask specifics about their reaction to the allergens.
- The following are the components of a past medical history:
  ○ **History of physical or mental health conditions:** Ask whether ever diagnosed with specific conditions (e.g., heart disease, elevated blood pressure, cancer, diabetes, depression, arthritis, asthma); clarify whether the conditions are current or past health problems.
  ○ **History of hospitalizations and surgeries:** Clarify reason and dates.
  ○ **Recent changes in health:** Ask about recent illness, accidents, injuries, or exposures, as well as ED or urgent care visits.
  ○ **Immunization status**: Clarify dates and record of vaccines.
  ○ **Individualized health considerations:** Ask about sexual and reproductive health history (menstrual, gynecologic, obstetric, gender identity, sexual orientation concerns), pediatric health history (birth history, growth, development), and older adult health history (polypharmacy, history of falls, functional and cognitive status).
  ○ **Medications:** Ask about prescribed and OTC medications and supplements, including dose and frequency.
  ○ **Allergies:** Ask about allergies to medications, or seasonal, environmental, and/or food allergies, including reactions.

FAMILY HISTORY

- Family history is the review of the immediate family members' history related to medical events, illnesses, and hereditary conditions that place the patient's current and future health at risk.
- Immediate family includes parents, grandparents, siblings, children, and grandchildren.
- As details are provided during the family history, inquire whether the relative is alive or deceased. If the person is deceased, ask about the age at death and the cause of death, especially for first-degree relatives.
- Assess for the following during family history:
  ○ **Chronic diseases:** Hypertension, heart disease, obesity, diabetes, cancer, epilepsy, and asthma

- ○ **Acute or recent episodic illnesses:** Infectious diseases, allergies, and environmental exposures
- ○ **Mental health disorders:** Anxiety, depression, bipolar disorder, severe and persistent mental illness, substance use disorders, and developmental delays
- ○ **Genetic or hereditary conditions**
- Family history provides valuable insight into an individual's health risks and allows clinicians to assess risks for certain diseases, such as cancer, heart disease, or inherited disorders. Family history can identify red flags that may warrant further investigation or testing, and supports recommendations for referrals that may include genetic counseling (**Box 1.1**). Assessing family history provides the foundation for understanding personalized risk for diseases caused by a single gene (genetics) or for recognizing complex diseases caused by multiple genes and environmental factors (genomics).

SOCIAL HISTORY

- Social history provides information regarding one's health beliefs and behaviors, including support systems; it also allows the clinician to identify risk factors that may impact well-being. Note that the influence of culture on health beliefs, behaviors, practices, perceptions, and approaches is vast; this component of history requires a sensitive and humble approach that respects cultural, family, community, and personal values and norms. The following are the components of social history:
  - ○ Substance use history
    - ♦ Tobacco use in any form (pipe, snuff, chewing tobacco, e-cigarettes, hookah, vaping, cigars, cigarettes)? If yes, assess smoking history and readiness to quit.
    - ♦ Alcohol use? If yes, screen for binge drinking and problematic use.

BOX 1.1 Red Flags in Subjective History
That Indicate a Need for Genetic Counseling

- Early age of onset (<50 years)
- Rare cancers (e.g., male breast cancer, retinoblastoma)
- Cancer diagnosis or related cancers in more than one generation or more than one individual; cancer occurs in every generation
- Paired cancers in a family, including breast, ovarian, prostate, colon, melanoma, pancreatic, or other cancers
- Bilateral cancer, or multiple primary cancers in one individual
- Predisposition to certain genetic disorders (e.g., Ashkenazi Jewish ancestry or known family genetic mutation)

- - Other substances (e.g., medications not prescribed, illicit drugs)?
    - Ask whether the patient has ever taken medications not specifically prescribed for them.
    - Ask whether the patient has ever taken substance for how it would make them feel.
  - Relationships, including marital status, and living arrangements
    - Family dynamics
    - Friends and social support system
    - Strengths, including spiritual, religious, and ethnic/cultural support systems
    - History of trauma, victim of violence, and adverse childhood events
  - Safety of home, work, and/or school environments
    - Ask about exposure to hazards (e.g., fumes, radiation, chemicals, viruses).
    - Ask about risk or current exposure to violence, trauma, and stressors.
    - Ask about behaviors involving risk-taking and risk of falls.
    - Ask about safe participation in sports and physical activities.
    - Screen for use of seat belts and bicycle/motorcycle helmets.
    - Screen for smoke detectors in the home.
    - Screen for access to guns in the home, neighborhood, and at work.
    - Assess social determinants of health.

Social Determinants of Health

Asking about the environments in which an individual resides, works, learns, plays, worships, and connects socially offers important insight into the determinants of their health. Key areas to consider related to the determinants that impact an individual's health include the following:

- **Economic stability:** Access to employment, career counseling, and high-quality childcare; access to resources to meet daily needs, including food
- **Neighborhood and built environment:** Access to safe, affordable housing in the neighborhood without exposure to violence, toxic substances, or other safety hazards
- **Healthcare access and quality:** Availability of quality healthcare services; access to clinicians with linguistic and cultural competency; access to insurance coverage and care meeting health literacy needs
- **Social and community context:** Availability of resources and support within communities for recreation, worship, work, learning, and meeting basic needs; experiences of discrimination, isolation, bullying, and loss
- **Education access and quality:** Access to quality education, including early childhood education; broadband access to internet and emerging technologies

PREVENTIVE CARE CONSIDERATIONS

Assess an individual's participation in behaviors that prevent disease and illness.

- Healthy lifestyle behaviors, including diet/nutrition, physical activity/exercise, and sleep
- Management of stress and coping with stressors
- Recent/needed health screenings based on age, medical history, and family history

REVIEW OF SYSTEMS

- ROS is the inventory of symptoms obtained by a series of questions that are organized by body systems.
- ROS offers essential information about current/potential disease processes or health problems that may otherwise go unnoticed.
- ROS includes pertinent positive and negative findings. Important: ROS is a subjective information provided by the patient, and not the clinician's observation or findings.
- Clinicians choose the depth of the ROS based on the acuity of the individual presenting to them, whether the patient is established or new, and according to the level of diagnostic decision-making that is required during a visit. ROS can be focused, extended, or complete. The following are examples of ROS history questions:
  - **General/constitutional:** Weight gain or loss? Unusual fatigue? Changes in sleep pattern? Night sweats? Fevers? Frequent infections? Difficulty in recovering from illnesses?
  - **Integumentary:** Lesions or rashes? Changes in skin, hair, nails? Itching? Changes in moles?
  - **Head, neck:** Headaches? Neck pain? Recent head trauma or falls? History of concussion, loss of consciousness, or head injury?
  - **Lymphatic/hematologic:** Swollen or tender lymph nodes? Bruise or bleed easily?
  - **Eyes, ears, nose, and throat:** Eye drainage or redness? Vision changes? Itchy eyes/ears/nose? Ear pain? Hearing loss? Rhinorrhea or congestion? Sinus pressure or pain? Sore throat? Trouble chewing or swallowing? Bleeding gums? Dental pain? Painful or painless sores in mouth or throat?
  - **Cardiovascular:** Chest pain? Palpitations? Exercise intolerance? Orthopnea? Edema?
  - **Respiratory:** Cough? Dyspnea or shortness of breath? Wheezing? Hemoptysis? Snoring?
  - **Breast/chest:** Tenderness? Palpable lumps or masses? Skin changes or discharge?
  - **Gastrointestinal:** Abdominal pain? Change in bowel habits? Blood in the stool? Nausea? Vomiting? Heartburn? Change in appetite?

- ○ **Genitourinary:** Urinary frequency? Pain with urination? Nocturia? Urgency? Hematuria? Unusual discharge or odor? Pelvic or groin pain? Dyspareunia?
- ○ **Musculoskeletal:** Back pain? Muscle aches? Joint swelling? Limitations of function?
- ○ **Neurologic:** Numbness or tingling? Syncope? Memory loss? Restlessness? Changing level of consciousness? Loss of coordination? Tremors?
- ○ **Endocrine:** Increased thirst? Heat or cold intolerance? Thyroid tenderness or enlargement?
- ○ **Psychiatric/mental health:** Worry? Nervous or anxious? Sadness, helplessness, hopelessness? Insomnia? Change in mood? Irritability? Difficulty coping with stress? Trouble concentrating? Previous or current thoughts of harm to self or others?

HISTORY TAKING FOR A WELLNESS EXAM

KEY CONSIDERATIONS

- Wellness exams can be an important health promotion and disease prevention strategy; goals include early identification of health risks and/or detection of health problems.
- Sports physicals, well-child exams, work physicals, and annual exams are examples of wellness exams; these visits require age- and gender-appropriate history and physical exam.
- Because patient history taking during wellness exams is not problem-oriented, the history will not include a CC, although the reason for the visit can be listed. In addition, there is not likely to be a need to collect HPI. Rather, a wellness exam should include a comprehensive history and physical examination appropriate to the patient's age and sex, counseling and anticipatory guidance, risk reduction interventions, ordering or administration of vaccine-appropriate immunizations, and ordering of appropriate laboratory and/or diagnostic testing.
- The wellness exam differs from the episodic visit and chronic care management visit because the components of the wellness exam are based on age and risk factors, not a presenting problem.

COMPONENTS OF WELLNESS EXAMS

- Patient history, that is, past medical history, family history, social history, preventive health practices, and ROS
- Physical exam, including general survey and additional components, informed by patient history, age (e.g., child or older adult), and clinician judgment
- Anticipatory guidance regarding risks to health and wellness, and developmental and safety needs

- Evidence-based recommendations for immunizations, screenings, and diagnostic testing
- Health counseling or coaching for reaching health and wellness goals

HISTORY TAKING AND CHRONIC CARE MANAGEMENT

KEY CONSIDERATIONS FOR CHRONIC CARE MANAGEMENT VISITS

- More than half of all adults in the United States have a chronic condition; chronic diseases are among the leading causes of death and disability.
- Common chronic diseases include heart disease, cancer, chronic lung disease, stroke, Alzheimer disease, diabetes, arthritis, obesity, epilepsy, and chronic kidney disease.
- Having a chronic disease is associated with increased likelihood of depression, anxiety, isolation, fatigue, and disabilities.
- Key considerations regarding chronic disease management that are important for clinicians to prioritize include the following:
  - **Early detection and diagnosis:** This is critical to preventing or delaying progression of the disease. Regularly screen patients who are at risk.
  - **Patient-centered care:** Patients should be actively involved in their own care. Respect patient needs and preferences. Identify barriers to care. Prioritize partnership with patients, caregivers, and families.
  - **Multidisciplinary approach:** Involve healthcare professionals from different specialties, including primary care providers, specialists, nurses, social workers, dietitians, counselors, and pharmacists. Collaborative team-based care improves the quality, safety and reliability of care.
  - **Education and support:** Provide patients with resources to support self-management. Recognize health literacy needs and any misinformation. Offer support, health coaching, written educational materials, and digital tools appropriately.
  - **Care coordination:** Collaborate with other healthcare professionals to coordinate care and ensure that individuals with chronic conditions receive necessary screenings, testing, treatments, referrals, and follow-up care.
  - **Use of technology:** Technology can play a significant role in chronic disease management, from remote patient monitoring to telehealth visits. Recommend tools that can help improve patient outcomes and streamline care delivery.
  - **Social determinants of health:** Address determinants of health, such as housing and food insecurity. Assess barriers to care. Support community partnerships to increase access to care and health equity.

THERAPEUTIC COMMUNICATION

- Regardless of the type of patient visit, the goal during history taking is to be attentive to the patient and receptive to their needs.
- Conducting patient history requires patient-centered interviewing skills, which include skillful use of therapeutic communication. Therapeutic communication techniques include the following:
  - **Open-ended questions:** The use of open-ended questions allows the patient to express their concerns. Example: "You've reported you have shortness of breath, can you tell me more about that?"
  - **Active listening:** Providing an opportunity for an individual to share their history and concerns without interruption and with full engagement communicates nonverbally that what is being said is being heard. Example: The clinician nods their head and maintains eye contact while the patient is sharing the reason why they made the visit.
  - **Reflection:** The use of reflection demonstrates active listening and acknowledges the patient's response. Example: "I can see the news has been upsetting to you."
  - **Empathy:** The patient's emotions are central to effective decision-making. Affirming the patient's emotions demonstrates that the clinician appreciates how the patient is feeling. Example: "You are experiencing lots of changes in your health; it's understandable that this would be difficult to accept right now."
  - **Seeking clarification:** Asking follow-up questions to history statements is helpful in obtaining an accurate history and with establishing trust with the patient. Example: "You said that you were unable to quit smoking; tell me more about that."
  - **Summary or restatement:** Summarizing the patient's statement to demonstrate an understanding of their values and preferences allows the clinician to develop a partnership with the individual. Example: "I hear you say that you value your time with your family, and your preference is to receive treatment for your breast cancer."
- In each chapter of this text, history questions specific to each system are listed; many are specific to the patient's CC. The questions are intended to be asked in a confidential, sensitive manner and will reveal the patient's perspectives about health, wellness, and illness. As each chapter is reviewed, remember to spend time in self-reflection and consider how to sensitively ask and respond to patient assessments. Implementing evidence-based, patient-centered assessment requires sensitivity and openness to the patient's responses as specific details of their history and perspectives are shared.

REFERENCES

References for this chapter draw from Chapter 3, Evidence-Based History Taking, Approach to Patient Visits, and Documentation, and Chapter 4, Evidence-Based, Culturally Sensitive, Therapeutic Communication, of the textbook *Evidence-Based Physical Examination: Best Practices for Health and Well-Being Assessment (Second Edition).* The references may be accessed in the digital version of the handbook at connect.springerpub.com/content/book/https://connect.springerpub.com/.

2

Evidence-Based General Survey Including Vital Signs

CLINICAL CONSIDERATIONS

- Evidence-based assessment begins with observation. Skilled, systematic observation is essential for accurate clinical evaluation.
- The components of a general survey are primarily observational and include assessment of physiologic stability; observations of appearance, behavior, and mobility; a focused assessment of mental status; and measurement of vital signs.
- As a clinician approaches an individual to complete the general survey, they should first assess the situation to ensure their own personal safety and to note any risks related to completing the assessment. Immediate observations should include noting signs of anger or confusion in an individual, and an environmental assessment for exposures to toxins, chemicals, extreme heat, cold, electric currents, or infectious agents.
- Clinician considerations include whether gloves, gown, eye/face shield, or mask needs to be worn to avoid exposures and/or whether additional support is needed for a patient with an unstable mental status.

SUBJECTIVE HISTORY

COMMON REASONS FOR SEEKING CARE

- Evidence-based history and physical exam as a component of clinician visits for episodic concerns, follow-up, wellness, or chronic care management begins with a general survey.
- Urgent or emergent problems noted during a general survey include the following:
  - Syncope, loss of consciousness
  - Choking, wheezing, respiratory distress, hypoxia, tachypnea
  - Chest pain, dizziness, hypertension, hypotension, bradycardia, tachycardia
  - Pulselessness
  - Diaphoresis, cyanosis
  - Fever

○ Pain, whether acute, recurrent, episodic, or chronic
○ Underweight, overweight, obesity, weight gain, weight loss, malnutrition
○ Inattention, impulsivity, distraction, anxiety
○ Confusion, disorientation, depressed mood

INITIAL STEPS TO DETERMINE PHYSIOLOGIC STABILITY

- The initial assessments of a general survey are completed to determine whether the individual being evaluated is in distress. Observing whether the patient is well or unwell is essential and can be completed quickly.
- Use the ABCDE mnemonic to determine whether an individual has physiologic stability: **A**irway, **B**reathing, **C**irculation, **D**isability, **E**xposure.
- **Box 2.1** lists the red flags (signs and symptoms) for emergent or urgent medical problems.
- For the patient who is physiologically unstable, experiencing emergent distress, and is unconscious, unresponsive, or not breathing normally, the clinician should respond to the situation appropriately, which may require initiating CPR while continuing to assess.
- For the patient who is physiologically and functionally stable, the clinician's next steps include completing the history and physical exam.
- This chapter includes a significant review of vital signs, pain, and mental status, which are key assessments in determining patient stability and function. Subsequent chapters will review additional priority assessments, including signs and symptoms of respiratory distress, hypoxia, heart failure, and neurologic disorders.

BOX 2.1 Red Flags in Initial General Survey That May Indicate Physiologic Instability (Emergent Distress)

- **Airway:** Paradoxical chest and abdominal movements with respirations, cyanosis, diminished breath sounds, noisy breath sounds, wheezing, stridor
- **Breathing:** Wheezing, stridor, cyanosis, dyspnea, hypoxia, retractions, inability to speak in full sentences, apnea
- **Circulation:** Chest pain, dyspnea, bleeding, decreased perfusion, tachycardia, bradycardia, pulselessness
- **Disability:** Confusion, irritability, vomiting, seizure, loss of consciousness, nonresponsiveness, sudden change in neurologic status
- **Exposure:** Trauma that may have caused functional instability; panic, feelings of impending doom, restlessness

- Completing the initial general survey allows the clinician to determine an appropriate, subsequent history and physical exam.

HISTORY OF PRESENT ILLNESS

- **Onset:** When did the symptoms start? Did they occur suddenly, or have they been developing gradually? When did the patient or the caregiver first notice this problem?
- **Location:** Does the individual have pain or discomfort? If so, where is the discomfort located? Multiple sites?
- **Duration:** How long do the symptoms last? Are the symptoms worsening? Persistent?
- **Characteristics:** Describe the symptoms being experienced.
- **Aggravating factors:** What actions, activities, exposures, or positions make the symptoms worse? Is the problem associated with a particular activity, food, or place? Additional temporal factors, such as recent illness, infection, or travel?
- **Relieving factors:** What actions decrease the symptoms? If relieved, how long does the relief last?
- **Treatment:** What medications have been taken to help with the symptoms? Clarify the dosage and frequency of any medications.
- **Severity:** How severe are the symptoms on a scale of 0 to 10? Do the symptoms limit participation in activities, interrupt sleep, or impact work or school attendance? Are there associated symptoms? Is the individual feeling anxious or fearful?

HEALTH HISTORY

Past Medical History
- Chronic illnesses (physical, mental/behavioral)
- Recent injury, trauma; ED or urgent care visits
- Hospitalizations, surgeries

MEDICATIONS

- Prescribed and over-the-counter (OTC) medications or supplements, including dose and frequency

Allergies
- Are there allergies to medications, or seasonal, environmental, and/or food allergies? If "yes," clarify reactions.

Preventive Health Behaviors
- Physical activity and exercise
- Typical diet, access to fruits and vegetables, food handling and cooking
- Adequate sleep and rest

- Stress reduction/coping strategies
- Vaccine history

FAMILY HISTORY
- Chronic illnesses such as cardiac disease, hypertension, obesity, diabetes, cancer, epilepsy, and asthma
- Genetic disorders and developmental delays
- Mental health disorders such as anxiety, depression, bipolar disorder, attention deficit hyperactivity disorder (ADHD), and learning disorders
- Infectious diseases or immune disorders

SOCIAL HISTORY
- Home situation and relationships
  - Married/single/divorced/widowed/partnered?
  - Who lives in the home? Composition of family? Caregivers?
  - Substance use in the home?
  - Is housing/home/neighborhood safe?
  - Social support system? Close friends? Pets?
  - Sexual history (including risk factors for sexually transmitted illnesses)?
- Substance use
  - Smoking/vaping history/history of tobacco use/exposure to secondhand smoke?
  - Alcohol use? Times in the last year when more than four to five drinks were consumed in a day?
  - Other substances (e.g., medications not prescribed, illicit drugs)?
- Safety (including work or school environment)
  - Trauma history, including adverse childhood events, trauma, grief, isolation?
  - Risk or current victim of violence?
  - Stress, anxiety, depression/suicidal risk, burnout?
  - Financial or career concerns?

REVIEW OF SYSTEMS
- **General:** Fatigue, fever, weight changes, pain
- **Integumentary:** Dryness, itching, bruising, rashes, lesions, hair loss
- **Head, eyes, ears, nose, throat:** Headache, congestion, eye or ear pain, sore throat
- **Lymphatic:** Bruising, bleeding, lymphadenopathy
- **Cardiovascular:** Chest pain, shortness of breath, rapid pulse
- **Respiratory:** Dyspnea, wheezing, cough, breathlessness
- **Gastrointestinal/genitourinary:** Appetite changes, dysphagia, nausea, vomiting, constipation, diarrhea, abdominal pain, dysuria, pelvic pain

- **Mental health:** Sadness/depression, helplessness, hopelessness, suicidal ideation, worry, insomnia, hypersomnia; changes in memory, concentration, or mood
- **Neurologic:** Weakness, numbness, fainting, falls, dizziness, confusion

NUTRITIONAL ASSESSMENT

- While not routinely included in the general survey, the clinician may determine that a more in-depth assessment of nutritional status is needed, based on observations and the patient's reason for seeking care. The primary determinants of nutritional status are food and nutrient intake, which can be assessed by estimating the energy and protein intake of the individual. Estimates can be obtained through the history (e.g., verbal report, food diary, food tracking app) or, when feasible, by direct observation.
- There are many valid/reliable nutritional assessment tools for screening malnutrition in adults. The Malnutrition Screening Tool and the Mini Nutritional Assessment (www.mna-elderly.com/forms/mini/mna_mini_english.pdf) are two screening tools that should be considered if the patient presents with recent weight loss, recent poor intake/appetite, and/or a low body mass index (BMI). Both tools have high sensitivity and specificity.

ASSESSMENT OF PAIN

- While not routinely included in the general survey, the clinician may determine that a more in-depth assessment of pain is needed, based on observations and the patient's reason for seeking care. Verbalization of pain (subjective) is the most common way to assess pain. Although the patient may demonstrate nonverbal, objective signs that indicate pain (e.g., increases in heart rate, blood pressure [BP], respiratory rate), assessing subjective experience is best practice.
- Noting symptom characteristics and responsiveness to treatment allows the clinician to appreciate whether pain is nociceptive or neuropathic, somatic, or visceral.
  - **Neuropathic pain:** Results from within the nervous system; described as sharp, shooting, tingling, and burning; may respond poorly to traditional analgesic medications
  - **Nociceptive pain:** Usually responsive to medications, can be somatic or visceral
    - *Somatic pain* originates from the musculoskeletal tissue, is sharp or dull, and is usually well localized.
    - *Visceral pain* originates from the internal organs, is poorly localized, and is accompanied by symptoms of autonomic nervous system stimulation (nausea, vomiting, diaphoresis).

- Evidence-based tools are effective in assessing pain and monitoring response to treatment.
    - **Initial Pain Assessment Tool:** Eight questions regarding the onset, location, duration, quality, intensity, aggravating triggers, relieving factors, and effects of pain
    - **Numeric rating scales:** A number is chosen that best indicates current level of pain, with 0 being no pain and 10 being the worst pain that can be imagined
    - **Descriptor scales:** Keywords that describe different levels of pain intensity (e.g., no pain, moderate pain, severe pain)
    - **Visual Analog Scale:** Combines a numeric scale and descriptor words; uses a red-yellow-green color scheme depending on the level of pain
    - **Wong–Baker FACES Scale:** A series of faces with different expressions to demonstrate varying levels of pain; used for children who can verbalize their pain level but may not be able to correlate it with a number
- Understanding is crucial before attempting to use any self-reporting pain scale or tool. The commonly held belief that people overexaggerate their pain is prevalent and is unsupported by evidence.
- For younger children and older adults who are not developmentally or cognitively able to describe pain, be aware that interruptions in appetite, sleep, elimination, and/or activity may be indicators of pain intensity.

PHYSICAL EXAMINATION
- Assessment always begins with observation to determine whether the individual being evaluated is well or ill, and if ill whether they are experiencing distress.
- Review **Box 2.1** for signs and symptoms that require emergent or urgent action.
- Once the clinician has determined that the individual is not experiencing acute distress, the next steps involve observation of their appearance, behavior, and cognition. Much of these assessments are completed while the clinician assesses the patient's history; additional mental status assessments may also be considered part of the physical exam.

MENTAL STATUS ASSESSMENT
- An assessment of the individual's mental status provides the basis for identifying signs and/or symptoms related to their overall mental health functioning. The general survey includes assessment of appearance, behavior, and mobility; a focused mental status exam; and measurement of vital signs.
- Chapter 16, Evidence-Based Assessment of Mental Health Including Substance Use Disorders, contains information about

completing a comprehensive mental health exam, including interpretation of findings. A focused mental status exam can be remembered using the mnemonic ABSATTC, or All Best Students Are Taught to Care:

- **Appearance:** Eye contact, hygiene, dress, body habitus, posture
- **Behavior:** Verbal and nonverbal expressions, interactions toward the clinician or others, activity level, body movements and mobility
- **Speech:** Amount, rate, rhythm, volume, and tone; includes language
- **Affect:** Outward expressions of feelings, emotions, or mood
- **Thought process:** Flow of thoughts (may be coherent/incoherent, logical/illogical)
- **Thought content:** Ideas, concerns, and fears (may include obsessions, hallucinations)
- **Cognition:** Orientation to time, person, place, and situation; attention and concentration; judgment, memory, and insight

MEASUREMENT OF VITAL SIGNS

Measurement of Temperature

- There are multiple routes to measure temperature: oral, rectal, axillary, temporal artery, tympanic membrane, and infrared.
- Consider the advantages/disadvantages of each route when selecting the best method.
- Temperature elevation that is considered "abnormal" can depend on age, site of measurement, and clinical condition of the patient; in general, body temperature elevated above 100.4°F (38°C) rectally is considered a fever.
- The average body temperature is 98.6°F (37°C), with a normal range of 95.4°F to 99.3°F (35.2°C–37.4°C). Body temperature fluctuates 1°F to 1.5°F (0.6°C–0.9°C) over the course of a day, with temperature at its lowest early in the morning and highest in the evening.

Oral Temperature

- Oral temperature is generally considered a reliable means of measuring body temperature.
- The thermometer probe is positioned either in the right or left posterior sublingual pocket, which has a rich blood supply and offers an indirect reflection of core temperature.
- Ask the individual to close their mouth around the probe during measurement. Most electronic thermometers will alert with an audible tone once the body temperature is registered.
- Disposable sheaths or probe covers offer protection from transmission of infection between patients.

Rectal Temperature
- Rectal temperature is considered the best reflection of core temperature; however, it is used less frequently in practice because it is more invasive.
- Do not use oral thermometers rectally as these can cause injury. Rectal thermometers have a security bulb designed specifically for safely taking rectal temperatures.
- Place the patient in the Sims position. Lubricate the tip of the thermometer's probe cover. While wearing gloves, insert the thermometer probe 1 to 1½ inches into the adult rectum (½ inch for babies); hold it in place until the temperature is registered. Care should be given to ensure patient privacy throughout the procedure.

Axillary Temperature
- Axillary temperature is most commonly conducted using an electronic thermometer.
- The probe is placed in the middle of the axilla and the corresponding arm is held against the body to keep it in place until the audible tone is heard and the temperature is recorded.
- The axilla provides greater surface vasculature in newborns and infants than in adults, making it a better reflection of core temperature and a more appropriate site for temperature assessment.
- Axillary temperatures are about 1° lower than oral temperature readings; however, as axillary temperatures can vary widely, no standard conversion to core temperature exists.

Temporal Artery Temperature
- Temporal artery temperature is measured using an infrared scanning thermometer. Accuracy is dependent on user technique.
- Place the thermometer probe flat on the center of the patient's forehead. Press and hold the scan button. Keeping the sensor flat against the skin, slide the thermometer across the forehead to the hairline.
- If perspiration is present on the forehead, continue to depress the scan button, lift the probe from the forehead, and touch the probe to the neck behind the earlobe. This will account for the potential cooling effect of perspiration. Release the scan button to display the reading.

Tympanic Temperature
- Tympanic thermometers use infrared scanning to measure the temperature at the tympanic membrane in the ear.
- Gently pull the ear back to help straighten the canal (pull up and back for adults; pull down and back for children under 3). Insert the thermometer probe into the ear to seal the canal. Press and hold the scan button until an audible tone is noted (1–3 seconds). Remove from the ear canal; the thermometer will display the patient's temperature.
- Disposable probe covers should be used to prevent cross-contamination between patients.

Noncontact Infrared Temperature

- Infrared "no-touch" thermometers use the same type of technologies as tympanic thermometers.
- The advantage is the reduction of cross-contamination risk; strict adherence to manufacturer guidelines and instructions is required for accuracy.
- Ensure the environment is appropriate; use a draft-free space, away from direct sunlight and radiant heat sources. The test area of the forehead should be uncovered, clean, and dry. Hold the sensing area perpendicular to the forehead, instruct the patient to remain stationary, and press the scan button.
- Normal temperature readings should be below 99.0°F (37.2°C).

Assessment of Pulse Rate

- The clinician should note the pulse rate (number of beats per minute), rhythm (pattern or regularity of the beats), and amplitude (strength of the pulse).
- To determine the rate, the clinician should count the number of beats for a full 60 seconds, or for 30 seconds and multiply by 2. The normal pulse rate for an adult is 60 to 100 beats per minute or bpm. If the rhythm of the pulse is irregular, default to using the full 60 seconds to calculate the rate.
- Peripheral pulses can be assessed at multiple locations, including over the carotid, brachial, radial, femoral, popliteal, dorsalis pedis, and posterior tibial arteries. See Chapter 3, Evidence-Based Assessment of the Heart and Vascular System, for a review of the locations for palpating peripheral pulses. The most common site for determining the pulse rate in adults is over the radial artery. Gently compress the radial artery with the fingertips of the middle and index fingers; this allows for easy assessment of the pulse rate.
- Apical pulse is located over the apex of the heart at the fifth intercostal space left of the midclavicular line. Place the bell of the stethoscope over this area and listen, noting the rhythm and amplitude of the heartbeats, as well as the heart rate. Chapter 3, Evidence-Based Assessment of the Heart and Vascular System, delineates placement locations on the chest wall for additional, more thorough evaluation of heart sounds.

Assessment of Respiratory Rate

- Observe the rise and fall of the chest; count the number of breaths that occur in 1 minute. In practice, clinicians do not always count respirations for a full minute, but instead count for 30 seconds and multiply by 2. This practice should be avoided as it decreases the accuracy of the respiratory assessment, especially in younger populations.

- The normal rate of respirations depends on age, recent physical activity, and level of alertness (e.g., waking/sleeping states). Respiration rates may increase with fever, illness, or medical conditions.
- The normal respiratory rate for an adult is 12 to 20 breaths per minute. Clinicians should assess for tachypnea, an elevated respiratory rate; and bradypnea, an abnormally slow breathing rate. If either condition exists, further assessment is needed. Chapter 4, Evidence-Based Assessment of the Lungs and Respiratory System, includes a review of abnormal respiratory findings.

Blood Pressure Measurement

- BP measurement/monitoring can be completed using home, ambulatory, or office-based methods.
- In the United States, office-based BP monitoring is the standard of care for screening, diagnosis, and management of elevated BP (hypertension).
- The correct measurement of an office-based BP requires attention to the time of day, type of device, cuff size, cuff placement, technique of measurement, and recent use of nicotine or caffeine. The following are considerations for accurate measurement:
  ○ **Select the equipment:** The length of the BP cuff bladder should be 80% of the circumference of the upper arm; the width should be at least 40% of the circumference of the upper arm. A cuff that is too small will result in artificially high BP readings; a cuff that is too large will result in artificially low readings. Measurement also requires an available, functioning manometer.
  ○ **Assess the circumstances:** The patient should have had no caffeine in the hour preceding the BP reading, no smoking in the 30 minutes prior, and no recent use of decongestant. The environment should be quiet and warm.
  ○ **Posture and positioning:** Proper patient positioning is essential for accuracy. The patient should be seated with their back supported, legs uncrossed, and arm supported at the level of the heart (**Figure 2.1**). They should be allowed to sit quietly for 5 minutes before the BP is measured. Factors that can influence measurement include bladder distention, background noise, and talking. The patient's arm should be free of clothing; do not roll the sleeve up as this can create a tourniquet effect and alter the reading. Place the midline of the cuff bladder over the palpated brachial artery pulsation. The lower end of the cuff should be 2 to 3 cm above the antecubital fossa to minimize artifact noise from the stethoscope rubbing the cuff. The cuff should fit snugly on the patient's arm. Once the cuff is placed, the arm should remain supported at the level of the heart; neither the patient nor the clinician should talk.

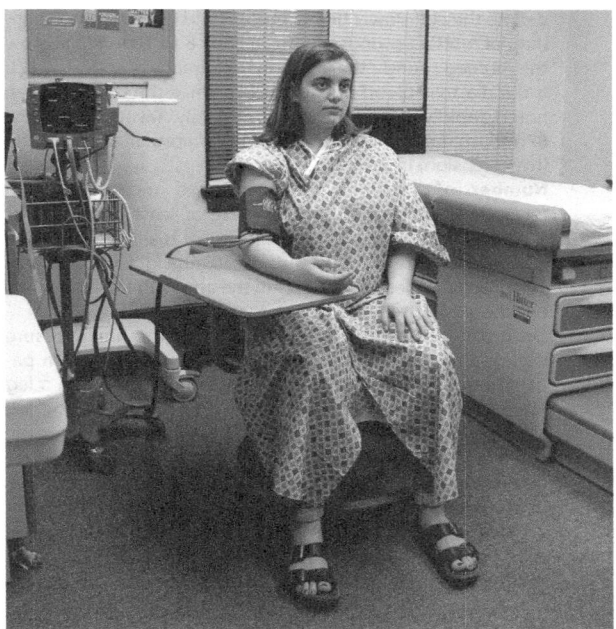

FIGURE 2.1 In-office blood pressure measurement.

○ **Technique:** The estimated systolic blood pressure (SBP) should be palpated initially to avoid misinterpretation of the BP, which is more likely if the patient has an auscultatory gap. An auscultatory gap is a period of diminished or absent Korotkoff sounds during BP measurement, which can be missed if the cuff is inflated without first palpating the SBP. To palpate the SBP, place the fingers of one hand over the brachial or radial artery and feel for the pulsation. Rapidly inflate the cuff with the hand bulb 30 mmHg above the point at which the pulse was not palpable. Slowly deflate the cuff at a rate of 2 to 3 mmHg/sec until the pulse is palpated again, which is the estimated SBP, then quickly deflate the cuff completely. Once the palpable SBP has been determined, place the bell of the stethoscope lightly over the brachial artery and inflate the cuff quickly to 30 mmHg above the palpable SBP. Slowly release the cuff at a rate of 2 to 3 mmHg/sec; listen for the first audible pulse (Korotkoff sound), which is the SBP. Continue to deflate the cuff slowly below the SBP and listen for the beginning of muffled sounds; approximately 8 to 10 mmHg below the muffled sounds, there is a disappearance of sound, which is the diastolic blood pressure (DBP). Once the DBP has been noted, rapidly deflate the cuff completely. **Table 2.1** lists the BP measurements that are considered normal and elevated (hypertension) in adults.

○ **Number of readings:** Evidence-based recommendation for accurate measurement is to take at least two readings (1–2 minutes apart), while the individual is seated, one from each arm. If there is a substantial (>10 mmHg) and consistent SBP difference between the arms, the arm with the higher values should be used for future measurements.

○ **Optional assessment using leg cuff:** If the arm pressure is elevated, take the pressure in one leg, particularly in patients under 30 years of age. The principles to obtain a leg BP reading are the same as in the arm. The SBP in the leg is expected to be 10% to 20% higher than when using the brachial artery.

○ **Optional assessment of postural changes:** Check for postural changes by taking readings after the individual has been supine for 5 minutes, then immediately and 2 minutes after standing. This is particularly important for older adults, individuals with diabetes, or patients taking antihypertensive medication.

TABLE 2.1 Blood Pressure Measurements in Adults Including Hypertension Staging

Blood Pressure	ACC/AHA 2017	JNC8
<120/<80	Normal	Normal
120–129/80	"Prehypertension"	"Elevated"
130–139/80–89		Stage 1 HTN
140–159/90–100	Stage 1 HTN	Stage 2 HTN
≥169/≥100	Stage 2 HTN	

ACC/AHA, American College of Cardiology/American Heart Association; HTN, hypertension; JNC8, Eighth Joint National Committee.

Life-Span Considerations for Measurement of Vital Signs
Pediatric Vital Signs

- Vital signs for infants and children can vary greatly in comparison with the normal range for adults. Normal vital signs are listed in **Table 2.2** by age.
- The technique for temperature measurement is age-dependent. Rectal temperature is preferred for infants and young children; oral temperature can be obtained when the child is developmentally able to hold/maintain the thermometer under the tongue. In general, fever is defined by a temperature ≥100.4°F. Newborns and some children with neurologic conditions may demonstrate a lower than normal temperature, even in the presence of a serious infection.

TABLE 2.2 Pediatric Vital Signs			
Age	Heart Rate (Beats Per Minute)	Blood Pressure (mmHg)	Respiratory Rate (Breaths Per Minute)
Premature	110–170	SBP 55–75, DBP 35–45	40–70
0–3 months	110–160	SBP 65–85, DBP 45–55	35–55
3–6 months	110–160	SBP 70–90, DBP 50–65	30–45
6–12 months	90–160	SBP 80–100, DBP 55–65	22–38
1–3 years	80–150	SBP 90–105, DBP 55–70	22–30
3–6 years	70–120	SBP 95–110, DBP 60–75	20–24
6–12 years	60–110	SBP 100–120, DBP 60–75	16–22
>12 years	60–100	SBP 110–135, DBP 65–85	12–20

DBP, diastolic blood pressure; SBP, systolic blood pressure.

- For older children and adolescents, heart rate can be assessed in a manner similar to adults, by auscultation of the apical pulse or palpation of the radial pulse. In infants, assess the brachial or femoral pulse; each femoral pulse should be palpated simultaneously with a brachial or radial pulse. A delayed or diminished femoral pulse in comparison with the brachial or radial pulse is suggestive of coarctation of the aorta.

- Respiratory rate varies not only with age but also with activity or distress. It is most accurately assessed for a full minute while the infant or young child is calm or sleeping.

- BP measurement in children not only varies with age but is also evaluated against a standard reference population of sex and height percentile. Annual, routine BP monitoring begins at 3 years of age. At any age, BP is taken in response to other findings suspicious for underlying cardiac or renal disease. It is imperative to use an appropriately sized BP cuff to obtain an accurate measurement for children. The cuff should cover approximately two-thirds of the upper arm.

- Many young children are fearful of the measurement of vital signs. To facilitate measurement and alleviate fear, the clinician can allow the child to touch and examine the equipment first and should be mindful of the language used for children who are concrete thinkers.

Vital Signs During Pregnancy

- BP and heart rate measurements are assessed during prenatal visits to identify early signs of arrhythmias, heart disease, and/or hypertension in pregnancy. Hypertension during pregnancy is a major health concern that can have significant complications and consequences for mothers and babies. Recognition is complicated by the normal physiologic changes in vital signs during pregnancy and a lack of evidence supporting long-held beliefs that BP decreases significantly and heart/respiratory rates increase significantly during the first 28 weeks of gestation.

- Evidence-based recommendations for normal range of vital signs during pregnancy include the following: no change in the reference range for BP during pregnancy, a heart rate of 120 per minute for the high-risk threshold, and a respiratory rate of 25 per minute as indicative of high risk.

- Changes in vital signs during pregnancy are primarily a result of increased blood volume and cardiac output. Clinicians are advised to individualize recommendations for each pregnant person based on personal risk and health status. Note that Black women are at increased risk of hypertensive disorders of pregnancy and cardiovascular (CV) diseases.

Considerations for Measurement of Vital Signs in Older Adults
- With advanced age, the body's thermoregulatory measures and kinetic heart rate recovery are less effective. Older adults are less capable of adapting to extreme environmental temperatures, putting them at risk for both hypothermia and heat-related illness. Older adults are also less likely to develop a fever with infection, making body temperature a less reliable indicator of health status.
- Allow the older adult to rest after a period of activity before measuring their pulse rate. Because the heart takes longer to recover from activity and stress as individuals age, if the older adult presents with an abnormally rapid heart rate the clinician should review the activities that preceded the assessment to determine possible cause.
- Older adults have risks for both elevated BP (hypertension) and low BP (hypotension). Age-related increases in BP are a leading risk factor for ischemic heart disease and stroke. Although strict or aggressive BP management does reduce the overall mortality rate, this population is more likely to experience adverse effects from medications. Orthostatic hypotension is more common in the geriatric population partly due to their diminished baroreceptor sensitivity.

PHYSICAL EXAMINATION OF BODY HABITUS

Height
- *Height (stature)* is defined as the distance from the plantar surface of the foot to the crown of the head. It is measured in the standing position once the individual reaches 2 years of age and is able to stand independently. Measurement is completed using a *stadiometer*, which consists of a vertical ruler and a sliding horizontal piece with a flat bottom.
- To measure height with a stadiometer, make sure the patient's shoes, any hat, and excess or bulky clothing are removed prior to measurement; ask the patient to keep their eyes looking straight ahead, stand straight with their feet together, and place their heels and back against the vertical measuring surface (**Figure 2.2**).

Weight
- Weight represents total body mass. Body weight alone is a poor predictor of health because it is strongly correlated with height and not reflective of body composition. To evaluate health risks that may be related to an individual's weight, it must be considered in relation to height.
- Scales must be placed on a solid, flat surface and should be balanced appropriately (consult the operating manual for the device). Weight should be measured to the nearest 0.1 kg (or nearest 0.1 lb). Ensure the patient's shoes and any excess or heavy clothing are removed. Ask the patient to remove any belongings

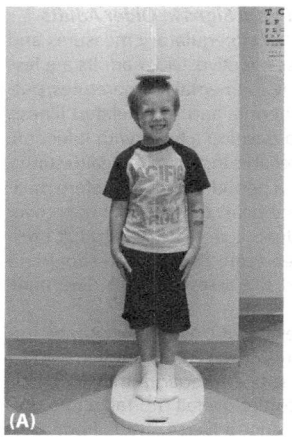 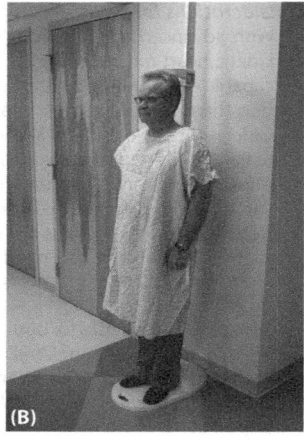

FIGURE 2.2 Correct measurement of height using a stadiometer. (**A**) Child. (**B**) Adult.

from their pockets, including wallets, keys, and phones. Have the patient place both feet in the center of the scale and avoid movement during measurement.

Body Mass Index Calculation

- Weight may be evaluated relative to height by calculating the BMI. Divide weight in kilograms by height in meters squared (expressed as kg/m²; if measuring in inches and pounds, it may be calculated as [lb/in²] × 703). Online BMI calculators can be accessed for ease of calculation: https://www.nhlbi.nih.gov/health/educational/lose_wt/BMI/bmicalc.htm.
- BMI status may be classified according to standard cut-points outlined by the National Heart, Lung, and Blood Institute (**Table 2.3**).
- Despite widespread use in clinical practice, the BMI metric has limitations. It does not capture information on the distribution of body fat, and in general:
  - At the same BMI, women tend to have more body fat than men.
  - At the same BMI, Blacks have less body fat than Whites.
  - At the same BMI, older adults tend to have more body fat than younger adults.
  - At the same BMI, athletes have less body fat than nonathletes.

Waist Circumference

- Presence of elevated waist circumference and/or elevated waist:hip ratio is an indicator of proportionally more adipose tissue distribution around the abdomen compared with the hip and thigh. Distribution of adiposity around the abdomen is referred

TABLE 2.3 Classification of Body Mass Index in Adults	
Classification	Adults (kg/m²)
Underweight	<18.5
Normal	18.5–24.9
Overweight	25.0–29.9
Obesity	≥30.0

Note: Adult obesity may be further classified in increments of 5 kg/m²: class I, 30.0 to 34.9 kg/m²; class II, 35.0 to 39.9 kg/m²; class III, >40.0 kg/m².

to as an *android distribution*, as opposed to a *gynoid distribution*. The android pattern of adiposity is associated with increased risk of adverse health outcomes, including CV diseases and diabetes, and remains so even after statistically accounting for BMI.

- To measure waist circumference, have the patient remove any constricting clothing from their waistline. Tell the patient to breathe normally and avoid "sucking it in." The clinician should use their hands to walk up both sides of the patient's hips. Place the tape measure at the top of the iliac crest (**Figure 2.3**). Use

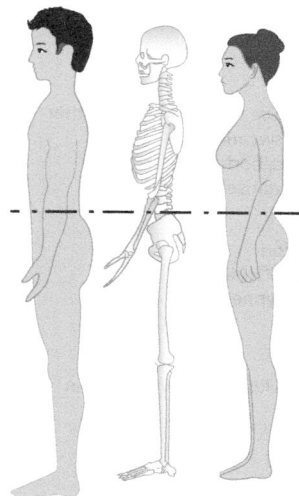

FIGURE 2.3 Correct placement of tape measure for measurement of waist circumference.

a flexible tape measure that measures in inches or centimeters. Make sure that the tape measure is snug but does not compress the skin and that it lies parallel to the floor. Have the patient relax and exhale.
- It is not necessary to do a waist circumference on any patient with a BMI of 35 or greater or any individual with a height of under 5 feet because of inaccuracies. Monitoring changes in waist circumference over time may be helpful, in addition to measuring BMI, since it can provide an estimate of increased abdominal adipose tissue even in the absence of a change in BMI. In obese patients with metabolic complications, changes in waist circumference are useful predictors of changes in CV risk factors.

Pediatric
Growth and Developmental Assessment
- Growth and development are closely monitored in children as key markers of health and well-being. See Chapter 17, Evidence-Based Considerations for Assessment Across the Life Span, for evidence-based assessment of growth and developmental milestones in infants and children.

ABNORMAL FINDINGS

FEVER
An elevation in body temperature above 100.4°F (38°C) in response to internal and/or external factors

Hyperthermia
History
- Prolonged exposure to hot, humid weather
- Flushing, excess sweating
- Chills or shivering, body aches
- Loss of appetite, nausea, vomiting
- Weakness, fatigue

Physical Examination
- Fever above 104.0°F (40.0°C)
- Tachycardia, tachypnea
- Delirium

Consideration
- Increased risk with older age, certain illnesses, and certain medications

Hypothermia
History
- Prolonged exposure to cold air or water
- Drowsiness, confusion, loss of coordination

Physical Examination

- Body temperature <95.0°F (35.0°C)
- Respiratory distress
- Bradycardia, slow weak pulse

Considerations

- Assessment of temperature in newborns is a priority. Cold stress in a newborn can lead to hypoglycemia, hypoxia, and hypothermia.
- Fever can be induced to manage certain medical conditions.

HYPERTENSION: ELEVATED BLOOD PRESSURE

History

- Patient may be asymptomatic.
- Severe hypertension may result in headaches, blurred vision, and chest pain.
- Modifiable risk factors include smoking, obesity, poor diet including excessive alcohol and sodium intake, or physical inactivity.
- Nonmodifiable risk factors include older age, family history, and race/ethnicity.

Physical Examination

- Elevated BP (may be the only sign; review **Table 2.3** for BP measurements associated with diagnosis of hypertension)
- Obesity
- Retinal changes including papilledema, arteriovenous (AV) nicking, and exudates
- Carotid and/or abdominal bruits, adventitious heart sounds
- Peripheral edema

Considerations

- Secondary hypertension is caused by a specific medication or disease state.
- Medications that can elevate BP include oral contraceptives, nonsteroidal anti-inflammatory drugs (NSAIDs), decongestants, and stimulants.
- Medical conditions that cause hypertension include obstructive sleep apnea, primary renal disease, pheochromocytoma, Cushing syndrome, hyperthyroidism, and coarctation of the aorta.

SHOCK

Shock is a life-threatening condition caused by lack of blood flow that leads to hypotension and hypoxia. Identifying the cause is essential.

- **Septic shock:** Response to overwhelming infection
- **Systemic inflammatory response syndrome:** Results from noninfectious conditions like burns, amniotic fluid embolism, air embolism, and crush injuries
- **Neurogenic shock:** Result of severe traumatic brain or spinal cord injury

- **Anaphylactic shock:** Results from severe allergic reactions
- **Cardiogenic shock:** Result of myocardial infarction
- **Hypovolemic shock:** Occurs from hemorrhagic or nonhemorrhagic fluid loss
- **Endocrine shock:** Associated with adrenal failure
- **Drug- and toxin-induced shock:** Associated with drug overdoses, snakebites, transfusion reactions, and poisonings

MALNUTRITION
Defined as imbalances, deficiencies, or excesses in intake of energy and/or nutrients

Undernutrition
Lack of adequate nutrition, caused by not having enough food or by not eating enough foods that contain the nutrients needed for proper growth and development

History
- Loss of appetite, or weight loss with normal appetite
- Dental pain or problems
- Unbalanced diet, lack of specific nutrients
- Pagophagia, compulsive craving, chewing, or consumption of ice and iced drinks
- Diarrhea, steatorrhea, change in stooling pattern
- Fatigue, weakness, dizziness, paresthesia
- Older adult, resident of a nursing home or rehabilitation facility
- May have functional decline, dementia, or Alzheimer disease
- May have history of malabsorption syndrome(s) and/or cancer(s)

Physical Examination
- Anemia, glossitis, cheilosis, or angular stomatitis
- Pallor
- Weight loss, wasting, muscle atrophy
- Growth delay
- Dermatitis or dermatoses
- Low bone density, pathologic fractures

Consideration
- Very young and very old at higher risk

Overweight/Obesity
A multifactorial chronic disease, defined by BMI, which increases risks for chronic conditions, including CV disease, diabetes, cancer, stroke, sleep apnea, and mental illnesses

History
- Imbalance in caloric intake and caloric expenditure
- Reported diet high in sugar, trans fats, saturated fats

- Sedentary lifestyle, little to no exercise
- Menstrual cycle changes
- Fatigue, sluggishness
- May have associated changes in body image, mental health, metabolism
- May have modifiable risk factors related to diet choices, dietary patterns, excessive alcohol intake, physical inactivity, stress
- May have nonmodifiable risk factors, including older age, genetics, comorbid chronic conditions

Physical Examination

- **Adults:** BMI of 25 or greater (overweight) or 30 or greater (obese)
- **Children:** BMI from the 85th to 94th percentile (overweight) and at or above the 95th percentile (obese); note: percentiles determined by age and gender

Consideration

- It is possible to be both overweight and micronutrient-deficient.

Weight Gain

Similar to obesity, weight gain may arise from one of many causes. Consider secondary causes if weight gain cannot be attributed to alterations in diet or activity, or is associated with dyspnea, edema, headache, substance use, or changes in mental health.

Weight Loss

Weight loss results from energy expenditure that is in excess of energy intake. It may also result from a change in dietary habits and/or physical activity, or more complex causes, including medications, endocrine factors, psychosocial factors, and other illnesses.

History

- Imbalance in caloric intake and caloric expenditure
- Reported reduction in energy intake; diet low in fats, protein, calories
- Reported increase in physical activity
- Medications
- Diarrhea, abdominal pain
- Decreased appetite (anorexia), nausea, dyspepsia, dysphagia

Physical Examination

- Poor dentition
- Generalized muscle wasting
- Decreased hand/grip strength

Consideration

- Can result from decreased intake, decreased absorption, increased metabolic requirements, and/or increased loss of nutrients

Cachexia

A multiorgan syndrome that is characterized by anorexia, a dramatic loss of skeletal muscle mass and adipose tissue, substantial weight loss, and inflammation

History

- Anorexia, dramatic weight loss
- Fatigue, weakness
- Often associated with advanced cancers, AIDS, certain autoimmune diseases, and other chronic conditions like heart failure and chronic kidney disease

Physical Examination

- Weight loss in adult or growth failure in children
- Insulin resistance
- Increased muscle protein breakdown, decreased muscle strength
- Low fat-free mass index (FFMI)
- Increased inflammatory markers
- Significant anemia, low serum albumin

Consideration

- Cancer data strongly suggest that cachexia hinders treatment responses and patients' ability to tolerate treatment. Inflammatory cytokines, in particular, have been closely associated with cachexia and mortality in cancer patients.

Sarcopenia

A complex and multifaceted process that involves the degenerative (involuntary) loss of skeletal muscle mass, quality, and strength; most often a result of healthy aging

History

- Loss of muscle mass, strength, and function
- Difficulty performing activities of daily living (ADLs)
- Most commonly seen in inactive people but can also affect those who remain physically active throughout their lives

Physical Examination

- Loss of balance, slowed gait
- May require assistive devices

Consideration

- It is one of the most important causes of functional decline and loss of independence in older adults; adequate nutrition and targeting exercise remain gold standard for prevention and treatment.

PHYSICAL EXAMINATION DOCUMENTATION

Documentation of physical exam includes appraisal of illness and wellness, vital signs, and body habitus; and growth and developmental assessment in children.

EXAMPLE DOCUMENTATION OF GENERAL SURVEY: ADULT

Height 5'5", weight 185 lb, body mass index 30.8; temperature 98.6°F orally; pulse rate 72 per minute, respiratory rate 12 per minute; blood pressure 144/88 right arm, 140/82 left arm, both after 5 minutes, seated; repeat blood pressure right arm, 138/84.

A 70-year-old White female. Affect pleasant. Oriented to time, person, and place. Nontoxic appearance. Respirations easy without distress. Pulse regular in rate and rhythm. Mucosa pink. Thoughts coherent; able to articulate health history with clarity. Steady gait; ambulates without assistive devices or abnormal movements. Transfers to table easily. Seated upright.

EXAMPLE DOCUMENTATION OF GENERAL SURVEY: 19-YEAR-OLD ATHLETE

Subjective

Jasmine is a 19-year-old female who presented to the clinic for a sports physical. Reports no current concerns or symptoms. Denies a history of concussions. Reports history of ankle sprains, but is currently asymptomatic. No recent injuries, ED visits, or hospitalizations. Family and personal health history unremarkable; no history of heart disease, sudden cardiac death, or hypertension. Has played tennis since she "could hold a racket" and has an athletic scholarship. A college freshman. Denies feeling down, depressed, helpless, or hopeless. Denies worry or anxiety. Maintaining above 3.7 grade point average (GPA).

Objective

Height 5'7", weight 150 lb, body mass index 23.5; temperature 98.6°F orally; pulse rate 52 per minute, respiratory rate 12 per minute; blood pressure 102/68.

A 19-year-old Black female. Affect pleasant. Oriented to time, person, and place. Nontoxic appearance. Respirations easy without distress. Pulse regular in rate and rhythm. Mucosa pink. Thoughts coherent; able to articulate health history with clarity. Steady gait; ambulates without assistive devices or abnormal movements. Ankles bilaterally without swelling or instability.

Assessment

Jasmine is a healthy 19-year-old female athlete with a history of ankle sprain. Cleared for participation on her college tennis team. Recommendations for injury prevention provided, including proper warm-up and stretching techniques before physical activity, wearing appropriate footwear, and maintaining proper hydration.

REFERENCES

References for this chapter draw from Chapter 7, Evidence-Based General Survey Including Assessment of Vital Signs, and Chapter 8, Evidence-Based Assessment of Body Habitus, Body Mass Index, and Nutrition, of the textbook *Evidence-Based Physical Examination: Best Practices for Health and Well-Being Assessment (Second Edition)*. The references may be accessed in the digital version of the handbook at connect.springerpub.com/content/book/https://connect.springerpub.com/.

3

Evidence-Based Assessment of the Heart and Vascular System

CLINICAL CONSIDERATIONS

- Understanding the structure and function of the heart and vascular system provides the foundation for evidence-based assessment.
- Completing a comprehensive, evidence-based history and physical examination when an individual presents with concerns, symptoms, and/or risks related to the cardiovascular (CV) and peripheral vascular (PV) systems provides a clinician with the opportunity to identify and distinguish between normal and abnormal findings.
- Early recognition of acute coronary syndrome (ACS), acute myocardial infarction (AMI), arrhythmias, heart defects, heart failure (HF), and cardiovascular disease (CVD) can reduce costs, improve quality of life, and save lives.
- Auscultation is a sensitive, specific, and effective method of detecting how the heart is functioning. S1 indicates the beginning of systole and coincides with the apical pulse. S2 indicates diastole, closure of the aortic and pulmonic valves, and is heard best at the base.

SUBJECTIVE HISTORY

COMMON REASONS FOR SEEKING CARE
Chest pain, palpitations, lower extremity edema, leg pain (**Box 3.1**)

HISTORY OF PRESENT ILLNESS
- **Onset:** When did the symptoms start? What was the individual doing when they became symptomatic? Did this occur suddenly, or has it been developing gradually?
- **Location:** Does the symptom have associated pain or discomfort? If so, where is the discomfort located? Does the pain radiate? Is there pain in the left jaw, neck, or arm? Is the edema in one or both legs?
- **Duration:** How long do the symptoms last? Do the symptoms come and go? Over what period of time have the cardiac symptoms developed?

> **BOX 3.1** Red Flags in Subjective History Indicating Urgent Risk of Vascular Disorder
>
> - Family history of premature atherosclerotic cardiovascular disease, sudden death, and bleeding disorders
> - Chest pain
> - Unstable angina
> - Calf pain or unilateral lower extremity edema
> - Sudden, severe headache
> - Dyspnea
> - Hemoptysis
> - Trauma to the chest, abdomen, or extremities

- **Characteristics:** Describe the pain/discomfort. Is the pain aching, burning, sharp, shooting, squeezing, crushing, tight, or dull?
- **Associated symptoms:** Presence or absence of numbness, tingling, weakness, nausea, vomiting, fever, heaviness in the arms or chest, neck pain; heartburn/reflux, hemoptysis, shortness of breath, unusual fatigue, feeling clammy or sweaty?
- **Aggravating factors:** What actions, activities, or body positions make the symptoms worse? If exertion worsens symptoms, clarify the level of exertion that causes exacerbation. Are the symptoms worse at night or in the early morning?
- **Relieving factors:** Does rest decrease the symptoms? If relieved, how long does the relief last? Does elevating the legs or wearing compression hose/socks relieve the edema?
- **Treatment:** What medications or other treatments has the individual taken to help with the symptoms? Do any of the medications or treatments provide relief?
- **Severity:** How severe are the symptoms on a scale of 0 to 10? Do the symptoms limit participation in activities? Are the symptoms worsening? Is the individual feeling anxious or fearful about them?

HEALTH HISTORY

Past Medical History

- History of CVD throughout the life span
  - Premature birth history or fetal heart defect diagnosed during the prenatal, infancy, or childhood periods (including treatments and correctional surgeries)
  - Hypertension (HTN) or history of elevated blood pressure (BP) readings

- ○ Hyperlipidemia (HLD)
- ○ Stroke or transient ischemic attacks (TIAs)
- ○ Blood clots, including pulmonary embolism
- ○ ACS
- ○ AMI
- ○ Lower extremity edema, peripheral vascular disease (PVD)
- ○ HF
- ○ History of stress tests, echocardiograms, EKGs, Holter monitors (including results)
- Comorbidities or risk factors related to CV/PVD
  - ○ Diabetes (insulin- or noninsulin-dependent)
  - ○ Obstructive sleep apnea (including use of continuous positive airway pressure [CPAP])
  - ○ COVID-19
  - ○ Kidney disease
  - ○ Erectile dysfunction
  - ○ Depression
  - ○ Anxiety
  - ○ Stress (acute or chronic)
  - ○ History of pregnancy-associated conditions that increase later CVD risk (e.g., preeclampsia, eclampsia, gestational HTN)
  - ○ History of premature menopause
  - ○ Previous surgeries, ED visits
  - ○ Adverse childhood experiences

Medications
- Prescribed medications with dose, frequency, side effects, consistency of taking medications, and barriers to medication adherence (including antihypertensive medications, statins, nitroglycerin, antiarrhythmic medications, diuretics, and anticoagulants including warfarin)
- Over-the-counter (OTC) medications or supplements, including aspirin, fish oil, coenzyme Q10, garlic, niacin
- Use of nitroglycerin, frequency and timing of use
- Chemotherapy (past or present)

Allergies
- Allergies to medications, or seasonal, environmental, and/or food allergies? If "yes" to being allergic to any substance or environmental trigger, clarify reactions.

Pediatric Considerations
- Birth history
  - ○ Any respiratory distress after birth? Any apneic episodes? Did the child require oxygen, pulse oximetry monitoring, or support for breathing as an infant? Apgar scores at birth?

- Mother's health during pregnancy? Exposures during pregnancy? Maternal illnesses, illicit drug use, and medication use when pregnant?
- Fetal abnormalities identified during the prenatal stage?
- Growth and development history
  - Meeting the developmental milestones?
  - Suboptimal growth or poor weight gain (based on pediatric growth charts)?
- Eating and nutritional history
  - Is the child exhibiting intolerance to feeding? Note vomiting, diarrhea, decreased intake, little interest in feeding, easily fatigued or perspiring during feeding, and/or any color changes including cyanoses during feeding.

FAMILY HISTORY

- AMI (especially if it occurred at a young age), congenital heart disease (CHD), coronary artery disease (CAD), congestive heart failure (CHF), long QT syndrome, sudden cardiac death
- Stroke
- Depression
- Diabetes
- Down syndrome
- HLD
- HTN
- Inherited hypercoagulable conditions, including factor V Leiden, prothrombin gene mutation, and/or deficiencies of natural proteins that prevent clotting (such as antithrombin, protein C, and protein S)

SOCIAL HISTORY

- Tobacco use (type, pack-years)
- Alcohol intake (type, amount, daily intake)
- Substance use (specifically cocaine, opioids, and whether use was in the past or present)
- Stress level (acute vs. chronic)
- Sleep (patterns, duration, snoring)
- Diet (specifically sodium intake, trans fats, red meat consumption)
- Exercise (frequency, duration, type, tolerance)
- Home monitoring of BP and/or daily weight

REVIEW OF SYSTEMS

- **General:** Fever, fatigue, dizziness, weight changes, recent travel (long car or plane ride)
- **Head, eyes, ears, nose, throat:** Visual disturbances/visual difficulty, periodontal disease, recent strep infections, or history of untreated/undertreated strep infections
- **Respiratory:** Shortness of breath, orthopnea, snoring with or without witnessed apneas

- **Cardiovascular:** Chest pain (with activity, at rest, or both); left arm, jaw, or neck pain; use of nitroglycerin; palpitations; skipping beats; racing heart rate; lower extremity edema; pain in lower extremities during activity; hair loss on the lower legs; history of stress test or EKG with results
- **Gastrointestinal:** Abdominal pulsations, abdominal pain, gastro-esophageal reflux disease (GERD)
- **Genitourinary:** Use of oral contraceptives
- **Neurologic:** Weakness, numbness, and tingling; syncope, headache, falls, and dizziness
- **Musculoskeletal:** Weakness, recent activity, or overuse
- **Mental health:** Depression, anxiety; changes in mentation, memory, or mood; current stress level and coping mechanisms

PHYSICAL EXAMINATION

- A systematic approach to the heart and vascular exams should be taken to ensure that all components of the exam are completed.
- CV exam is completed with the patient in the seated, supine, or left lateral position, and in some cases the standing/squatting position.
- The CV and PV exams follow the order of most system exams: inspection, palpation, and auscultation. Some techniques are not completed in all positions or for all portions of the exams.
- Keep in mind the location of the heart valves and chambers: the second right (aortic valve) and left (pulmonic valve) intercostal space (ICS), the left lower sternal border (LSB; mitral valve and right ventricular area), and the fifth ICS midclavicular line (MCL; mitral valve and left ventricular [LV] area). See **Figure 3.1** for depiction of these sites.

GENERAL SURVEY

- The following are important general observations:
  - Does the patient appear comfortable? Those presenting with chest pain or shortness of breath should especially be observed for an urgent or emergent situation.
  - Observe skin color, respiratory effort, and mental status. Abnormalities in these parameters may indicate CV compromise.
  - Discoloration or ulceration of the skin of exposed extremities may indicate PVD.
  - Refer to Box 2.1 in Chapter 2, Evidence-Based General Survey Including Vital Signs, for a reminder of assessments to determine physiologic stability. If the patient's status is unstable, immediate intervention is warranted.

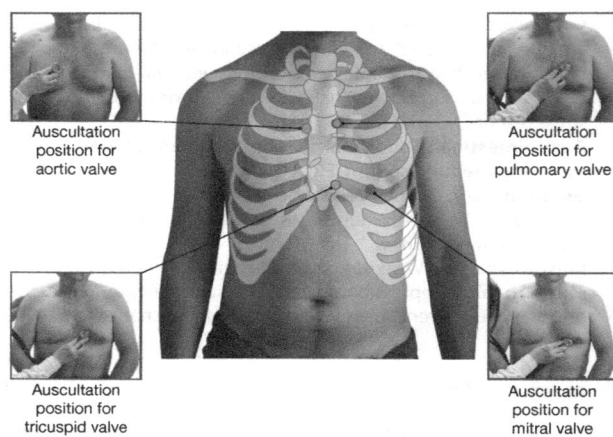

Auscultation position for aortic valve

Auscultation position for pulmonary valve

Auscultation position for tricuspid valve

Auscultation position for mitral valve

FIGURE 3.1 Auscultatory sites for heart sounds. Positioning for the aortic valve, pulmonary valve, tricuspid valve, and mitral valve.

CARDIOVASCULAR EXAMINATION OF THE PATIENT: SEATED POSITION

General Survey Assessment Including Vital Signs

- BP, pulse and respiratory rates, temperature, and pulse oximetry are all indices of the CV and PV systems. An accurate BP reading in both arms is imperative to the assessment of the heart and vascular system. See Chapter 2, Evidence-Based General Survey Including Vital Signs, for more information on vital signs and taking an accurate BP.
- Observational assessment of appearance, behavior, and mobility may reveal significant nonverbal expressions of pain or mental status change. In addition, an increase in an individual's weight over a relatively short time frame may be due to vascular congestion and volume retention due to conditions such as HF; assess for associated dyspnea, wheezing, activity intolerance, weakness, and/or edema.

Inspection

- Inspect the chest surface. Note the skin color, scars (which may be evidence of prior surgery or an implanted cardiac pacemaker or defibrillator), apparent heaves and lifts, or abnormal pulsations. Heaves and lifts are abnormal outward thrusting or focal movement of the chest wall during the cardiac cycle that may indicate enlarged chambers, aneurysm, or an underlying valvular disorder.
- The apical impulse is visualized at the same anatomic location where the point of maximal impulse (PMI) is palpated. This normal pulsation is observed, in normal-sized hearts, in the left fifth ICS

at or just medial to the MCL. Reference any abnormalities to the known cardiac anatomic landmarks so that consideration is given to the area during palpation of the chest wall.

Palpation
- Palpation is typically done during the supine portion of the exam. This is discussed in the text that follows.

Auscultation
- Auscultate the apical pulse, noting the heart rate and rhythm. The rhythm should be regular, and the rate should be between 60 and 100 impulses per minute. For any irregular rhythm, note whether there is a regular or irregular pattern. Assess the radial pulse in conjunction with auscultation of the apical pulse. Any difference between the apical rate and the radial pulse rate is noted as a pulse deficit and may indicate an abnormal cardiac rhythm.
- Identify S1 and S2. These heart sounds will allow the clinician to identify systole and diastole and assist in identifying the timing of abnormal heart sounds. S1 indicates the beginning of systole and is heard as a "lub." S1 also coincides with the carotid artery pulse.
- Auscultate the apical pulse while gently palpating the carotid artery (refer to Peripheral Vascular Exam of the Patient later in this chapter for the correct technique for carotid palpation) to ensure the sound is S1. S1 is heard with each pulsation of the carotid artery. S2 indicates diastole, follows S1, and is heard as "dub." S1, representative of the closure of the mitral and tricuspid valves (atrioventricular [AV] valves), is heard best at the apex and is louder than S2 at this location. S2, indicating the closure of the aortic and pulmonic (semilunar) valves, is heard best at the base and is louder than S1 here.
- Listen to the two sounds individually, denoting systole from diastole. A split in the S1 sound (heard best along the LSB) and a physiologic S2 split (heard best in the left second and third ICS) are normal. Persistent S2 splitting may indicate underlying conduction or valvular disorder. A fixed S2 split with no variation with respiration may indicate an atrial septal defect (ASD) or a ventricular septal defect (VSD).
- The auscultatory exam may start at the apex or the base of the heart. Regardless of the approach used, follow a "Z" pattern inching along the path, listening throughout systole and diastole at each site. Starting at the base of the heart, from the second right ICS, move the stethoscope in turn to the second left ICS, the right sternal border (RSB), and the apex in the fifth ICS near the MCL. The order is reversed if starting at the apex. Listen with the bell first, then repeat the pattern listening with the diaphragm.
- Before completing the seated portion of the exam, the patient is asked to lean forward and hold their breath after full exhalation

while the clinician uses the diaphragm to listen along the left LSB. This position brings the LV outflow tract closer to the chest wall and enhances the high-pitched sounds of the semilunar valves.

- At each precordial site, listen first for systole and then diastole relative to S1 and S2. Once these are identified, listen carefully for abnormal or extra heart sounds, such as the third (S3) and fourth (S4) heart sounds or murmurs. S3 and S4 may be auscultated in diastole and can be normal or abnormal. A pathologic S3 is also referred to as a ventricular gallop and indicates decreased compliance of the ventricle and volume overload, as might occur in HF or high cardiac output (CO) states. Although not often detected in the outpatient setting, evidence strongly supports the utility of an S3 in the diagnosis of HF. S4, occurring immediately before S1, is a soft sound with low pitch. It is heard best with the bell of the stethoscope when the patient is in the left lateral position. A pathologic S4, or atrial gallop, may occur as a result of decreased compliance of the ventricle and increased afterload.

- A variety of abnormal heart sounds may be auscultated over the precordium. These can include a variety of murmurs and pericardial friction rubs. Murmurs may be heard as a whooshing, clicking, snapping, vibrating, rumbling, or blowing sound. Murmurs can be benign (physiologic) or pathologic, related to congenital or acquired abnormalities, such as valvular disease and CHD. Murmurs are described according to eight characteristics: timing, loudness, pitch, pattern, quality, location, radiation, and posture (**Table 3.1**).

CARDIOVASCULAR EXAMINATION OF THE PATIENT: SUPINE POSITION

Inspection

- The precordial exam is also completed with the patient supine. Lower the head of the bed (HOB) so that the patient's head and chest are at a 30° to 45° angle. Young patients and healthy patients with no known or suspected cardiopulmonary disease may be examined lying flat.

- Visual inspection of the chest with the patient in the supine position replicates the inspection completed while in the seated position.

Palpation

- Palpating with the palm of the hand and then the pad(s) of the finger(s), locate the apical pulse (**Figure 3.2A**). It is <2.5 cm in diameter, approximately the size of a quarter. Note the location, size, amplitude (upstroke), intensity (strength/force), and duration of the pulse. The apical impulse represents the brief contraction of the LV and as such is located at the apex of the heart,

TABLE 3.1 Characteristics of Heart Murmurs

Type of Murmur	Precordial Location	Timing in Cardiac Cycle	Radiation	Pitch	Sound Quality	Special Maneuvers
Aortic stenosis	Right second and third intercostal spaces	Midsystolic	Toward the carotid arteries	Crescendo–decrescendo; medium	Harsh	It is best heard with the patient sitting and leaning forward.
Mitral stenosis	Apex	Diastole	None	Decrescendo; low	Rumbling	Use the bell of the stethoscope at the PMI; it is best heard with the patient in left lateral decubitus position.
Aortic regurgitation	Left second to fourth intercostal spaces	Diastole	Toward the apex	High	Blowing	It is best heard with the patient sitting and leaning forward with their breath held following exhalation.
Mitral regurgitation	Apex	Holosystolic	Toward the left axilla	Medium/high	Harsh	Murmur should not vary with respiration.
Tricuspid regurgitation	Lower left sternal border	Holosystolic	Toward the xiphoid process	Medium	Blowing	Murmur will increase with inspiration.
Pulmonic stenosis	Left second and third intercostal spaces	Midsystolic	May radiate to the left shoulder	Crescendo–decrescendo; medium	Harsh	None

PMI, point of maximal impulse.

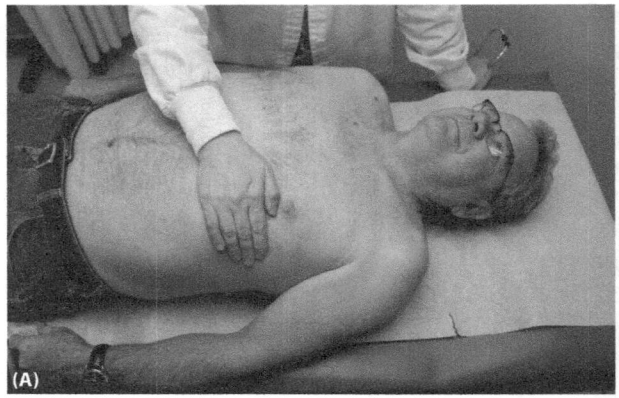

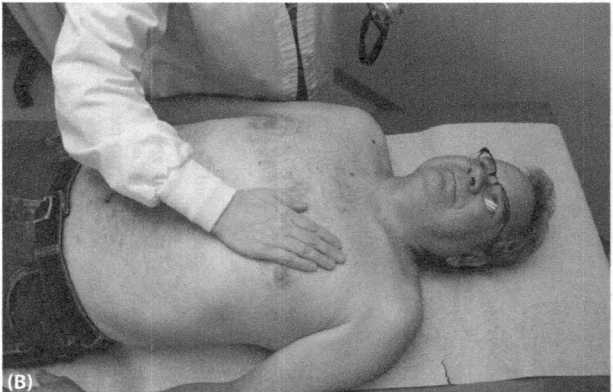

FIGURE 3.2 Palpation of the chest. (**A**) Palpation with palm of the hand to locate the apical pulse. (**B**) Palpation over the heart region to determine thrills, lifts, or heaves.

approximately the fifth ICS MCL. The apical impulse is the PMI in patients with normal-sized hearts and surrounding anatomy. PMI locates the left border of the heart and is typically in the fifth ICS, 7 to 9 cm lateral to the midsternal line (MSL). Palpation of the apical impulse and PMI provides information about the size of the heart. Displacement of the apical impulse suggests increased left ventricular end-diastolic volume (LVEDV) and LV mass. The apical impulse is palpated with the patient in the supine position, but can also be performed in the left lateral position if there is difficulty identifying it while the patient is supine.

- Palpate over the heart region to determine any thrills, lifts, or heaves (**Figure 3.2B**). A *thrill* is a palpable murmur, and any grade 4/6 murmur or louder will have an accompanying palpable thrill. Evidence demonstrates a systolic thrill to be strongly suggestive of significant valvular disease.

Auscultation

- Auscultation of the heart with the patient in the supine position is identical to the exam completed in the seated position, listening over all auscultatory sites with both the bell and the diaphragm. In addition, the patient is asked to turn to the left lateral position and the clinician auscultates over the apex of the heart, the left fifth ICS MCL, with the bell. In this position, the LV is closer to the chest wall, accentuating S3, S4, and mitral murmurs, specifically mitral valve stenosis.
- Patients in whom a systolic murmur has been identified should be examined in additional positions in an attempt to further delineate the origin of the murmur. Examining a patient in the squatting and standing positions can help distinguish between the systolic murmurs of aortic stenosis (AS) and hypertrophic cardiomyopathy (HCM). AS is best heard in the second right ICS, while the murmur of HCM is best heard in the third to fourth left ICS. With the patient in the standing position, and preferably using the exam table for balance, the clinician stands next to the patient and places the stethoscope on the chest. The clinician asks the patient to squat and then stand while auscultating the heart. The patient is asked to momentarily pause while in the squatting position, then rise. The murmur of AS intensifies while the murmur of HCM decreases in intensity during the squatting phase as a result of increased arterial BP, stroke volume, and LV volume. The standing phase decreases arterial BP, stroke volume, and LV volume, thus decreasing the intensity of the AS murmur and intensifying the murmur of HCM. Patients may also be asked to perform the Valsalva maneuver (bear down as when having a bowel movement) while supine. The murmur of HCM intensifies during the Valsalva.

PERIPHERAL VASCULAR EXAMINATION OF THE PATIENT: SUPINE POSITION

- This portion of the exam includes evaluation of the carotid artery, jugular venous pressure (JVP), and vascular aspects of the abdomen and extremities.
- As noted previously, the PV exam of the extremities may be performed with the patient seated. For individuals in whom vascular disease is suspected, it is important to examine the legs supine and seated as color changes can indicate certain disorders.

Inspection

Jugular Venous Pressure

- Identify the jugular vein to be used for measurement of JVP. The internal jugular vein lies deep in the sternomastoid muscle and can be difficult to see. Its pulsation is best visualized in the sternal notch. The top of the external jugular vein is visualized where it overlies the sternomastoid muscle.

- Raise the HOB 30° to 45° for visualization of the jugular vein and measurement of JVP. The angle may be more or less depending on at what elevation or height the jugular column (venous meniscus) is visualized. For patients suspected of hypovolemia, the HOB may need to be lowered for visualization of the jugular pulsation. For those suspected of fluid overload, the HOB may need to be raised higher.

- Use a folded pillow or blanket behind the patient's head to elevate the head off the mattress while maintaining the shoulders on the mattress. Turn the patient's head away and elevate the jaw slightly. Shine a tangential light across the neck to help visualize the venous motion.

- If jugular venous pulsations are not visualized in the neck, JVP is likely normal. Lower the HOB until a pulsation is visualized to ensure that the pressure is not so high that it cannot be visualized.

- If JVP is elevated, perform the hepatojugular reflux (HJR). With the patient supine, place the right hand over the midabdomen below the right costal margin and push firmly for 10 to 15 seconds, observing the right jugular. If the jugular rises for a few seconds and then returns to baseline, the central venous pressure (CVP) is considered normal. Sustained elevation of the jugular is consistent with elevated CVP. In conjunction with an elevated JVP, positive HJR increases the likelihood (likelihood ratio+ 8.0) of elevated venous pressure.

Palpation

- Palpate the right and left carotid arteries, located just medial to the sternomastoid muscle. The patient should be in the supine position with the HOB elevated to 30° to 45°. Do not apply firm pressure or palpate both carotids at the same time; this can compromise blood flow to the brain, causing syncope. Using several fingers, palpate the artery at the level of the cricoid cartilage. Use the right fingers to palpate the left carotid pulse and vice versa. Avoid palpating near the top of the thyroid cartilage, the location of the carotid sinus, as pressure on this may cause slowing of the heart rate. Note the symmetry, rhythm, rate, amplitude (or upstroke), and intensity (or strength, force) of the pulse. It should be smooth and symmetric with a brisk upstroke.

- Palpation of the carotid artery may be done in conjunction with cardiac auscultation during identification of S1 and S2. Palpation of the carotid and femoral arterial pulses simultaneously is done for suspected coarctation of the aorta. With this condition, there is delayed transmission and amplitude of the femoral pulse as compared with the carotid.

Auscultation
- Carotid artery auscultation is completed after palpation, when there is an indication of neurologic signs or symptoms consistent with decreased cerebral blood flow, as occurs with carotid artery stenosis, or when a palpable bruit is identified.
- Place the bell of the stethoscope over the identified carotid artery (**Figure 3.3**). Ask the patient to take a breath, exhale, and hold the breath. Holding the breath helps avoid interpreting tracheal sounds as turbulent blood flow. This technique also avoids contraction of the levator scapulae muscle in the neck from dampening the sound. As when listening for other turbulent blood flow, note a blowing or swishing sound, a carotid bruit. Cardiac murmurs may be transmitted from the heart to the carotids. To avoid interpreting a heart murmur for a bruit, perform a complete precordial exam.

ABDOMEN
Refer to Chapter 12, Evidence-Based Assessment of the Abdomen and Gastrointestinal and Urological Systems, for information on completing the PV exam for the abdomen, including inspection, auscultation, and palpation of the aortic, renal, and femoral arteries.

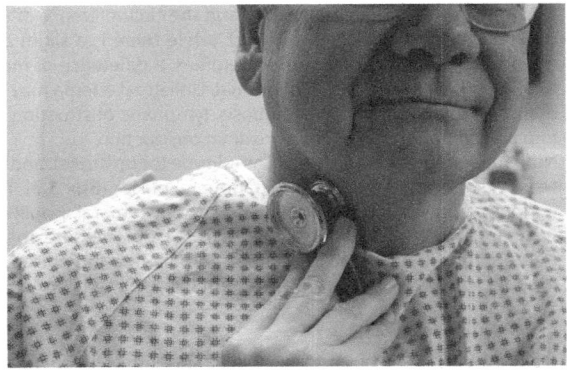

FIGURE 3.3 Auscultation of carotid artery.

EXTREMITIES

Inspection

- Inspect the extremities. Note the skin color (keeping in mind the patient's ethnicity). Assess the color of the nails, noting any cyanosis. Check for capillary refill (see Chapter 4, Evidence-Based Assessment of the Lungs and Respiratory System).
- Examine the lower extremities for skin color, hair distribution, lesions, and edema. The arms and legs should be symmetric in size. Decreased hair distribution, cool skin, skin ulcerations, pale legs on elevation, and dusky red skin in the dependent position may be signs of peripheral artery disease (PAD). Brown pigmentation or petechiae of the skin, cyanosis with leg dependency, stasis dermatitis (dry, scaling, hyperpigmented skin), and ulcerations may indicate venous insufficiency. Note any varicosities (engorged veins) of the legs. Note edema of the lower extremities as this may indicate poor venous return (as in venous insufficiency) or fluid retention, as occurs in HF.

Palpation

- Palpate the arms and legs for skin temperature, texture, turgor, and edema. Lower extremity edema is identified as either pitting or nonpitting, with pitting edema graded 1 to 4. Press firmly and gently with the thumb over the dorsum of the foot and pretibial area of the lower leg (shin). Hold the pressure for 5 seconds. Pitting is present if an indentation remains in the tissue after the thumb is removed (**Figure 3.4**). Grade the pitting and note the extent to which the edema ascends the extremity. See **Box 3.2** for information on grading and documenting edema.
- If unilateral edema is present, use a tape measure to document the difference between the two extremities. Measure at the smallest and largest difference of the calf and the circumference of the mid-thigh (if edema is present here). While there is a slight difference in the measurement of extremities, a difference of more than 1 to 2 cm is considered abnormal. Unilateral edema may be due to an injury, a venous thrombosis, lymphatic obstruction, or impaired venous return from a proximal obstruction.
- Note the symmetry, rate, rhythm, amplitude (or upstroke), and intensity (strength or force) of the peripheral pulses (**Box 3.3**). The peripheral pulses include the radial, brachial, femoral, popliteal, posterior tibial (PT), and dorsalis pedis (DP). Light pressure on the pulse is important as firm pressure may obliterate the pulsation. In some adults, this pulse may be absent bilaterally (**Figure 3.5**).

PEDIATRIC CONSIDERATIONS

- Many aspects of the physical exam in infants and children are the same as adults.

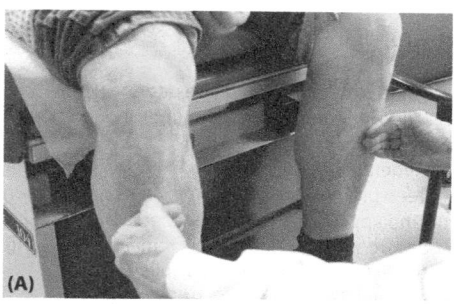

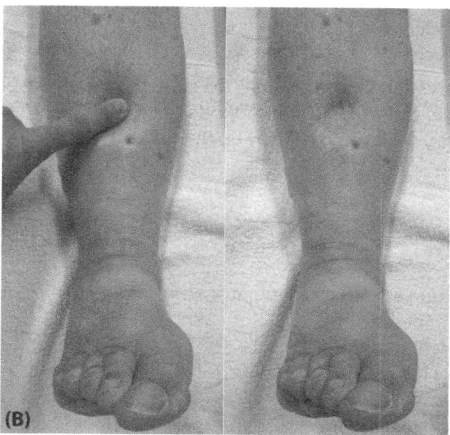

FIGURE 3.4 (**A**) Palpation of the legs. (**B**) Pitting edema.
Source: Part B image courtesy of James Heilman, MD.

- Auscultation of heart sounds may indicate different disease processes in the pediatric population; however, they occur at the same landmarks and are described and classified in the same fashion.
- General appearance of the infant or child (happy or cranky) as well as nutritional and respiratory status are very important. Subtle changes in these systems can signal warning signs for CHD.
- Palpation of pulses is another very important exam technique in infants and children as differentials in pulses between extremities can be indicative of a coarctation of the aorta while bounding pulses may be indicative of a shunt lesion.

BOX 3.2 Documenting Edema

The following scale is used to grade pitting edema:
- **1+:** Mild pitting; there is only slight indentation and no appreciable extremity edema.
- **2+:** Moderate pitting; thumb indentation resolves rapidly.
- **3+:** Deep pitting; indentation remains for a brief period of time and appreciable extremity edema is present.
- **4+:** Severe pitting; indentation remains for a long time and the extremity is obviously swollen.

Nonpitting edema is graded according to severity:
- Mild
- Moderate
- Severe

Documentation also includes the extent to which the edema ascends the extremity (e.g., moderate nonpitting edema of the feet, ankles, and halfway up the calf).

BOX 3.3 Grading Scale for Pulses

Pulses are graded on a 3-point scale according to the strength or force of the pulse:
- **3+:** Bounding
- **2+:** Normal
- **1+:** Weak
- **0:** Absent

- BP evaluation in children is just as important as it is in adults and can help screen for heart diseases. Clinicians should be familiar with appropriate techniques for obtaining BP, as well as normative BP ranges for infants and children by age. See Table 2.1 in Chapter 2, Evidence-Based General Survey Including Vital Signs, for normal BPs by age.

CONSIDERATIONS FOR THE OLDER ADULT
History questions and the physical exam for older adults presenting with cardiac symptoms are not different from those used for the adult. However, age itself is an independent risk factor for CVD, so the likelihood of CVD being present is much higher in the older adult (**Box 3.4**).

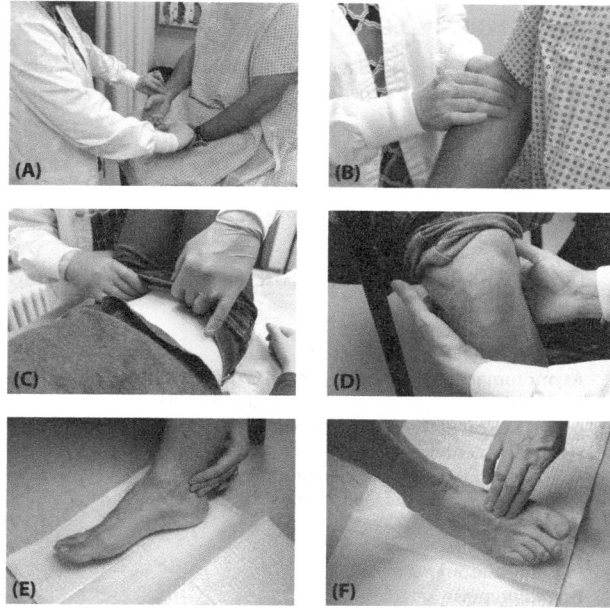

FIGURE 3.5 Palpation of peripheral pulses. (**A**) Radial pulse. (**B**) Brachial pulse. (**C**) Femoral pulse. (**D**) Popliteal pulse. (**E**) Posterior tibial pulse. (**F**) Dorsalis pedis pulse.

BOX 3.4 Red Flags in Objective Exam Indicating Urgent Risk of Vascular Disorder

- Diaphoresis with reported chest pain, nausea/vomiting
- Bleeding
- Tachycardia or bradycardia
- Pulselessness
- Sudden confusion, change in mental status
- Unilateral weakness, facial drooping
- Slurred speech
- Sudden trouble walking or seeing
- Cold with color changes to extremity

ABNORMAL FINDINGS

The abnormal findings and differential diagnoses listed in this section are in alphabetical order, rather than in order of prevalence. The list is not exhaustive.

ABDOMINAL AORTIC ANEURYSM
A ballooning or weakening of the aortic wall that is predisposed to rupturing

History
- History of atherosclerosis and/or HTN, family history of aneurysms
- Older age
- History of smoking
- Caucasian males more affected
- Asymptomatic in the majority of patients; if symptomatic but not ruptured, pain typically near the position of the aneurysm (epigastric region of the abdomen, back, flank, or pelvic region)
- Has an indolent onset
- Pain unchanged with position or movement
- History of syncope or feeling faint

Physical Examination
- Pulsatile abdominal mass
- Bounding pulse
- Ruptured abdominal aortic aneurysm (AAA) triad, that is, severe acute pain, a pulsatile abdominal mass, and hypotension, which occurs in approximately 50% of patients

Consideration
- Most often diagnosed with an ultrasound

ACUTE CORONARY SYNDROME
A constellation of symptoms caused by a prolonged period of decreased myocardial oxygenation due to decreased blood flow in the coronary arteries

History
- Older age
- Smoking
- History of HTN, atherosclerosis, PAD, diabetes, HLD
- Lack of exercise, unhealthy diet
- Recent cocaine use
- Overweight/obese
- Family history of heart disease
- History of an abnormal stress test

- Chest pain that is described as aching, pressure, squeezing, tightness, or burning; occurs at rest and with activity; does not change with respiration or position; change in pain pattern over the past 24 hours and pain unrelieved with nitroglycerin; pain radiating to both arms, left arm, jaw, or neck
- Nausea/vomiting
- Shortness of breath
- Fatigue
- Dizziness, lightheadedness, syncope
- Feeling of impending doom

Physical Examination
- Diaphoresis
- General appearance of distress and unrest
- Changes in BP (hypotension, HTN, or can be normotensive)
- Changes in pulse (tachycardia or bradycardia)
- EKG abnormalities (ST depression)
- Elevated cardiac serum markers (troponin)
- HEART score range of 7 to 10. HEART is an acronym of scoring components: **H**istory, **E**KG, **A**ge, **R**isk factors, and **T**roponin. Each component is scored with 0, 1, or 2 points.
- Thrombolysis in Myocardial Infarction (TIMI) risk score of 5 or higher

Considerations
- Patients with a history of ACS experience a decrease in their ability to perform ordinary activities and experience other comorbidities and mental health issues that affect their quality of life.
- About 10% of patients who present with acute chest pain are diagnosed with ACS.

ATHEROSCLEROSIS AND CORONARY ARTERY DISEASE
Atherosclerosis is a condition that causes thickening and loss of elasticity of the arterial wall due to plaques. Atherosclerosis causes CAD. See **Box 3.5** for the American Heart Association (AHA) and American College of Cardiology (ACC) risk calculator for estimating 10-year risk for atherosclerotic cardiovascular disease.

History
- HLD, HTN, metabolic syndrome, intermittent claudication, TIAs, heart attacks, angina, and/or stroke
- Smoking
- Diabetes
- Asymptomatic in mild disease
- Chest pain in the middle or left side (can extend into the left arm, jaw, or neck pain); pain worsening with activity or emotional stress
- Shortness of breath

BOX 3.5 Risk Calculator for Estimating 10-Year Risk for Atherosclerotic Cardiovascular Disease[a]

Calculation information:

- Age, sex, race
- Systolic and diastolic BP
- Total cholesterol, HDL, and LDL
- History of diabetes, smoking (current, former, never)
- Current (yes/no) medications for HTN, statin, or on aspirin therapy

Factors that increase ASCVD risk included in clinician–patient risk discussion:

- Family history of premature ASCVD
- Primary hypercholesterolemia
- Metabolic syndrome
- Chronic kidney disease
- Chronic inflammatory conditions
- History of premature menopause
- History of pregnancy-associated conditions that increase later ASCVD risk (e.g., preeclampsia)
- High-risk race/ethnicity (e.g., South Asian ancestry)
- Lipids/biomarkers associated with increased ASCVD risk

10-Year risk for ASCVD:

- Low risk (<5%)
- Borderline risk (5%–7.4%)
- Intermediate risk (7.5%–19.9%)
- High risk (≥20%)

ASCVD, atherosclerotic cardiovascular disease; HDL, high-density lipoprotein; HTN, hypertension; LDL, low-density lipoprotein.

[a]Calculations are for those without ASCVD only. The calculator can be found online at http://tools.acc.org/ASCVD-Risk-Estimator-Plus/#!/calculate/estimate.

Physical Examination
- High BP
- Abdominal obesity
- Weak pulses
- Bruits
- Decreased BP in the limbs

- Elevated inflammatory biomarkers (C-reactive protein)
- Coronary artery calcium score >100 (moderate disease), >300 (severe disease)
- Ankle-brachial index <0.9 or >1.4

Considerations
- Signs and symptoms of transient ischemia (e.g., stable angina, TIAs) may appear when lesions decrease blood flow by narrowing the arterial lumen by 70% or more and/or by rupturing and acutely occluding a major artery.
- Atherosclerosis and CAD can also lead to aneurysms, arterial dissection, or sudden death without any prior symptoms of angina.

ATRIAL SEPTAL DEFECT
ASD is an opening between the right and left atria, or the upper two chambers of the heart. ASD is common in combination with other heart defects and is often critical to blood flow and oxygenation in some CHDs.

History
- Patient has family history of ASD.
- Patient has genetic syndrome, such as Holt–Oram syndrome, trisomy 21, or Noonan syndrome.
- Young infants and children are often asymptomatic.
- Occasionally an infant with isolated ASD may present as symptomatic with signs of CHF.
- Older children may present with mild fatigue or dyspnea.
- Adults with an unrecognized or untreated ASD may develop right-sided HF, pulmonary HTN, or Eisenmenger syndrome.

Physical Examination
- Wide, fixed split S2, a hallmark finding
- Systolic ejection murmur at the left parasternal area (midway between the sternal border and the MCL); may have very soft murmurs in early childhood
- Those with long-standing left to right shunting, including left precordial bulge and prominent right ventricular impulse
- Abnormalities on chest x-ray, transesophageal echocardiogram, and occasionally on EKG. Likely has normal sinus rhythm (NSR), but may have prolonged QRS

Considerations
- ASD is common in combination with other heart defects and is often critical to blood flow and oxygenation in some CHDs.
- As an isolated heart defect, ASD accounts for approximately 8% to 10% of congenital heart defects in children.

CHRONIC VENOUS INSUFFICIENCY
A condition caused by stasis and reflux of venous blood flow

History
- History of prolonged sitting or standing throughout the day
- Obesity, physical inactivity
- Older age
- Female
- Prior injury to the extremity
- Pregnancy
- Can be asymptomatic, especially early in the disease
- Aching in the lower legs the most commonly reported symptom
- Heaviness and itching in the lower legs

Physical Examination
- Pitting edema in the lower legs (cardinal sign)
- Varicose veins
- Will often see combined edema and hyperpigmented skin, sometimes called brawny edema
- Reduced ankle motion
- Hyperpigmentation and lipodermatosclerosis (inflamed and thickened skin) are signs of more advanced disease
- Lower extremity ulcerations
- Normal sensory and motor exams (helps exclude diabetic neuropathy)
- Normal abdominal exam (helps exclude abdominal mass as the cause of venous insufficiency)

Considerations
- Chronic venous insufficiency (CVI) exists along a continuum that progresses from small telangiectasic "spider" veins to varicose veins, and in severe cases venous ulcers.
- CVI can occur at various anatomic levels, including superficial, deep, and perforating veins. The location of venous ulcers can be a clue to the location of the disease.

COARCTATION OF THE AORTA
A defect of the aortic arch involving a narrowing of the arch often occurring at the insertion site of the ductus arteriosus

History
- Patient has family history of coarctation.
- Patient has genetic syndrome, such as Turner syndrome or 22q11.2 (DiGeorge) syndrome.
- Many infants will present with symptoms within the first week of life as the ductus arteriosus closes, hence limiting blood flow past the obstruction.
- Infants with a critical obstruction to blood flow will present with acute symptoms of shock, metabolic acidosis, renal failure, and necrotizing enterocolitis.

Physical Examination
- Systolic ejection murmur is heard along the left sternal border.
- Gallop rhythm is common.
- Older children or adults may present with systemic HTN and a murmur.
- Signs of CHF, which include the following:
  ○ Pulse abnormalities, including weak or absent femoral pulses; a delay between upper and lower extremity pulses
  ○ Tachypnea and tachycardia
  ○ Skin mottling, delayed capillary refill, and peripheral cyanosis
  ○ Chest x-ray abnormalities
- EKG abnormalities, which include the following:
  ○ In infants, normal right ventricular dominance with right axis deviation
  ○ In older child or adult, left ventricular hypertrophy (LVH)
- Echocardiogram shows the location and degree of coarctation as well as velocity measurements to determine severity.

Considerations
- Coarctation can present in varying degrees depending on the amount of narrowing.
- Critical coarctation in the infant is a life-threatening condition if not quickly recognized and treated. Coarctation can be repaired with surgery or by stenting the narrowed segment.
- Children or adults with repaired coarctation require lifelong cardiology follow-up as they can have recoarctation or complications arising from the initial surgical repair.

CONGESTIVE HEART FAILURE/HEART FAILURE
A complex syndrome caused by ventricular dysfunction and results in the inability of the heart to sufficiently meet the body's metabolic needs required to sustain life (see **Figure 3.4**)

History
- Fatigue, anorexia, nausea, and weakness
- Medical history of AMI, LVH, diabetes, obesity, and/or HTN
- Smoking and sedentary lifestyle
- Nocturia
- Chest pain, heaviness, or tightness (if caused by an AMI)
- Dyspnea at rest or with exertion
- Difficulty completing activities of daily living (ADL)

Physical Examination
- Arrhythmia or tachycardia
- Abdominal fluid accumulation (ascites)
- Jugular venous distention (JVD)
- Cough with white or pink blood-tinged exudate
- Edema, swelling

- Displacement of PMI
- Weight gain (can be rapid from fluid retention)
- Elevated atrial natriuretic peptide (ANP) and B-type natriuretic peptide (BNP); elevated Gal-3 and sST2 proteins

Considerations
- HF has a significant impact on health-related quality of life (HRQoL), including higher rates of depression, higher body mass index (BMI), low perceived control, and uncertainty about prognosis.
- The term *heart failure* is not the same as *cardiomyopathy* or *LV dysfunction* because the latter two terms describe structural or functional abnormalities that cause HF.
- There are two main classifications of HF based on ejection fraction (EF) of LV: heart failure with preserved ejection fraction (HFpEF) and heart failure with reduced ejection fraction (HFrEF; Yancy et al., 2013). HFrEF is defined as HF with left ventricular ejection fraction (LVEF) ≤40%, and HFpEF is HF with LVEF ≥50% EF. More recently, patients with an LVEF between 40% and 50% have been classified as heart failure with midrange ejection fraction (HFmrEF; Yancy et al., 2013).
- HF classification is important because it helps describe the severity and development of disease progression. It can also guide therapy choices. There are several different classification systems. The New York Heart Association functional classification system and the ACC/AHA classification are two of the most widely used.

DEEP VEIN THROMBOSIS
Occurs when clots develop in the deep venous systems of the extremities

History
- Active cancer
- History of recent immobilization, bed rest, or surgery
- Recent travel
- Mostly occurs in the lower extremities but can occur in the upper extremities
- History of prior deep vein thrombosis (DVT) or coagulation disorders
- Estrogen use (including birth control pills)
- Pregnancy

Physical Examination
- Unilateral leg edema
- Visible collateral superficial veins
- Pitting edema in the leg
- Leg size greater than the opposite leg
- In the outpatient, reduced probability of DVT to <2% if scores 1 or less on the Wells' criteria (**Table 3.2**) combined with a negative D-dimer test

TABLE 3.2 Wells' Clinical Prediction Tool	
Criteria	Point
Active cancer	1
Immobilization or paralysis of the lower extremity	1
Recent bed restrictions	1
Tenderness along the deep venous system	1
Leg swelling (ankle to thigh)	1
Symptomatic leg swollen >3 cm compared with asymptomatic leg	1
Pitting edema of the symptomatic leg greater than the asymptomatic leg	1
Prior DVT	1
Visible collateral superficial veins other than varicose veins	1
Other diagnosis than DVT more or as likely	−2
Low pretest probability of DVT = score of 1 or less; high pretest probability = score of 2 or higher	

DVT, deep vein thrombosis.

Source: From Wells, P. S., Anderson, D. R., Bormanis, J., Guy, F., Mitchell, M., Gray, L., Clement, C., Robinson, K. S., & Lewandowski, B. (1997). Value of assessment of pretest probability of deep-vein thrombosis in clinical management. *The Lancet, 350*(9094), 1795–1798. https://doi.org/10.1016/S0140-6736(97)08140-3.

Considerations
- There is risk for serious sequelae, like pulmonary embolus, especially if the diagnosis is missed.
- The Wells' Clinical Prediction Tool, which can be used to determine the need for further imaging, can be found in **Table 3.2**.

HYPERTENSION
See Chapter 2, Evidence-Based General Survey Including Vital Signs, for information on HTN.

INFECTIVE ENDOCARDITIS
An infection of the endocardial surface of the heart, which may include one or more heart valves, the mural endocardium, or a septal defect that causes severe valvular insufficiency, which may lead to intractable CHF and myocardial abscesses

History
- Fever, chills, malaise
- Dyspnea, cough
- Arthralgias
- History of dental disease
- History of intravenous (IV) drug use

Physical Examination
- Petechiae, which are a common, but nonspecific, finding
- Subungual (splinter) hemorrhages, which are dark-red, linear lesions in the nailbeds
- Osler's nodes, which are tender subcutaneous nodules usually found on the distal pads of the digits
- Janeway lesions, which are nontender maculae on the palms and soles
- Focal neurologic deficits, including paralysis, hemiparesis, and aphasia
- Delirium
- Gallops
- Rales
- Cardiac arrhythmias
- Pericardial or pleural friction rub

Consideration
- Many organisms have been identified as causative agents; however, *Staphylococcus aureus* has become the primary pathogen of endocarditis. Untreated, it is often fatal.

MITRAL VALVE PROLAPSE
Displacement or prolapse of the mitral valve leaflets into the LA during systole

History
- Family history of mitral valve prolapse (MVP)
- History of Graves disease, sickle cell, or rheumatic heart disease (RHD)
- Can be asymptomatic
- Chest pain
- Fatigue
- Dyspnea on exertion
- Anxiety
- Heart palpitations or arrhythmias

Physical Examination
- Midsystolic click on auscultation of the heart
- Mitral valve leaflet thickness ≥5 mm by echocardiography

Considerations
- There is evidence that suggests a good prognosis exists with MVP; however, there are instances of serious complications such as sudden cardiac death, endocarditis, or severe MVP.

- The degree of leaflet thickness can help ascertain the severity of disease as it is associated with a 14-fold higher risk of complications, including sudden death.

PERICARDITIS
An inflammation of the pericardium, which is the fibroelastic membrane that surrounds the heart

History
- History of acute trauma or infection
- Autoimmune disease
- Can be acute or chronic
- Chills or weakness
- Chest pain that worsens with breathing and lying down
- Chest pain that improves with sitting upright or leaning forward

Physical Examination
- Tachypnea and nonproductive cough
- Fever >100.4°F
- Pericardial friction rub
- Additional signs (rare) including cool extremities, cyanosis, hypotension, and decreased systolic BP >10 mmHg during inspiration, if cardiac tamponade (pressure on the heart secondary to accumulation of fluid in the pericardial sac) occurs

Considerations
- Pericarditis may be secondary to a systemic disease process or a primary process unrelated to another systemic disease.
- The disease can cause cardiac tamponade, which is the presence of fluid in the pericardial sac.

PERIPHERAL ARTERY DISEASE
An atherosclerotic disease that affects the arteries of the lower extremities (**Figure 3.6**)

History
- Past or present smoking history
- African American race
- History of HTN, HLD, chronic kidney disease, diabetes, or metabolic syndrome
- Older age (>65)
- Pain in the calves or other parts of the lower extremity (iliac, femoral, popliteal, peroneal, and/or tibial arteries), exacerbated by exercise
- Can be bilateral or unilateral
- Can be asymptomatic in 20%

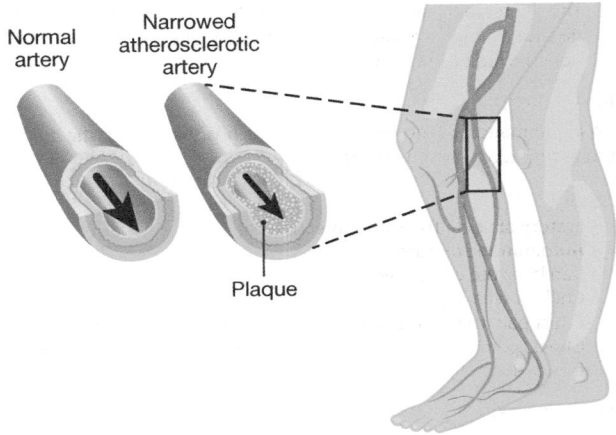

FIGURE 3.6 Peripheral artery disease.

Physical Examination

- Femoral and iliac bruits (present in advanced and/or proximal disease)
- Weak or no PT and/or DP pulses
- Asymmetric temperature to the feet
- Hairless lower extremities and atrophic skin
- Lower extremity ulcers/wounds usually found on the toes and feet and have a well-demarcated border
- Ulcers painful and lack edema

RAYNAUD PHENOMENON

Occurs from a vasomotor dysfunction that affects the distal arterial circulation of the fingers, toes, earlobes, face, nipples, or nose

History

- Females more affected than males
- Family history of Raynaud
- History of co-occurring vascular diseases like PAD and CVI
- Vasospasms that last a few minutes to a few hours
- Fingers (index, middle, and ring fingers) most often affected, followed by the toes
- Can affect a single digit or only part of a digit
- Triggered by cold or stress
- May experience pain, numbness, and tingling, with the affected extremities becoming hyperemic, as recovery of pallor ensues

Physical Examination
- Thinner patients
- Color change of the digits, "tricolor" phase of symptoms (from white to blue to red)
- Sclerodactyly, or thickening and tightness of the skin of the affected areas, highly associated with Raynaud phenomenon

Consideration
- It is primarily diagnosed through history and physical exam; however, diagnostic tests can be used.

RHEUMATIC HEART DISEASE
RHD is a sequela of rheumatic fever (RF) characterized by permanent damage to the heart valves. RF is an inflammatory response in the body that is a result of untreated strep throat and/or scarlet fever.

History
- History of suspected RF or untreated or undertreated strep throat
- Living in poverty or of lower socioeconomic status
- Little access to healthcare
- Joint pain and/or arthritis symptoms
- May not have any initial symptoms in children

Physical Examination
- Pathologic heart murmur (mitral or aortic valve stenosis or regurgitation)
- Chest pain or swelling due to myocarditis or pericarditis
- Flat or slightly raised, painless rash with a ragged edge
- Small, painless bumps beneath the skin

Considerations
- Symptoms of RHD show up 10 to 20 years after the original illness.
- Most often, the mitral valve is damaged, but the aortic valve can also be affected.
- Usually, RHD can be prevented by preventing strep infections or treating them with antibiotics when they do occur.

TETRALOGY OF FALLOT
A cyanotic congenital heart defect that comprises four different defects: VSD, overriding aorta, pulmonary stenosis (PS), and right ventricular hypertrophy

History
- Family history of CHD
- 70% diagnosed prenatally with 90% accuracy on ultrasound
- Genetic syndromes including 22q11.2 deletion (DiGeorge syndrome); trisomy 21, 18, and 13; Holt–Oram syndrome; and Alagille syndrome

- Reports irritability and/or prolonged crying
- Reports tiring easily during play or exercise
- Episodes of loss of consciousness and "tet spells"

Physical Examination
- "Tet spells" (an acute decrease in blood across the right ventricular outflow tract, causing the infant to suddenly develop deep blue skin, nails, and lips after crying or feeding)
- Poor weight gain
- Systolic ejection murmur at the left LSB with a single S2
- Clubbing
- Cyanosis of varying degrees
- Abnormalities on chest x-ray, EKG, and echocardiogram

Consideration
- Most infants with Tetralogy of Fallot do well with surgical intervention and survive into adulthood.

VENTRICULAR SEPTAL DEFECT
VSD is an opening between the right and left ventricles. It often occurs in combination with other heart defects as well as in isolation.

History
- Family history of VSD
- Genetic syndromes including trisomy 13, 18, and 21, and Holt–Oram syndrome
- Maternal use of marijuana, cocaine, and paint stripping
- Poor eating
- Failure to thrive
- Easy tiring, fatigue, and weakness

Physical Examination
- Tachypnea
- Murmur, dependent on the size of the defect
  - **Large defect:** May not have a significant murmur or may have a short systolic ejection murmur
  - **Small defect:** Loud holosystolic murmur often recognized in early infancy
- Abnormalities on chest x-ray, EKG, and echocardiogram

Considerations
- Small VSDs are pressure-restrictive and infants do not develop volume overload or CHF symptoms. Smaller defects may spontaneously close over time.
- Large VSDs that are left untreated can result in the development of CHF, pulmonary vascular disease, and Eisenmenger syndrome.

PHYSICAL EXAMINATION DOCUMENTATION

HEART AND CARDIOVASCULAR SYSTEM

Documentation should include results of inspection, palpation, and auscultation.

Example of Normal Findings

Skin on chest and back without lesions, rashes, or erythema. No visible heaves, or lifts over the precordium; apical impulse visualized in the fifth intercostal space (ICS) of the left chest at the midclavicular line (MCL). No palpable heaves, lifts, or thrills over the precordial area, apical impulse palpable in the fifth ICS of the left MCL. Auscultation: S1 and S2 distinct, with S1 more prominent at the heart's apex, S2 more prominent at the base; rate and rhythm regular without extra heart sounds, murmurs, gallops, clicks, or friction rubs audible.

PERIPHERAL VASCULAR SYSTEM

Documentation should include results of inspection, palpation, and auscultation.

Example of Normal Findings

Skin on extremities without lesions, rashes, varicosities, or stasis changes. No visible pulsations noted on the chest or abdomen. Carotid artery pulsations symmetric, brisk; no bruits auscultated bilaterally. Jugular venous distention absent. Extremities warm, nonedematous, and nontender to palpation. Capillary refill brisk less than 2 seconds in the upper and lower extremities. Radial, brachial, femoral, popliteal, dorsalis pedis, and posterior tibial pulses 2+ bilateral. No abdominal or femoral bruits noted.

REFERENCES

References from this chapter draw from Chapter 9, Evidence-Based Assessment of the Cardiovascular System, and Chapter 10, Evidence-Based Assessment of the Vascular System of the textbook *Evidence-Based Physical Examination: Best Practices for Health and Well-Being Assessment (Second Edition)*. The references may be accessed in the digital version of the handbook at connect.springerpub.com/content/book/https://connect.springerpub.com/.

4

Evidence-Based Assessment of the Lungs and Respiratory System

CLINICAL CONSIDERATIONS

- Assessing respiratory status is a key factor in determining the extent or severity of an illness.
- The best practice for examining the respiratory system is not to assess over clothing.
- Clean the entire surface of a stethoscope after use, including the ear tips.
- Pertinent health history includes assessment for recent travel and illness exposures.
- Ask about smoking status and exposure to secondhand smoke. Advise individuals that it is never too late to quit smoking.
- Always consider any environmental factors that could be contributing to the respiratory symptoms or conditions.

SUBJECTIVE HISTORY

COMMON REASONS FOR SEEKING CARE
Shortness of breath or dyspnea, cough, chest congestion

HISTORY OF PRESENT ILLNESS
- **Onset:** When did the symptoms start? What was the individual doing when they became symptomatic? Did this occur suddenly, or has it been developing gradually?
- **Location:** Does the symptom have associated pain or discomfort? If so, where is the discomfort located?
- **Duration:** How long do the symptoms last? Over what period of time has the respiratory symptom developed?
- **Characteristics:** Is the patient winded, unable to take air in, feeling short of breath, wheezing, or coughing? If coughing, is the cough deep, barking, whooping, spasmodic, or productive? If productive, is sputum frothy, foul-smelling, thick, of large volume, blood-streaked, or with frank bleeding? Is the patient experiencing or noticing any color changes in the lips, mucosa, or nails associated with the symptom(s)?

- **Aggravating factors:** What actions, activities, or body positions make the symptoms worse? If exertion worsens symptoms, clarify the level of exertion that causes exacerbation. If lying flat worsens symptoms, clarify the number of pillows needed to rest easy. Has exposure to smells, dust, pollen, smoking, or activities caused an increase in symptoms?
- **Relieving factors:** What actions, activities, or body positions decrease the symptoms? If relieved, how long does the relief last?
- **Treatment:** What medications has the individual taken to help with the symptoms? Did the patient use any breathing treatments or inhaled respiratory medications? Clarify the dosage and frequency of any medications.
- **Severity:** How severe are the symptoms on a scale of 0 to 10? Do the symptoms limit participation in activities? Are there associated symptoms? Are the symptoms worsening? Is the individual feeling anxious or fearful?

HEALTH HISTORY
Past Medical History

- History of respiratory illnesses throughout the life span
  - Premature birth history or lung disease diagnosed during childhood
  - Previous diagnoses of asthma, bronchiolitis, bronchitis, pneumonia, emphysema, and COVID-19
  - Previous ED visits or hospital stays for respiratory problems
  - History of need for intubation, mechanical ventilation, or respiratory resuscitation
  - Previous thoracic procedure or surgery
  - Recurrent respiratory illnesses that caused shortness of breath, wheezing, or cough
  - History of eczema or allergic rhinitis
  - Similar symptoms (note circumstances)
- Comorbidities or risk factors related to pulmonary disease
  - Recent travel (note mode of transportation, location, and length of stay)
  - Recent exposure to individuals with flu, flu-like symptoms, or COVID-19
  - Known or suspected pulmonary, cardiac, or renal disease
  - History of malignancy
  - Recent surgery, hospitalization, or immobility
  - Pregnancy status (note likelihood of pregnancy or if currently or recently pregnant)

Medications
- Prescribed and over-the-counter (OTC) medications or supplements, including dose and frequency
- Use of inhalers, nebulizers, and/or spacers, and how they are being used
- Recent antibiotic and/or oral steroid use
- Recent start of angiotensin-converting enzyme (ACE) inhibitors

Allergies
- Allergies to medications, or seasonal, environmental, and/or food allergies? If yes to being allergic to any substance or environmental trigger, clarify reactions.
  - Nausea, intestinal upset? Vomiting?
  - Skin rashes, itching? Hives?
  - Swelling of tongue, lips, face?
  - Dyspnea, wheezing, dizziness?

Immunizations
- **Risks for vaccine-preventable illnesses:** Vaccine status; date of last COVID-19, influenza, pertussis, and pneumococcal vaccinations; risks for tuberculosis (TB), flu, pertussis, and pneumonia

Pediatric Considerations Related to Health History
- Additional assessments for children under 3 years of age and/or presenting with respiratory symptoms
  - Birth history
    - Delivery eventful or uneventful, vaginal or Cesarean section, prolonged or abrupt?
    - Any respiratory distress after birth? Any apneic episodes? Did the child require oxygen, pulse oximetry monitoring, or support for breathing as an infant? Apgar scores at birth?
    - Mother's health during pregnancy? Exposures during pregnancy?
    - Fetal abnormalities identified during the prenatal stage?
  - Growth and development history
    - Meeting developmental milestones?
    - Suboptimal growth or poor weight gain (based on pediatric growth charts)?
  - Eating and nutritional history
    - How has the child been eating? Specifically for the infant, is the infant breast- or bottle-fed? Has the child's eating patterns changed?
    - Is the child exhibiting intolerance to feeding (which can be associated with COVID-19 and other illnesses)? Note vomiting, diarrhea, decreased intake, little interest in feeding, easily fatigued or perspiring during feeding, and/or any color changes including cyanoses during feeding.

FAMILY HISTORY

- Asthma, reactive airway, allergies, or breathing problems
- Chronic bronchitis, lung cancer, asbestosis, or lung problems
- Cystic fibrosis (CF), congenital anomalies, or respiratory illnesses related to genetics

SOCIAL HISTORY

Environmental Exposures

- Exposure to pollutants and/or irritants in the work environment
- Low-level chronic exposure to hazardous substances at work or at home
- Safety/protective measures, including handwashing practices and wearing masks at work, at home, or in public
- Air quality and exposures where the individual lives
- Exposure to secondhand or thirdhand smoke

Lifestyle Behaviors (Including Substance Use)

- Typical use of alcohol, episodes of binge drinking, alcohol misuse
- Use of prescription medications or illicit substances for nonmedical purposes
- Use of OTC drugs for reasons other than health, especially inhalants
- Use of tobacco, including cigarettes, smokeless tobacco, e-cigarettes or vapes, cigars (note the amount of use and the length of time to determine *pack-years*; use the 5 As as steps to intervene in response to positive tobacco use history for every individual; **Box 4.1**)

BOX 4.1 The 5 As: Steps to Intervention in Tobacco Use Disorder

1. **Ask:** Identify and document tobacco use status for every patient at every visit.
2. **Advise:** Support the self-efficacy of every person who uses tobacco to quit.
3. **Assess:** Determine each individual's willingness and readiness to quit.
4. **Assist:** Individuals willing to make a quit attempt should be offered options, including counseling and pharmacotherapy, as appropriate.
5. **Arrange:** Schedule follow-up, in person or by phone, within the first week of a quit date.

REVIEW OF SYSTEMS

- **General:** Fever, fatigue, chills, night sweats, weight changes, appetite changes
- **Skin, hair, nails:** Rashes, lesions, changes in mucosa, changes in skin and hair
- **Lymphatic:** Generalized or localized lymph node swelling and/or tenderness
- **Head, eyes, ears, nose, throat:** Headache, throat pain, ear pain, eye drainage or redness, congestion
- **Respiratory (additional review):** Orthopnea, snoring, hemoptysis, postural dyspnea
- **Cardiovascular:** Chest pain, palpitations, edema; if positive for chest pain, note whether pleuritic (i.e., sudden, intense, stabbing, sharp, or burning pain exacerbated by deep breathing, coughing, or sneezing)
- **Gastrointestinal:** Nausea, heartburn, abdominal pain, epigastric discomfort, vomiting
- **Neurologic:** Weakness, numbness and tingling, tremors, dizziness, syncope
- **Musculoskeletal:** Weakness, chest wall tenderness or pain, myalgias, leg pain or swelling
- **Mental health:** Sadness; insomnia; uncontrolled worry; changes in mentation, memory, or mood; current stress level and coping mechanisms; history of panic attacks

RED FLAGS IN SUBJECTIVE HISTORY

- Shortness of breath, difficulty breathing, breathlessness, wheezing, confusion, "coughing up blood," drooling, and/or any swelling of the lips or throat indicate the need for immediate physical exam and intervention.
- Key symptoms in individuals with pulmonary disease include pleuritic chest pain, dyspnea, and cough. Clarify the characteristics of these symptoms and review the individual's history of chronic lung disease and smoking.
- See **Box 4.2** for red flags that indicate risk for pulmonary embolus.

BOX 4.2 Red Flags in Subjective History That Indicate Risk for Pulmonary Embolus

- Sudden onset of pleuritic chest pain
- Breathlessness
- Dizziness or syncope
- Recent long-distance travel
- Prolonged immobility

(continued)

> **BOX 4.2** Red Flags in Subjective History That Indicate Risk for Pulmonary Embolus (*continued*)
>
> - History of trauma to the lower extremities or pelvis surgery in the last 3 months
> - Previous deep vein thrombosis, emboli, and malignancy
> - Comorbid heart failure or chronic lung disease
> - Pregnancy
> - Use of hormonal contraception
> - History of smoking and/or vaping

PHYSICAL EXAMINATION

GENERAL SURVEY

- Vital signs including temperature, pulse rate, respiratory rate, blood pressure, and pulse oximetry
- Rate, rhythm, depth, and effort of breathing
- Posture and position
- Ability of the patient to speak in full sentences
- Wheezing or audible breath sounds
- Tracheal deviation, nasal flaring, or retractions (suprasternal, substernal, or intercostal)
- Presence of head bobbing
- Central cyanosis, which can present as a generalized bluish, grayish, or purplish cast to the skin and/or the mucous membranes depending on the severity of the hypoxemia and/or the skin tone of the individual; typically not present until the arterial blood concentration is <80% to 85%
- Assessment of the lips for pursing, which is a sign of increased expiratory effort
- Note: If the patient is exhibiting any signs and symptoms of respiratory distress, including tracheal deviation, nasal flaring, retractions, central cyanosis, head bobbing, or use of accessory muscles, immediate interventions may be needed.

INSPECTION

Peripheral Assessment

- Observe the lips, oral mucosa, and conjunctiva for cyanosis or pallor.
- Assess for purse-lipped breathing (i.e., exhaling through tightly pressed lips).
- Evaluate the nailbeds for color and capillary refill; assess for clubbing (**Figure 4.1**). Normally, the angle between the skin and the nailbed is 160°, which creates a diamond-shaped window (Schamroth's window) when opposing fingers are held back to back.

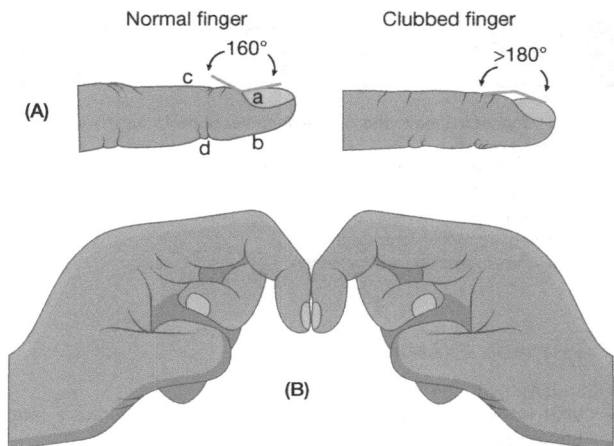

FIGURE 4.1 Assessment for clubbing. (**A**) Assessment of nailbed angle.
(**B**) Schamroth's window.

Inspection of the Thoracic Cage and Chest Movement

- Observe the rate, rhythm, and depth of respirations for a full minute.
  - The rate of respirations depends on several factors, including age, recent physical activity, and level of alertness. Adult respiratory rate is normally 12 to 20 breaths per minute. Infant and child respiratory rate varies with age. Refer to Chapter 2, Evidence-Based General Survey Including Vital Signs.
  - The rhythm of breathing at rest should be even, with occasional sighs.
  - The depth and ease of breathing should be unlabored and quiet, without use of accessory muscles.
- Inspect the anterior and posterior chest wall.
  - Inspect for presence of any skin lesions, masses, or discolorations.
  - Inspect shape and symmetry, noting the presence of chest or spine deformities. The anteroposterior (AP) diameter of the chest is ordinarily half of the lateral diameter, or 1:2. The thoracic cage is described as being a barrel chest when the AP diameter is equal to or greater than the lateral (transverse) diameter, or 1:1.

PALPATION

- Palpate the entire chest wall using the palmar surface of the hands to assess for tenderness, depressions, masses, deformities, or crepitus.

- Palpate the spine to identify any tenderness.
- Palpate the posterior thorax for symmetric chest expansion (**Figure 4.2**). Ask the patient to take a deep breath in and then exhale. During inspiration, the thumbs should separate and each hand should move away from the midline equally. Asymmetric chest wall expansion is suggestive of unilateral lung pathology, and limited movement is associated with poor diaphragmatic excursion and hyperinflation, changes that occur with chronic obstructive pulmonary disease (COPD).
- *Tactile fremitus* refers to the palpable vibratory sensation transmitted to the surface of the chest during speech. Palpate the posterior and anterior chest wall for fremitus (**Figure 4.3**). Ask the patient to say "99" and to repeat this while palpating the entire chest wall. Increased or decreased tactile fremitus is a finding that is understood to be a component of a constellation of signs and symptoms indicating respiratory disorders and is not solely diagnostic of pathology. The degree of fremitus found will vary. Tactile fremitus is usually stronger in the anterior versus posterior thorax, stronger at the apex than at the bases, and notable in the right upper back because this area is closer to the bronchial bifurcation.

PERCUSSION

- Percuss the posterior, lateral, and anterior chest wall, comparing each area bilaterally.
- Place the nonstriking finger of the nondominant hand on the chest wall firmly, while the remaining fingers are lifted slightly off the chest wall. Then use a quick, sharp wrist motion to strike the pressed finger at the midpoint between the proximal and distal

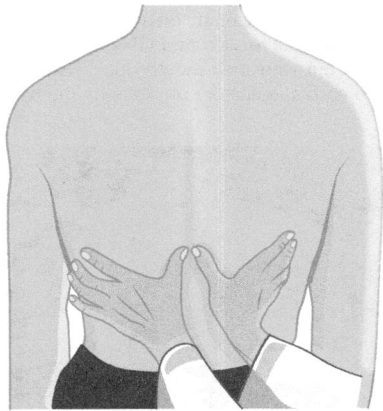

FIGURE 4.2 Palpation for symmetric chest expansion.

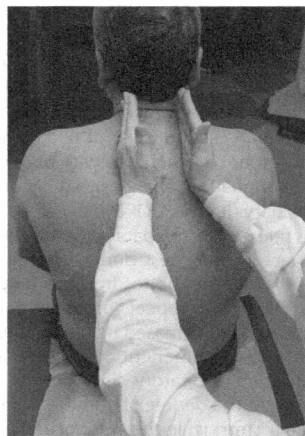

FIGURE 4.3 Palpation for tactile fremitus using the ulnar aspect of both hands.

interphalangeal joints with the plexor finger of the dominant hand to produce a sound. Strike the finger at least twice, lightly, sharply, and consistently, to produce a clear percussive sound (**Figure 4.4**).

- The landmarks used for percussion are illustrated in **Figure 4.5**; note that percussion is done in the same areas of the chest wall as auscultation.

AUSCULTATION

- Using a stethoscope, auscultate breath sounds.
- Instruct the individual to sit comfortably upright and take a deep breath in and out with their mouth open. Listen to at least one full breath in each auscultatory site. Caution the patient to do this

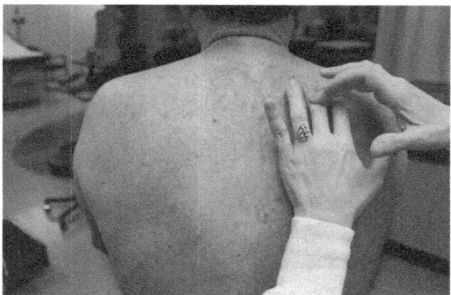

FIGURE 4.4 Percussion technique.

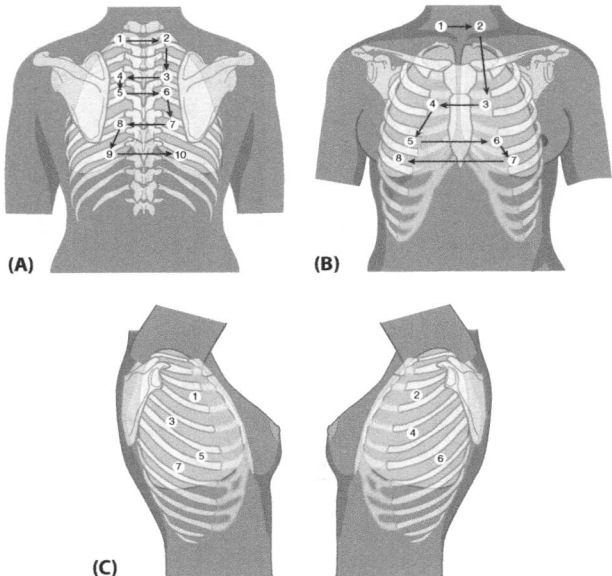

FIGURE 4.5 Landmarks for percussion and auscultation of lung fields.
(**A**) Anterior. (**B**) Posterior. (**C**) Lateral.

leisurely so as not to get fatigued or hyperventilate and to take breaks
as needed for comfort. Auscultate in a systematic manner from the
apex to the base, comparing breath sounds from side to side.
- The auscultatory sites of the posterior, lateral, and anterior chest
  wall are the same as those used for percussion (see **Figure 4.5**).
  To assess breath sounds in all the lobes of the lungs, being systematic is a priority. Note the anatomic location of the lobes of
  the lungs, as shown in **Figure 4.6**.
- Auscultate to assess the characteristics of the breath sounds. The
  following are normal breath sounds:
  - **Tracheal breath sounds:** Loudest and high-pitched, usually
    heard over the upper aspect of the trachea and best heard on
    the anterior aspect of the neck
  - **Bronchial breath sounds:** Louder and higher in pitch, usu-
    ally heard over the lower aspect of the trachea and best heard
    over the manubrium
  - **Bronchovesicular breath sounds:** Intermediate inten-
    sity and pitch, usually heard over the major bronchi in the
    mid-chest area anteriorly or between the scapulae posteriorly
  - **Vesicular breath sounds:** Soft in intensity and low-pitched,
    usually heard over the peripheral fields bilaterally

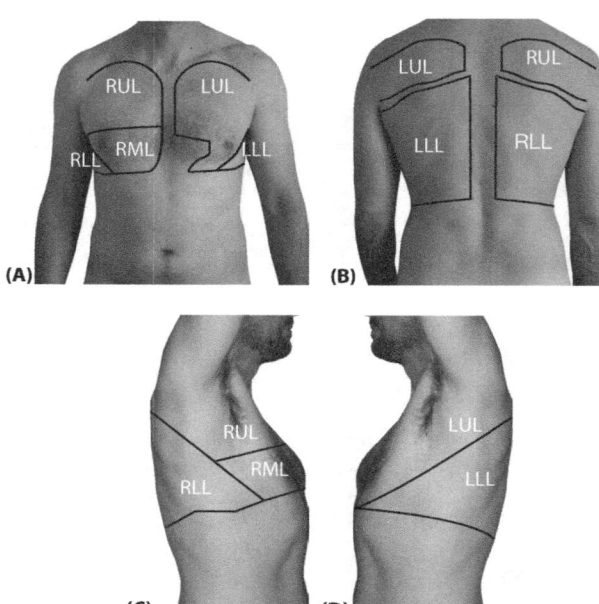

FIGURE 4.6 Lobes of the lungs. (**A**) Anterior lung fields. (**B**) Posterior lung fields. (**C**) Lobes of the right lung. (**D**) Lobes of the left lung. LLL, left lower lobe; LUL, left upper lobe; RLL, right lower lobe; RML, right middle lobe; RUL, right upper lobe.

- The following are abnormal breath sounds:
  - **Crackles:** Fine crackles are discontinuous high-pitched sounds that have a popping quality; these are usually inspiratory. Coarse crackles are discontinuous low-pitched sounds and are louder and longer. Crackles are heard as air passes through fluid-filled airways.
  - **Wheezes:** Continuous musical sounds, most likely to be heard during expiration. The tone of wheezing varies depending on the area(s) of the airways affected. If smaller airways are narrowed, resultant wheezes are musical in nature (polyphonic); if larger airways are narrowed, then wheezes sound hoarse (monophonic).
  - **Rhonchi:** Continuous low-pitched rattling sounds heard when larger airways are obstructed with secretions. The rattling sounds may mimic snoring. The unique feature of rhonchi is that they clear with coughing or suctioning.

- ○ **Stridor:** Loud and high-pitched sound caused by disrupted airflow, typically heard during inspiration, and associated with upper airway obstruction. Stridor may indicate impending respiratory distress and/or failure.
- ○ **Pleural rub:** Creaking or grating sound that can be heard during both inspiration and expiration as a result of friction (lack of lubrication or irritation) between the pleura. Described as two pieces of leather rubbing together, the sound of a pleural rub is not likely to stop with coughing, but will stop when the patient holds their breath.

PEDIATRIC CONSIDERATIONS

- For infants and children, the order of physical exam can be modified depending on their state of wakefulness and/or cooperativeness. The respiratory rate and rhythm can be assessed while the infant is sleeping in a parent's arms.
- The respiratory rate of infants can vary with temperature, activity, feeding, and even with sleep. When calculating respiratory rate, be sure to count for a full minute to calculate the normal respiratory rate because of these variations.
- When performing a physical exam on an infant, at some point during the exam, be sure to examine the baby on the exam table with only their diaper on so that their whole body can be viewed to get a better understanding of their respiratory effort. While the infant is lying down, inspect their chest for size and shape. Infants are likely to have periodic, irregular breathing. Assess that the infant's color does not change and that they are not using accessory muscles to breathe.

CONSIDERATIONS FOR THE OLDER ADULT

- As a person ages, the amount of mucus produced throughout the body decreases and this can be evident with dry mucous membranes in the nares, throat, and respiratory tract.
- Because of changes in the respiratory system of the older adult, expect to find an increased AP diameter of the chest wall and slight hyperresonance of the lung fields with percussion. There is also a decreased amount of chest expansion and more reliance on the diaphragm for breathing.

RED FLAGS IN OBJECTIVE EXAM

- The initial assessment of an individual to determine physiology stability includes measurement of vital signs; assessment of the rate, rhythm, depth, and effort of breathing; and observation for signs of respiratory distress. **Box 4.3** lists the key findings that indicate acute respiratory distress.

> ### BOX 4.3 Red Flags in Objective Exam That Are Indications of Acute Respiratory Distress
>
> · Labored or rapid breathing
> · Absent or diminished breath sounds
> · Suprasternal, substernal, or intercostal chest wall retractions
> · Hypoxia and cyanosis
> · Inadequate chest rise
> · Loss of consciousness
> · Additional population-specific signs:
>   · In infants, nasal flaring, grunting, head bobbing
>   · In children, drooling and stridor, extreme sleepiness
>   · In older adults, confusion with tachypnea and hypotension

ABNORMAL FINDINGS

VARIATIONS IN PATTERNS OF BREATHING

- **Tachypnea:** Abnormally increased respiratory rate associated with shallow breaths
- **Hyperpnea:** Increased rate and depth of breathing associated with elevated metabolic demand
- **Bradypnea:** Abnormally slow respiratory rate, may affect alveolar ventilation
- **Sighing respiration:** Normal respiratory rate with occasional deep, long breath; typically nonpathologic and associated with emotional state
- **Cheyne–Stokes breathing:** Abnormal breathing pattern; periods of progressively deeper breaths followed by gradual decrease resulting in temporary period of no breathing; pattern repeats, with each cycle usually taking 30 seconds to 2 minutes
- **Biot's breathing:** Clusters of respirations that alternate with periods of no breathing due to damage to the breathing center of the brain
- **Agonal breathing:** Occasional reflex-driven gasps, associated with anoxia, cardiac arrest, cerebral ischemia, or hypoxia
- **Apnea:** Absence of breathing that signals a life-threatening situation resulting in death if intervention is not immediate

COMMON RESPIRATORY DISORDERS

Acute Bronchitis

A lower respiratory tract infection most often of viral origin

History

- Initial common cold symptoms progress to productive cough, dyspnea, and pleuritic pain when coughing; cough persists for 2 to 6 weeks.

Physical Findings
- Mildly ill appearance
- Fever of <100.0°F in the first few days of illness; resolves
- May be normal on lung exam, or with wheezes and rhonchi, which clear with coughing

Consideration
- Differentiate from pneumonia. It is not typical for a healthy, immune-competent adult <65 years of age with normal vital signs and lung exam to have pneumonia.

Asthma
Disease of chronic airway inflammation with many variations

History
- Wheezing, dyspnea, chest tightness, and cough that vary over time and in intensity
- May be worse at night, on awakening; often triggered by exercise, laughter, allergens, or cold air; may occur with or worsen during viral infections

Physical Findings
- The most common finding during exacerbations is wheezing, especially with expiration.
- Head, eyes, ears, nose, throat (HEENT) and skin exams may show evidence of allergies and/or eczema.

Considerations
- Personal and family history of allergies as well as eczema increase the risk.
- Spirometry gives evidence of the variable expiratory airflow limitation through measurement of lung volumes and flow rates.
- It is important to assess pregnant women and those planning to become pregnant for history of asthma.

Bronchiolitis
An acute viral infection that most commonly presents in children under 2 years of age

History
- It most often occurs during the winter season.
- History often includes prodromal viral upper respiratory infection, followed by increased respiratory effort and wheezing; there is also presence of rhinorrhea and cough.

Physical Findings
- Tachypnea, wheezing, crackles
- Increased respiratory effort, such as grunting, nasal flaring, intercostal and substernal retractions

Considerations
- Less common in adults
- Most cases caused by respiratory syncytial virus (RSV)
- Increased risk with underlying conditions, prematurity, tobacco exposure

Chronic Obstructive Pulmonary Disease
A chronic inflammatory lung disease that causes obstructed airflow and decreased elasticity of the lungs

History
- Current or former tobacco smoking a primary risk factor
- Chronic cough, dyspnea, sputum production, recurrent lower respiratory tract infections, chest tightness (especially after exercise)

Physical Findings
- Varied exam findings depending on disease stage, such as inspiratory and expiratory wheezes, decreased lung sounds, limited chest expansion, fatigue, weight loss, and anorexia
- Clubbing of the nails
- Barrel chest

Considerations
- Spirometry is required for diagnosis. Persistent airflow limitation is confirmed when the forced expiratory volume in 1 second/forced vital capacity (FEV_1/FVC) is less than 0.70.
- The goal of COPD assessment is to determine severity, impact of disease, and risk of future exacerbations to guide therapy.

SARS-CoV-2 (COVID-19)
A highly contagious viral illness caused by the severe acute respiratory syndrome coronavirus 2 (SARS-CoV-2)

History
Highly associated symptoms include the following (CDC, 2022a):

- Known exposure to COVID-19 or sick contacts
- Fatigue
- Muscle or body aches
- Headache
- New loss of taste or smell
- Sore throat
- Congestion or runny nose
- Nausea or vomiting
- Diarrhea
- Can be asymptomatic, most often seen in the pediatric population; cough and fever the most common symptoms seen in children, but about half of the pediatric population are asymptomatic as suggested by evidence (CDC, 2020)

Physical Findings

- Physical exam for COVID-19 nonspecific and similar to other respiratory infections
- Positive COVID-19 nucleic acid amplification test (NAAT) and/or antigen test (CDC, 2022c)
- Fever or chills
- Dry cough
- Shortness of breath or difficulty breathing
- Abnormal chest x-ray
- Hypoxia

Considerations

- COVID-19 may result in complications such as pneumonia, sepsis, cardiac injury, or multiple organ failure.
- Additional complications specific to COVID-19 may include blood clots and multisystem inflammatory syndrome in children (MIS-C) and adults (MIS-A).
- Age is a strong risk factor associated with symptom progression.
- Other individuals at higher risk of complications include those with preexisting comorbidities such as asthma, cancer, cerebrovascular disease, chronic kidney disease, chronic lung disease, chronic liver disease, CF, diabetes, HIV, obesity, and primary immunodeficiencies.
- Most individuals who get COVID-19 will recover on their own.

Cystic Fibrosis

An inherited disorder caused by a mutation in the cystic fibrosis transmembrane conductance regulator (CFTR) protein.

History

- Infants with positive newborn screening; may have meconium ileus, respiratory symptoms
- In pediatric and adults, persistent, productive cough, wheezing, dyspnea, recurrent lung infections, pancreatic insufficiency, diabetes, infertility, anemia

Physical Findings

- Clinical features vary. Respiratory findings include chronic, productive cough; sinusitis; recurrent pneumonia, wheezing; and clubbing.
- Gastrointestinal findings include malabsorption, abdominal distention, and palpable masses
- Genitourinary findings include frequent urinary tract infections, amenorrhea in women, and undescended testicles in men

Considerations

- CF is a complex, progressive disease with a varying course, from mild symptoms to severe progressive airway and end organ damage.
- Improved therapies for airway clearance, pancreatic enzyme supplements, and medications have improved life expectancy.

Influenza
A highly contagious viral respiratory infection

History
- Cough, fever, sore throat, body aches, headache

Physical Findings
- Physical exam is nonspecific, except for the likelihood of fever.
- Abnormal breath sounds generally indicate other illnesses or complications of influenza.

Considerations
- Diagnostic testing is not necessary to make the diagnosis of influenza, especially in the midst of a community outbreak.
- Improved therapies for airway clearance, pancreatic enzyme supplements, and medications have improved life expectancy.

Lung Cancer
A malignancy that forms in the tissues of the lungs

History
- Lethargic
- Shortness of breath
- Chest pain
- Bone pain
- Weakness
- Headaches
- Confusion
- Nausea
- Constipation

Physical Findings
- Weight loss
- Vision changes
- Hoarseness
- Cough with or without hemoptysis
- Lymphadenopathy
- Pale, low-grade fever
- Tachypnea
- Hypoxia
- Jaundice
- Clubbing
- Lung findings including decreased or absent breath sounds, dullness to percussion
- Gastrointestinal findings including hepatomegaly, discomfort with abdominal exam

Considerations
- Screening guidelines vary.
- Individuals who have symptoms of lung cancer should have a diagnostic evaluation rather than a screening.

Obstructive Sleep Apnea
A syndrome of repeated episodes of reduced airflow during sleep

History
- Fatigue
- Reported daytime sleepiness

Physical Findings
- Obesity
- Loud snoring, frequent arousals, disruption of sleep
- Large neck circumference

Considerations
- Diagnostic testing is by polysomnography (PSG).
- Obstructive sleep apnea (OSA) is also associated with other poor health outcomes, such as cardiovascular disease, hypertension, metabolic abnormalities such as type 2 diabetes, and an increased risk of postoperative cardiac and respiratory complications.

Pertussis
A bacterial infection of the respiratory tract, also known as whooping cough.

History
- It begins with rhinorrhea and mild cough, progresses to severe coughing spasms, characteristic whoop sound to fill lungs, and postcough vomiting.

Physical Examination
- Assess for paroxysms of coughing, especially in unvaccinated individuals.

Consideration
- There are three stages: (1) catarrhal, 1 to 2 weeks; (2) paroxysmal, 1 to 6 weeks; (3) convalescence, 2 to 3 weeks.

Pneumonia
A bacterial infection of the lower respiratory tract

History
- Cough, dyspnea, pleural pain
- Sweating and night sweats
- Chills, myalgias

Physical Findings
- Fever greater than 100.6°F
- Tachycardia
- Tachypnea
- Crackles on auscultation
- Increased tactile fremitus

Considerations
- Consider chest x-ray for suspected pneumonia.
- The CURB-65 Pneumonia Severity Scale helps determine whether hospitalization is needed.

Pneumothorax
Pneumothorax occurs when air gathers outside of the lung but is confined within the pleural cavity. This air outside of the lung causes pressure on the lung, causing it to collapse.

History
- Chest pain, often described as sharp and severe and will radiate to the ipsilateral shoulder
- Shortness of breath

Physical Findings
- Respiratory distress
- Tachypnea
- Asymmetric lung expansion
- Decreased tactile fremitus on the affected side
- Hyperresonant percussion on the affected side
- Decreased or absent breath sounds on the affected side
- Imaging indicating pneumothorax (chest x-ray, CT scan, or ultrasound)

Considerations
- There are two types of pneumothoraxes: traumatic and atraumatic. A traumatic pneumothorax is caused by either a blunt force or penetrating trauma to the chest. There are two atraumatic subtypes: primary and secondary. The cause of a primary pneumothorax is unknown and happens spontaneously. A secondary pneumothorax is caused by an underlying pulmonary disease.

Tuberculosis
An infectious disease primarily caused by *Mycobacterium tuberculosis*.

History
- History of previous diagnosis or treatment
- Immunocompromising conditions
- Countries of origin or travel to countries with a high prevalence of TB
- Previous living conditions and possible contacts with TB
- Cough, possibly productive of blood or sputum
- Chest pain
- Fatigue
- Anorexia
- Chills
- Night sweats
- Dyspnea

Physical Findings
- Fever
- Weight loss, or in children growth delay
- Cutaneous lesions
- Lymphadenopathy
- Wheezing
- Respiratory distress
- Hepatosplenomegaly
- Positive tuberculin skin test (TST) or interferon gamma-release assay (IGRA)
- Nonspecific chest x-ray findings, but may include lymphadenopathy, especially in children, as well as nodular and fibrotic lesions, infiltrates, pleural effusions, and cavitations; normal chest x-ray findings also possible, but this does not rule out TB in a person with other signs and symptoms
- Positive acid-fast bacilli (AFB) smear
- Positive TB culture

Considerations
- No single symptom, physical finding, or chest x-ray result can diagnose active TB alone.

PHYSICAL EXAMINATION DOCUMENTATION

Documentation should include results of inspection, palpation, percussion, and auscultation.

EXAMPLE OF NORMAL FINDINGS
Respirations 14 breaths per minute, easy without retractions; regular rate and rhythm. O_2 sat with pulse oximeter at 99%. No lesions, masses, or skin discolorations of the anterior or posterior chest wall. Anteroposterior less than the transverse diameter. Chest expansion symmetric. Tactile fremitus equal bilaterally. No tenderness with palpation of thorax or intercostal cartilage. Lung fields resonant to percussion throughout. Breath sounds full, equal, and clear bilaterally; no adventitious sounds auscultated.

EXAMPLE OF ABNORMAL FINDINGS
Respiratory rate 28 breaths per minute, shallow, rapid breathing with slight intercostal retractions; sitting in the upright position and leaning forward. No audible adventitious breath sounds; no nasal flaring, no suprasternal or substernal retractions noted. Mucosa pale pink. O_2 sat with pulse oximeter at 94%. Chest expansion symmetric. No skin discolorations of the chest wall; no palpable tenderness. Tactile fremitus equal bilaterally. Hyperresonance to the lower lung fields bilaterally to percussion. Breath sounds diminished, equal with scattered expiratory wheezes noted at the bases bilaterally.

REFERENCES

References for this chapter draw from Chapter 11, Evidence-Based Assessment of the Lungs and Respiratory System, of the textbook *Evidence-Based Physical Examination: Best Practices for Health and Well-Being Assessment (Second Edition)*. The references may be accessed in the digital version of the handbook at https://connect.springerpub.com/content/book/978-0-8261-8852-6/chapter/ch04.

5

Evidence-Based Assessment of the Skin, Hair, and Nails

CLINICAL CONSIDERATIONS

- Be sure to ask about the patient's occupational history (e.g., exposure to chemicals, water, sun).
- Be consistent in the order in which the comprehensive skin exam is conducted. This will ensure a skin region is not missed.
- Integrate an exam of the surrounding skin when examining a specific body area.
- Include palpation of the skin in an attempt to feel abnormal areas on the skin that may be visually missed.
- During a total body skin exam, include an assessment of the mucous membranes of the oral cavity.
- There is assessment value in the use of smell during a skin exam to identify varied skin disorders.
- Always know red flags for the health history and clinical examination. (**Boxes 5.1** and **5.2**)

SUBJECTIVE HISTORY

COMMON REASONS FOR SEEKING CARE
- Rash
- Abnormal lesion(s)
- Changes in hair/nails

HISTORY OF PRESENT ILLNESS
- **Onset:** When did the rash start? When was the lesion first noticed? Did this rash/lesion occur suddenly, or has it been developing gradually?
- **Location:** Where is the rash located? Is there any rash noted on the rest of the skin? Are the hair changes on one side or both sides of the head?
- **Duration:** How long has the rash/lesion been present? Over what period of time has the rash/lesion developed?
- **Characteristics:** Are there any symptoms with this rash/lesion? Itching? Drainage? Tenderness or pain? Bleeding? Changes in color? Variations related to weather/season? Fever? Are there

---

BOX 5.1 Red Flags in Subjective History

- Immunosuppressed patient
- Severe pain
- Very old or very young age
- Associated photophobia, headache
- Start of a new medication

---

any contacts with a similar skin disorder? Have the rash/hair/nail changes happened in the past? Have there been any changes to the hair (loss, growth [slow or excessive], texture, or color)? Are the nails brittle or thin? Are the nails thickening or changing in color? Is there any discoloration in the nails?

- **Aggravating factors:** What action or activities make the rash worse? Are new skin care products or new household cleaning products being used? Are there any new exposures? Hot tubs, pools, lakes, and so on? Has there been any exposure to toxins or chemicals (environmental or occupational)? Are any commercial hair products used? Does the patient pull their hair? Do they bite their nails or pick their skin? Have they injured their nails or fingers? Are the hands/feet frequently in water?
- **Relieving factors:** How has the patient been treating the problem (e.g., medications such as steroids, antifungals, lotions)?
- **Treatment:** What medications or treatments have been tried to help with the rash/hair/nail changes?
- **Severity:** How severe are the symptoms on a scale of 0 to 10? Do the symptoms limit participation in activities or alter the quality of life? Are there associated symptoms? Are the symptoms worsening? How has this skin condition affected the patient (physical, psychological, or social)?

HEALTH HISTORY

Past Medical History

- History of allergic reactions, asthma, or allergic rhinitis
- Previous diagnoses of skin cancer, dysplastic nevi, or suspicious lesions
- History of any serious sunburns or childhood sunburns
- History of any chronic illnesses, mental health disorders, or autoimmune disorders
- History of tanning bed use, nail salons
- Previous diagnoses of alopecia or onychomycosis
- Any contact with a person who has a similar rash/lesion
- History of pregnancy or traumatic event(s)

- History of recent travel (If so, where, when, how long did they stay?)
- Sunscreen use (frequency, sun protection factor [SPF])

Medications
- Prescribed medications (oral and topical), including dose and frequency, specifically chemotherapy, psoralens, retinoids, tetracyclines, allopurinol, antiseizure medications, or antimalarials
- Over-the-counter (OTC) medications or supplements, including dose and frequency
- Recent or new antibiotic and/or medication use

Allergies
- Allergies to medications, or seasonal, environmental, and/or food allergies? If yes to being allergic to any substance or environmental trigger, clarify reactions, specifically previous reactions causing skin rashes, itching, or hives.

Immunizations
- **Risks for vaccine-preventable illnesses:** Vaccine status, including childhood vaccines (measles, mumps, rubella [MMR], varicella zoster, meningococcal, COVID-19, and human papillomavirus [HPV])

Pediatric Considerations
- Is the infant breast- or formula-fed? If formula, what type?
- Have foods been introduced? If so, what has been introduced and when?
- What is the skin cleansing routine with diaper changes? What types of diapers are used?
- What types of soaps, oils, and lotions are applied to the infant/child's skin?
- What types of food does your child eat? What are their usual eating habits?
- Are you aware of any infectious diseases to which your child may have been exposed?
- Has your child had any recent skin injuries? Frequent/recent falls or abrasions? Unexplained injuries?
- Does your child pull or twist their hair?
- Does your child bite or pick their nails or surrounding skin?

Considerations for the Older Adult
- Do you have increased or decreased sensation to touch?
- What is your level of lifetime sun or irritant exposures? Have there been any known occupational exposures?
- Do you fall frequently? Any recent falls?
- Do you have any limitations in your mobility?
- Are you taking any anticoagulants?

- Are you incontinent of bowel or bladder?
- Does your skin ever rip or tear?

FAMILY HISTORY

- Skin disorders (skin cancer, psoriasis, eczema, hives, hay fever, allergies, asthma, autoimmune disorders)
- Hair loss (receding hairline, baldness)
- Any chronic diseases, mental health disorders, or cancers

SOCIAL HISTORY

- Do you use alcohol, tobacco, or recreational drugs? If so, what type and how frequently?
- Have you ever been diagnosed with a sexually transmitted infection or disease?
- Do you consistently wear condoms during sexual encounters?
- Do you practice any cultural or special rituals that may affect your skin, hair, or nails?
- Have you experienced any recent stress?
- Do you paint your nails or apply artificial or gel nails?
- Do you dye your hair or get permanents?
- Can you describe your current living situation (who you live with and the type of residence)?
- Do you recall what you have eaten and drunk in the past 24 hours? Describe.

Occupation

- Are you required to wear a specific type of helmet, hat, goggles, gloves, or shoes?
- Do you use personal protective equipment at work?
- Does your work require you to perform repetitive tasks?
- Do you work with or around chemicals? If so, which ones?
- Do you work outdoors?
- Do you wear sunscreen or sun-protective clothing?
- Does your occupation place you at risk for chemical exposure to skin, hair, and nails? If so, how?

REVIEW OF SYSTEMS

- **General:** Fatigue, malaise, fever, weight loss or gain, pain anywhere in the body
- **Head, eyes, ears, nose, throat:** Hair loss or excessive growth, change of hair texture, ringing in the ears, decreased hearing, changes in vision, photosensitivity, blurred vision, dry eyes, runny nose, altered smell, sinus congestion, sore throat, hoarseness, dry mouth, changes in teeth or gums, enlarged lymph nodes on the head or neck
- **Respiratory:** Shortness of breath, cough (productive or dry), painful or altered breathing

- **Cardiovascular:** Chest pain; shortness of breath; palpitations; arrhythmias; hair loss on the lower extremities; swelling of hands, legs, or feet
- **Gastrointestinal:** Abdominal pain, bloating or distention, changes in bowel movements, heartburn, nausea, vomiting
- **Genitourinary:** Painful urination, urinary frequency, urinary retention, urinary urgency, incontinence, difficulty starting urine stream, blood in urine, vaginal or penile discharge, pain or swelling
- **Musculoskeletal:** Single or multiple joint pain, swelling of joints, decreased movement or strength, muscle pain and/or muscle weakness, skin changes over bony prominences
- **Neurologic:** Headaches, change in thinking or cognition, memory loss, tingling or numbness
- **Hematologic:** Easy bruising, bleeding, spider veins, prominent or painful blood vessels
- **Integumentary:** Changes in skin color; texture; thickness or thinning; excessive sweating or dryness; new lesions or rashes; temperature change; scar changes or nail changes; any loss of tissue in the face, arms, legs, or buttocks
- **Mental health:** Increased or persistent anxiety and/or depression, scratching or picking of skin or nails, pulling of the hair, self-harm behaviors

PHYSICAL EXAMINATION

GENERAL SURVEY
- Vital signs, including temperature, pulse rate, respiratory rate, and blood pressure
- Toxic versus nontoxic appearance
- Hygiene and odors

BOX 5.2 Red Flags in Objective Exam

- Toxic appearance
- Unstable vital signs
- Fever and a petechial/purpura or erythematous rash
- Scalded skin appearance
- Rash covering more than 90% of the body
- Nonblanching rash
- Mucosal lesions
- Rash or lesion that does not go away
- ABCDE for a mole

ABCDE, asymmetry, border, color, diameter, and evolving.

INSPECTION

- Inspect the skin in a head-to-toe sequence with the breast and genitalia examined last. Use the same assessment technique and order to maintain consistency and avoid omitting any portion of the patient's skin.
- Start with a general survey of the skin, including color, pigmentation, vascularity, bruising, lesions, color variations, and general hygiene.
- Inspect and measure all skin lesions (**Tables 5.1** and **5.2**). A dermatoscope can be helpful if it is available and the clinician is adequately trained in its use.
- Describe the findings, noting the number, location, size, color, shape, morphology, distribution, and configuration.
- Note distribution, texture, and quantity of hair.
- Inspect the fingernails and toenails, noting color and shape. Nail polish should be removed prior to examination.

PALPATION

- Palpate the skin and note the temperature, texture, moisture, and turgor.
- Palpate appropriate lesions, assessing the texture of the lesion, presence of tenderness or pain, temperature of the lesion and the surrounding skin, fluidity, and blanching capacity.
- Palpate the fingernails and toenails for texture and note capillary refill test (CRT).

PEDIATRIC CONSIDERATIONS

Preterm Infants

- Preterm infants' skin often appears ruddy, gelatinous, and almost transparent due to the decreased presence of stratum corneum and the small amount of fat present.
- Fine, silky hair called *lanugo* is more common in preterm infants and is usually present on the back and shoulders.
- The preterm and full-term infant's nails are soft and flexible.

Infants, Children, and Adolescents

- Approximately 50% of newborns experience physiologic jaundice, which is a normal phenomenon resulting from increased hemolysis of red blood cells following birth.
- Seborrheic dermatitis (cradle cap) appears as a scaly crust.
- There may be harmless markings on newborns, such as tiny, white facial papules (milia), vascular markings (salmon patches/stork bites), and Mongolian spots (congenital dermal melanocytosis).
- Bruising to lower legs may be present as the child becomes mobile.
- There are a variety of different rashes that typically occur only in childhood (**Table 5.3**).

TABLE 5.1 Primary Skin Lesions

Lesion	Description	Examples	Visual With Diagnosis
Macule	• Flat, nonpalpable • Smaller than 1 cm	• Freckles • Flat moles (nevi) • Measles • Petechiae[a]	Leukocytoclastic vasculitis 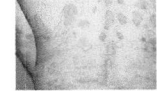
Patch	• Flat, nonpalpable • Larger than 1 cm	• Vitiligo • Mongolian spots • Port-wine stains • Chloasma • Café-au-lait patch	Tinea versicolor
Papule	• Elevated, solid palpable • Smaller than 0.5 cm	• Purpura[b] • Elevated moles • Warts • Insect bites • Lichens planus	Bedbug bites
Plaque	• Groups of papules • Larger than 5 cm	• Psoriasis • Seborrheic and actinic keratosis • Lichen planus	Psoriasis
Pustule	• Elevated, pus-filled vesicle or bullae • Varies in size	• Acne • Impetigo • Carbuncles	Pustules from fire ant bites 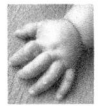
Cyst	• Elevated, encapsulated, fluid- or semisolid-filled, or solid mass in the dermis or subcutaneous layers • 1 cm or larger	• Sebaceous cyst • Epidermoid cyst • Acne	Inflamed sebaceous cyst 

(continued)

TABLE 5.1 Primary Skin Lesions *(continued)*

Lesion	Description	Examples	Visual With Diagnosis
Vesicle	• Elevated, fluid-filled, round- or oval-shaped with thin, translucent walls • Smaller than 0.5 cm	• Herpes simplex or zoster • Early chicken pox • Poison ivy • Small burn blister	Herpes zoster
Bullae	• Elevated, fluid-filled, round- or oval-shaped with thin, translucent walls • Larger than 0.5–1 cm	• Contact dermatitis • Friction or fracture blister • Large burn blister • Pemphigus vulgaris	Fracture blister
Nodule	• Elevated, solid, hard or soft, palpable mass deeper in the dermis • Smaller than 2 cm	• Small lipoma • Squamous cell carcinoma • Fibroma • Nevi • Erythema nodosum	Nodular melanoma
Tumor	• Elevated, solid, hard or soft, palpable mass deeper in the dermis with irregular borders • Larger than 2 cm	• Lipomas • Carcinoma • Hemangioma • Benign tumor	Basal cell carcinoma
Wheal	• Elevated, often reddish area with irregular borders caused by diffuse fluid in tissues (cutaneous edema) • Varies in size	• Insect bites • Hives (urticarial) • Allergic reaction	Urticarial drug reaction 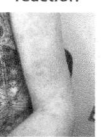

[a]Petechiae are unique in this list because they are nonblanching vascular lesions. They can be considered a subcategory of macules.
[b]Also a nonblanching lesion.

TABLE 5.2 Secondary Skin Lesions

Lesion	Description	Examples	Visual With Diagnosis
Atrophy	• Thinning or wasting of skin due to loss of collagen and elastin	• Striae • Aged skin	Pruritic urticarial papules and plaques of pregnancy (PUPPP) rash
Excoriation	• Absence of superficial epidermis, causing a moist, shallow depression	• Scratch marks • Abrasion • Scabies	Abrasion (bike wreck on asphalt)
Keloid	• Elevated area of excessive scar tissue that extends beyond the site of original injury (caused by excessive collagen formation during healing)	• Keloid for ear piercing or following surgery	Keloids from folliculitis barbae
Scale	• Flakes of greasy keratinized skin tissue • May be white, gray, or silver • Texture may be fine or thick • Varies in size	• Dry skin • Dandruff • Psoriasis • Eczema	Psoriasis
Crust	• Dried blood, serum, or pus on the epidermis from ruptured vesicles or pustules • Slightly elevated	• Eczema • Impetigo • Herpes • Scabs following an abrasion	Early impetigo

(continued)

TABLE 5.2 Secondary Skin Lesions *(continued)*

Lesion	Description	Examples	Visual With Diagnosis
	• May be red, brown, orange, or yellow • Varies in size		
Fissure	• Linear crack or break with sharp edges extending into the dermis • May be moist or dry	• Cracks at the corner of the mouth, on the fingers, or on the feet (athlete's foot)	Fissure caused by finger eczema
Lichenifi-cation	• A rough, thick-ened, hardened area of the epi-dermis resulting from chronic irritation such as scratching or rubbing (often involves flexor surfaces)	• Chronic dermatitis	Chronic dermatitis
Scar	• Elevated, irreg-ular area of con-nective tissue left after a lesion or wound has healed • May be red or purple if new scars • May be silvery or white if old scars	• Healed surgi-cal wound or injury • Healed acne	Surgical scar: knee replacement
Ulcer	• Irregularly shaped area of skin loss that extends into the dermis or sub-cutaneous tissue; concave • Varies in depth	• Stasis and de-cubiti ulcers • Aphthous ulcers	Aphthous ulcer

TABLE 5.3 Common Childhood Rashes

Disease State	History and Physical Findings	Visual
Fifth disease • Also called *erythema infectiosum* • Caused by parvovirus B19 • Transmitted through respiratory secretions and blood	• 4–14 days incubation period • Often have fever, rhinorrhea, myalgias, and headache • Facial rash that has a "slapped cheek" appearance • Can get a second itchy rash a few days after the facial rash that appears on the chest, back, buttocks, or arms and legs	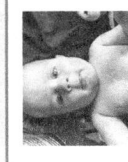
Hand, foot, and mouth disease • Caused by a virus called coxsackievirus A16 • Transmitted through respiratory secretions, fecal–oral route, or vesicle fluid	• Usually affects infants and children 5 years old or younger • Typically occurs in summer and early fall • Starts with fever, malaise, sore throat, and anorexia • Can develop painful macular or vesicular lesions in the mouth several days after the fever starts • May also develop rash on the palms of the hands and soles of the feet over 1 or 2 days as a macular and/or vesicular red rash; may also appear on the knees, elbows, buttocks, or genital area	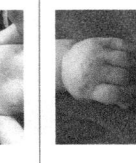 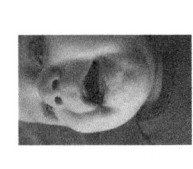

(continued)

TABLE 5.3 Common Childhood Rashes *(continued)*

Disease State	History and Physical Findings	Visual
Impetigo • Usually caused by *Staphylococcus aureus* or *Streptococcus pyogenes* • Bacteria introduced through a break in the skin • Three types of impetigo: bullous (large blisters), nonbullous (crusted), and ecthyma (ulcers)	• Most common in children between the ages of 2 and 6 • Can develop lesions anywhere, but usually occur on the face, around the mouth and nose, and on the hands/feet • Vesicular lesions, burst and develop honey-colored crusts • Can be spread to other areas of the body by fingers, clothing, and towels • If bullous impetigo, with larger blisters that are more likely to be on the trunk • If ecthyma impetigo, can form deep, painful ulcers	
Infantile seborrheic dermatitis • Commonly referred to as *cradle cap* when found on the scalp • Noncontagious	• Affects the oily areas of the body, including the scalp, face, sides of the nose, eyebrows, ears, eyelids, and chest • Typically presents with erythema and greasy scales • Usually benign and self-limited • Typically resolves within several weeks to several months	
Measles (rubeola) • Caused by the virus rubeola • Spread to others through respiratory secretions • Highly contagious • Vaccination available	• 7–14 days incubation period after a person is infected • Maculopapular rash that starts on the head and moves down the body • Other symptoms including malaise, high fever, cough, rhinorrhea, conjunctivitis, and Koplik spots (tiny white spots inside the mouth) • Conjunctivitis the main symptom that distinguishes measles from influenza, in addition to the rash	

Molluscum contagiosum

* Caused by a virus called the poxvirus
* Transmitted from direct person-to-person physical contact and through contaminated fomites

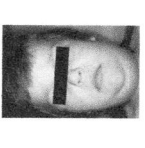

* White-, pink-, or flesh-colored papules that are umbilicated
* Often have a pearly appearance
* Usually smooth and firm
* Lesions ranging from about 2 to 5 mm in diameter
* May become pruritic, painful, erythematous, and/or swollen
* May occur anywhere on the body, including the face, neck, arms, legs, abdomen, and genital area
* Can occur alone or in groups

Mumps

* Caused by the mumps virus, which belongs to a family of viruses known as paramyxoviruses
* Transmitted through direct contact with saliva or respiratory droplets from the mouth, nose, or throat
* Vaccination available

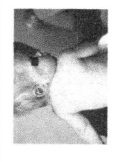

* Symptoms typically appearing 16–18 days after infection
* Puffy cheeks and a tender, swollen jaw due to swollen salivary glands on one or both sides (parotitis)
* Other symptoms including fever, headache, myalgias, malaise, and anorexia
* Can be asymptomatic in some

Roseola

* Caused by a virus called human herpes virus 6
* Transmitted by oral and respiratory secretions and direct person-to-person contact
* Vaccination available

* 9–10 days incubation period
* Common in children aged 3 months to 4 years (most commonly, 6 months to 1 year)
* Initial symptoms including acute-onset high fever, eye redness, sore throat, irritability, and rhinorrhea
* Presents pinkish-red, maculopapular rash once the fever resolves (after 2–4 days)

(continued)

TABLE 5.3 Common Childhood Rashes *(continued)*

Disease State	History and Physical Findings	Visual
Rubella • Also called German measles • Caused by the rubella virus (genus *Rubivirus* in the family Togaviridae) • Transmitted via direct or droplet contact with respiratory secretions • Vaccination available	• Rash starting on the trunk and spreading peripherally • Symptoms that may occur 1–5 days before the rash appears, including low-grade fever, headache, conjunctivitis, lymphadenopathy, cough, and/or rhinorrhea • Rash generally first appearing on the face, then spreading to the rest of the body, and lasts about 3 days • Can be asymptomatic • Typically mild presentation	
Scarlet fever • Also known as scarlatina • Caused by group A hemolytic *Streptococcus*	• Most common in children 5–15 years • Most commonly seen in conjunction with strep pharyngitis • Typically starts with a high fever and sore throat • Rash appearing after 1–2 days • Maculopapular exanthematous rash that looks like a sunburn and feels like sandpaper • Rash initially appearing on the neck and chest, then spreading over the body • Pastia's sign (linear bright red coloration of the creases in the axillary and inguinal folds) • Tongue that may appear white, with red, swollen papillae (white strawberry tongue), but by the fourth or fifth day becomes bright red (red strawberry tongue)	

- Rash caused by an erythrogenic exotoxin emitted by the streptococci
- Other symptoms including headache, chills, flushed face, nausea, and vomiting
- Rash usually fading in 4–5 days and followed by diffuse desquamation

Varicella
- Caused by the varicella zoster virus
- Transmitted mainly through close contact with someone who has chicken pox
- Highly contagious disease
- Vaccination available

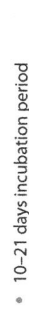

- 10–21 days incubation period
- Rash first appearing on the chest, back, and face, then spreading over the entire body
- Vesicular appearance of rash initially, followed by simultaneous occurrence of papular and macular rashes with crusting
- Rash highly pruritic
- Other symptoms including fever, malaise, anorexia, and headache
- Lasts 5–6 days
- Disease contagious until crusting appears

Sources: From Centers for Disease Control and Prevention (roseola, rubella, scarlet fever, varicella); Centers for Disease Control and Prevention and Heinz F. Eichenwald, MD (measles [rubeola]); Centers for Disease Control and Prevention, Patricia Smith, and Barbara Rice.

- The presence and characteristics of facial hair and body hair change considerably during adolescence. See Chapter 17, Evidence-Based Considerations for Assessment Across the Life Span, for the Tanner stages.
- Increased perspiration, oiliness, and acne are common in adolescents due to increased sebaceous activity.

CONSIDERATIONS FOR THE OLDER ADULT
- The clinician must be cognizant of signs of maltreatment by assessing for bruising, lacerations, pressure ulcers, dehydration, and poor hygiene.
- Skin may appear pale and to hang from the frame.
- Normal older adult skin variations may include solar lentigo (liver spots), seborrheic keratosis, and acrochordon (skin tag).
- Skin tears may also be present due to the fragility of the skin.
- The hair may be thin, gray, and coarse with symmetric balding in men.
- The amount of body hair decreases (body, pubic, and axillary hair).
- Men have an increase in the amount and coarseness of nasal and eyebrow hair. Women may develop coarse facial hair.

DERMATOLOGIC EXAMINATION CONSIDERATIONS FOR SPECIFIC POPULATIONS
- Hispanic, Asian, American Indian (including Pacific Islanders), African, and Black populations have differences and variations in skin color, tone, and rash presentations. A predisposition to scarring and pathogenesis of skin disorders is unique and common to these groups.
- Darker skin tones have a greater susceptibility to forming melasma, keloids, and dyschromia.
- Special clinical considerations and key features related to skin cancer exist for individuals with darker skin. Skin cancer occurs at a lower rate in darker skin compared with lighter white skin; however, the morbidity and mortality are significantly higher in persons of color due to delayed diagnosis.

ABNORMAL FINDINGS

ACNE
Chronic inflammatory dermatosis affecting the pilosebaceous follicles of the skin

History
- Typically seen in adolescents but can occur at any age
- History of polycystic ovarian syndrome (PCOS)
- May report pain, tenderness, and/or erythema in affected areas

Physical Examination
- Closed and open comedones (noninflammatory acne); papules, pustules, nodules, or cysts (inflammatory acne)
- May affect only the face, but the chest, back, and upper arms frequently involved due to the density of sebaceous glands
- Postinflammatory hyperpigmentation and/or atrophic scars (moderate to severe acne)

Considerations
- Acne may have a psychological impact.
- Assessment and examination should focus on the extent and severity of acne lesions, number of lesions, anatomic location of acne, scarring, and quality of life and other psychosocial metrics.
- Grading and classification systems may also be useful in patient care by specifically classifying acne (mild, moderate, or severe), directing treatment options, and assessing patient response to therapy.

ACTINIC KERATOSIS
Premalignant skin lesions that form from an abnormal production of keratinocytes after excessive prolonged UV exposure

History
- Frequently seen in people over 50 with excessive sun exposure
- History of sunburns
- Immunosuppression

Physical Examination
- Erythematous, hyperkeratotic scaly macules, papules, and plaques on sun-damaged skin (**Figure 5.1**)
- Typically located on the face, ears, scalp, neck, and extremities
- Six to eight average number of lesions identified
- Lesions ranging in color from white to yellow, pink, or red
- Feels rough on palpation

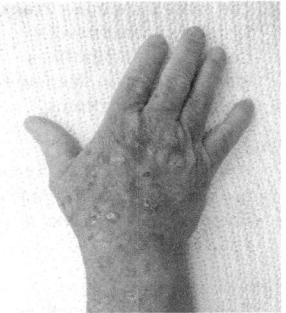

FIGURE 5.1 Actinic keratosis on the back of the hand.
Source: Image courtesy of James Heilman, MD.

Considerations
- Without treatment, can progress to squamous cell carcinoma
- Also known as *solar keratosis*

BASAL CELL CARCINOMA
Evolves from the basal cells found in the lower layer of the epidermis

History
- Most commonly develops on sun-exposed skin areas, history of sun damage
- Slow-growing, bleeds with trauma
- Fair-skinned patients disproportionately affected

Physical Examination
- A nonhealing sore that is friable and umbilicated
- Waxy papules with central depression, pearly, erosion, or ulceration
- Crusting
- Rolled border
- Translucency
- Surface telangiectasia

Consideration
- The most common malignancy in humans but usually does not metastasize

BED BUG BITES
Small, parasitic insects that feed on the blood of people and animals while they sleep

History
- Bite marks appearing anywhere from one to several days after the initial bite
- Bites mildly erythematous and pruritic
- Can cause insomnia and anxiety
- History of recent travel
- Contact with similar bites
- Identified bugs in sleeping environment
- No systemic symptoms

Physical Examination
- Bite marks can occur in a random distribution, a straight line, or in groups of three (see Papule in **Table 5.1**).
- Bites can cause additional skin problems that arise from intense scratching.

Consideration
- Can be difficult to eradicate from housing

CELLULITIS
A bacterial infection of the deeper dermis and subcutaneous tissues predominantly caused by group A *Streptococcus*, *Staphylococcus aureus* in adults, and *Haemophilus influenzae* type B in children less than 3 years old

History
- Those with a history of lymphedema, venous insufficiency, cellulitis, tinea pedis, and obesity at increased risk
- History of diabetes and peripheral vascular disease

Physical Examination
- Trauma to the skin
- Erythema
- Calor
- Edema of the skin
- Pain
- Fever
- Leukocytosis
- Mildly elevated sedimentation rate
- Unilateral
- Has indistinct borders

Considerations
- Cellulitis typically affects the skin on the lower legs, but can occur on any skin surface area (**Figure 5.2**).
- It can progress quickly to fulminant sepsis with necrotizing fasciitis especially in a patient with comorbidities.

CONTACT DERMATITIS
An eczematous inflammatory skin condition

History
- Painful or itchy skin
- Exposure to an allergen or irritants (poison ivy is most common)
- Common allergens including jewelry metals (e.g., nickel), cosmetic products, fragrances, and preservatives
- Common irritants including detergents, soap, cleaners, and acid
- Certain professions at higher risk, including construction workers, hair stylists, florists, landscapers, food handlers, healthcare clinicians, janitors, plumbers, and mechanics

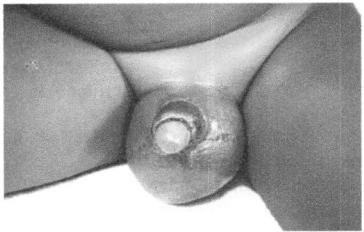

FIGURE 5.2 Cellulitis on the scrotum of an infant.
Source: Centers for Disease Control and Prevention/Robert S. Craig.

Physical Examination
- Dryness and scaling
- Pruritic papules, vesicles, and/or bullae with an erythematous base; crusting and oozing may be present
- If chronic presentation, may include lichenification, scaling, and fissuring
- Can occur on any part of the body that has come in contact with the offending agent

Considerations
- Irritant dermatitis accounts for 80% of contact dermatitis cases.
- Skin areas more vulnerable to contact dermatitis include hands, face, eyelids, neck, scalp, lower extremities, feet, and the anogenital region.
- Areas with thinner epidermis are at increased risk.

ECZEMA (ATOPIC DERMATITIS)

An inflammatory skin disorder characterized by pruritus and exacerbation and remission of dry, itchy, erythematous skin with no known etiology

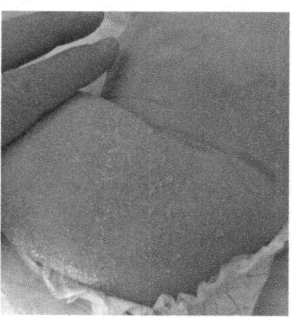

FIGURE 5.3 Atopic dermatitis (eczema) on the abdomen and thigh of an infant.
Source: Image courtesy of GZ.

History
- Occurs most commonly in infants 3 to 6 months of age (**Figure 5.3**)
- Often has a history of asthma, allergic rhinitis, urticaria, or acute allergic reactions to certain foods
- Pruritis

Physical Examination
- Scaly, erythematous patches
- Xerosis
- Lichenification
- Excoriation
- Possible erosions commonly appearing in creases of the elbows or knees or the nape of the neck

Considerations
- Scratching and rubbing further irritate the skin, increase inflammation, and make itchiness worse.
- Treatment for the condition aims to heal the affected skin and prevent flare-ups of symptoms.

EPIDERMOID CYST (SEBACEOUS CYST)
A benign encapsulated, subepidermal keratin-filled nodule

History
- Most commonly located on the face, neck, and trunk, but can develop anywhere
- Slow-growing
- History of chronic sun damage
- Asymptomatic

Physical Examination
- 0.5 cm to several centimeters, nonfluctuant, compressible, smooth, shiny, mobile nodule
- A central, dark comedone opening frequently present
- If the cyst ruptures, may look like a furuncle with tenderness, erythema, and swelling (see Cyst in **Table 5.1**)
- A foul-smelling, yellowish cheese-like discharge

Considerations
- Can be caused by imiquimod and cyclosporine

ERYTHEMA MIGRANS
A bull's-eye rash associated with the first stage of Lyme disease

History
- History of tick bite or being outdoors
- Appears 3 to 30 days after the bite occurred (average is about 7 days)
- Rarely itchy or painful
- Can also be associated with fever, myalgias, lymphadenopathy, fatigue, and malaise

Physical Examination
- Typically the rash occurs at the site of the tick bite.
- It has a distinct bull's-eye appearance (**Figure 5.4**).
- It expands in size gradually over a period of days reaching up to 12 inches or more (30 cm) across.
- It may have mild calor.

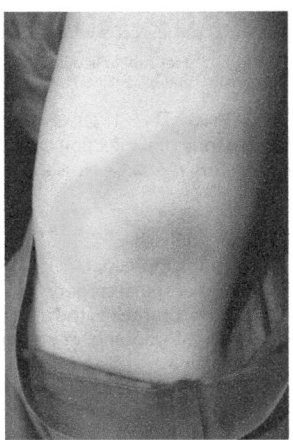

FIGURE 5.4 Erythema migrans.
Source: Centers for Disease Control and Prevention.

Considerations
- It is caused by the bacterium *Borrelia burgdorferi*.
- Approximately 70% to 80% of people with Lyme disease will have this rash.

FOLLICULITIS
An infection of the hair follicles caused by damage to the hair follicle or from blockage of the follicle

History
- Use of razor in the affected area
- Can cause itching or soreness
- History of hot tub, whirlpool, or swimming pool use

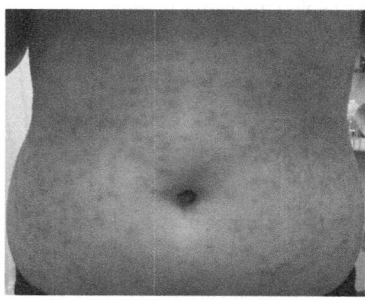

Physical Examination
- It can occur anywhere on the skin.
- Papules or pustules form around a hair follicle; it can look similar to acne (**Figure 5.5**).

Consideration
- Typically due to *S. aureus* bacteria but can also be caused by *Pseudomonas* aeruginosa

FIGURE 5.5 "Hot tub" folliculitis.
Source: Image courtesy of James Heilman, MD.

HERPES ZOSTER (SHINGLES)
A cutaneous viral infection caused by the reactivation of the varicella zoster virus, the same virus that causes varicella

History
- Older adults
- Immunosuppression
- History of spinal surgery
- Tingling, pruritus in the area prior to the eruption of the rash
- Burning, throbbing, or stabbing ("knife-like") pain in the dermatomal area
- Fatigue, malaise, and headache

Physical Examination
- Low-grade fever
- Dermatomal rash (thoracic and lumbar areas are the most common sites)
- Unilateral lesion eruption that is initially erythematous and maculopapular, then becomes clusters of clear vesicles

- Regional lymphadenopathy
- Lesions crusting within 7 to 10 days of eruption (see Vesicle in **Table 5.1**).

Consideration
- Vaccine available but efficacy decreases with age

MELANOMA
A malignancy of the pigment producing melanocytes in the basal layer of the epidermis

History
- Reports a spot or sore that burns, itches, stings, crusts, or bleeds, or any mole or spot that changes in size or texture, develops irregular borders, or appears pearly, translucent, or multicolored
- A new mole or lesion in adulthood (aside from pregnancy)

Physical Examination
- Lesion is typically black or brown, but can be skin-colored, pink, red, purple, blue, or white (see Nodule in **Table 5.1**).
- Lesion typically has one or more of the following: asymmetry, border irregularity, color variegation, diameter larger than 6 mm, and evolution of the lesion's growth.
- It is most commonly located in sun-exposed areas.
- Satellite lesions are present, which are new moles that grow near an existing mole.
- Pigment from the border of a spot spreads into the surrounding skin.
- Mole looks different from the surrounding moles (ugly duckling).

Considerations
- Melanoma is often diagnosed in later stages in Hispanic and African American populations, leading to poorer survival rates.
- In African American, Asian, Filipino, Indonesian, and Native Hawaiian populations, melanoma can occur on nonexposed skin with less pigment, with 60% to 75% of lesions presenting on the palms, soles, mucous membranes, and nails.

ONYCHOMYCOSIS
A disease of the nail(s) caused by yeast, dermatophytes, and non-dermatophyte molds

History
- History of diabetes, HIV
- Immunosuppression
- Obesity
- Smoking
- Older age

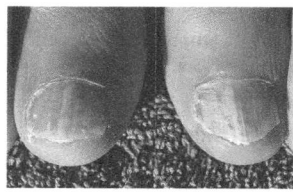

FIGURE 5.6 Onychomycosis of the toenails.
Source: Centers for Disease Control and Prevention/Edwin P. Ewing, Jr, MD.

Physical Examination
- Typically affects the toenails but can also occur on the fingernails
- Discoloration of the nail(s) (whitish, yellow, brown in color; **Figure 5.6**)
- Thickened and brittle nail(s), distortion of shape (ragged, crumbly)
- Onycholysis
- Can have an associated foul odor, pain, or paresthesia
- Microscopy consistent with fungus

Considerations
- *Candida* the most common type of yeast species involved
- Difficult to treat

PITYRIASIS ROSEA
An acute exanthematous disease that is associated with the endogenous systemic reactivation of human herpes virus (HHV-6 and/or HHV-7)

History
- Usually develops in healthy people who are 10 to 35 years old
- Mild and self-limiting; rash usually disappearing on its own without treatment
- May vary from 2 weeks to a few months in duration

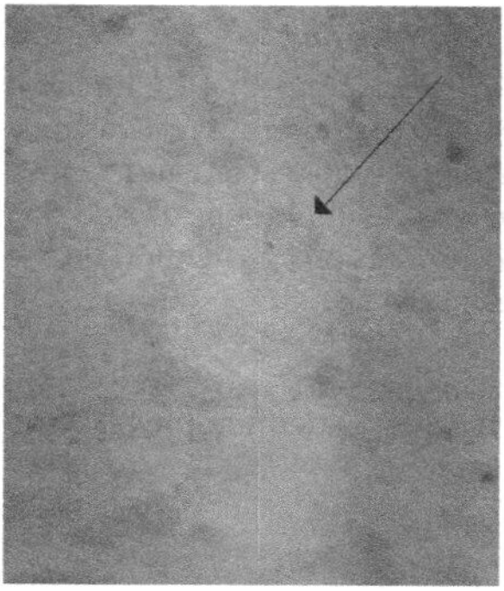

Physical Examination
- It begins with a single, circular, erythematous patch called a *herald patch* (**Figure 5.7**).
- Herald patch is followed by a secondary eruption with smaller patches on the cleavage lines of the trunk (configuration of a "Christmas tree").

Consideration
- Not thought to be contagious

FIGURE 5.7 Pityriasis rosea and associated erythematous "herald patch."
Source: Image courtesy of James Heilman, MD.

PSORIASIS
A complex, inflammatory, multisystem disease characterized by hyperproliferation of the keratinocytes in the epidermis, with plaque psoriasis the most common type

History
- Pruritic skin lesions often the most prominent and the only recognized feature of the disease
- Can have painful lesions
- Periods of exacerbations and remissions
- Family history of psoriasis
- Recent streptococcal throat infection, viral infection, immunization, or trauma
- Joint pain

Physical Examination
- Reddish pink, well-demarcated macules, papules, and plaques with a silvery scale (see Plaque in **Table 5.1**)
- Presence of Auspitz sign (pinpoint bleeding with removal of scales) a hallmark sign
- Usually form on the scalp, elbows, knees, and lower back, but can develop anywhere
- Worsening of a long-term erythematous scaly area
- Dystrophic nails
- Ocular symptoms including conjunctivitis and blepharitis

Considerations
- It appears to be induced by genetic, environmental, and immunologic factors.
- Psoriasis flares may result from systemic, psychological, infectious, and environmental influences.

ROSACEA (ACNE ROSACEA)
A common, chronic, and relapsing inflammatory skin condition involving the face and less often the neck and chest

History
- Can be triggered by UV light (most common), stress, exercise, wind, heat, spicy foods, dairy, and alcohol
- Fair-skinned European and Celtic individuals; most common in women aged 30 to 50 who are fair-skinned
- History of facial flushing

Physical Examination
- Nontransient erythema, telangiectasia, roughness of the skin, or papulopustular lesions
- Can resemble acne; comedones absent
- May also have erythema or flushing in the neck and upper chest
- Thickening of the skin of the nose (rhinophyma; **Figure 5.8**)
- May have ocular involvement

Consideration
- Cause of rosacea unknown

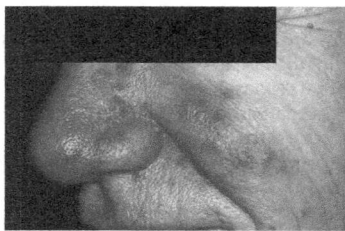

FIGURE 5.8 **Rosacea.**
Source: Image courtesy of Michael Sand, Daniel Sand, Christina Thrandorf, Volker Paech, Peter Altmeyer, and Falk G. Bechara.

SCABIES
A skin infestation caused by *Sarcoptes scabiei*, tiny parasites that burrow into the skin and lay eggs

History
- Can take 2 to 6 weeks to appear after exposure
- Institutionalized individuals at higher risk
- Intense, pruritic rash; pruritus worsens at night

Physical Examination
- Scabies is a maculopapular rash that can be found anywhere but tends to occur between the fingers and toes, under jewelry or watches on the wrist, and in armpits, skin folds, and genitalia.
- Lesions can arrange in linear patterns.

- It can also resemble pimples, eczema, and insect bites (**Figure 5.9**).
- Infants and young children may appear irritable, not wanting to eat or sleep, and have the rash in less common areas, including on their palms or the soles of their feet, face, scalp, and neck.

FIGURE 5.9 **Scabies.**
Source: Centers for Disease Control and Prevention/ Joe Miller.

Considerations
- Highly contagious
- Spread by direct, prolonged, skin-to-skin contact with another person who harbors the mites, but can also be spread indirectly by sharing articles such as clothing, towels, or bedding used by an infested person

SQUAMOUS CELL CARCINOMA
Arises from the epidermal keratinocytes

History
- History of radiation
- Older adults
- Fair skin
- History of sun damage or actinic keratosis
- Can itch, feel sore or tender, and/or feel numb

Physical Examination
- Most common on sun-exposed areas of the skin
- Generally slow-growing
- A raised, firm, skin-colored or pink, hyperkeratotic papule, or plaques (**Figure 5.10**)
- Can be an isolated lesion or multiple lesions; most occurring on the head and upper extremities

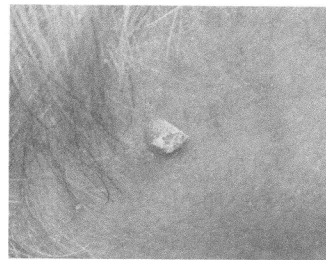

FIGURE 5.10 Squamous cell carcinoma.
Source: National Cancer Institute/Kelly Nelson, MD.

- A nonhealing sore or patch of rough skin
- Firm, dome-shaped growth; tiny rhinoceros horn-shaped growing from the skin; wart-like growth
- Black line under the nail

Considerations
- Second most common form of cancer
- Poses a substantial risk of morbidity, mortality, and impact on quality of life
- Most common skin cancer in Black populations

TINEA CORPORIS
A dermatophyte (fungal) infection of the face, trunk, and/or extremities

History
- Highest prevalence in children
- Contact sports participation, especially common in wrestlers
- History of diabetes or obesity
- Living or spending time in tropical, humid areas
- May be pruritic or asymptomatic lesions, occasionally burn, and vary in number

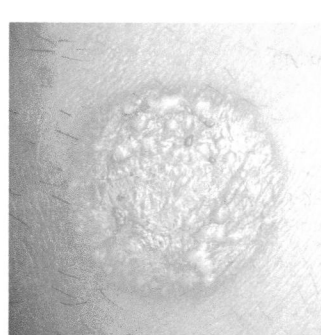

FIGURE 5.11 Tinea corporis.

Physical Examination
- A red, scaly patch with distinct annular borders and central clearing; can develop inflammation, scale, crusts, papules, vesicles, and bullae at the lesion's border (**Figure 5.11**).
- Size of lesions ranging from 1 to 5 cm, but varying size and distribution may occur
- Microscopy consistent with fungus

Consideration
- Highly contagious

TINEA VERSICOLOR
A benign fungal infection of the skin caused by the fungus *Malassezia furfur*

History
- Often diagnosed in summer
- Adolescents and young adults most susceptible
- People of all skin colors susceptible
- Can be pruritic

Physical Examination
- Multiple tan, brown, salmon, pink, or white scaling patches on the trunk, neck, abdomen, and occasionally face (see Patch in **Table 5.1**); patches may coalesce
- Budding and hyphae noted on a potassium hydroxide (KOH) wet mount

URTICARIA (HIVES)
A skin infection caused by the release of histamine and other inflammatory mediators from mast cells and basophils in the dermis

History
- May be acute or chronic and is often self-limited
- May cause significant pruritus (as a result of the histamine released in the dermis) and discomfort
- Usually resolves within 24 hours, but may persist depending on underlying etiology

Physical Examination
- Raised wheals that blanch with palpation (see Wheal in **Table 5.1**)
- May appear on any part of the body
- Can be linear, annular (circular), or arcuate (serpiginous)
- Lesions typically temporary on the affected skin and usually mobile

Considerations
- The most frequently identified cause of urticaria is infection.
- Urticaria that is recurrent is frequently associated with sun exposure, exercise, emotional or physical stress, and exposure to water.

VERRUCA VULGARIS (WARTS)
Benign epidermal growths that are caused by various types of HPV

History
- Common in children; will often resolve on their own
- Often asymptomatic
- Can be painful

Physical Examination
- Hyperkeratotic papules with a rough irregular surface; may vary in size (1 mm to larger)
- May occur anywhere on the epidermis, but commonly found on the fingers, hands, knees, and feet
- Can contain black dots that look like seeds
- Common where the skin is broken

Considerations
- Wart viruses are contagious and can spread by contact with the wart or something that touched the wart.
- There are several different types of warts.

PHYSICAL EXAMINATION DOCUMENTATION

EXAMPLE OF ABNORMAL FINDINGS
Documentation should include results of inspection and palpation.
When describing a lesion/rash, note the following:

- Primary morphology
- Size
- Demarcation
- Color
- Secondary morphology
- Distribution

○   **Skin:** Skin is clean, dry, and intact. Skin color and pigmentation are uniform. No lesions, rashes, or ecchymoses are present. Odor and hygiene are appropriate. Skin temperature is warm.

○   **Hair:** Hair is thick and blond. Hair distribution is equal and even with no signs of hair loss, hair thinning, infection, or infestation.

○   **Nails:** Nails are clean, smooth, and intact with the epidermis.

○   **Skin lesion:** 6-mm well-demarcated red plaque with dry serum/crusting, erosions, and scaling is located on the extensor surface of the left leg.

REFERENCES

References for this chapter draw from Chapter 12, Evidence-Based Assessment of the Skin, Hair, and Nails, of the textbook *Evidence-Based Physical Examination: Best Practices for Health and Well-Being Assessment (Second Edition)*. The references may be accessed in the digital version of the handbook at https://connect.springerpub.com/.

6

Evidence-Based Assessment of the Lymphatic System

CLINICAL CONSIDERATIONS

- The lymphatic system has many functions and plays a large role in immune system function.
- Palpable lymph nodes can be a normal part of an infectious process or a sign of underlying pathology.
- Multiple disease processes can cause lymphadenopathy.
- Lymph nodes greater than 1 cm in diameter or in the supraclavicular region should be further investigated.
- In both adults and children, enlarged lymph nodes that are present less than 2 weeks or more than 12 months without change in size have a very low likelihood of being neoplastic.
- Lymph nodes do not pulsate.
- Both edema and lymphedema can exist in the same patient.

SUBJECTIVE HISTORY

COMMON REASON FOR SEEKING CARE
- Enlargement of the lymph nodes (generalized or regional lymphadenopathy)

HISTORY OF PRESENT ILLNESS
- **Onset:** When did you first notice the lymph node(s)? Was it a sudden or insidious onset?
- **Location:** Is it one lymph node versus one region of the lymph nodes versus multiple regions of the lymph nodes that are affected? Are the lymph nodes unilateral or bilateral?
- **Duration:** Is the enlargement of the lymph node(s) recent, intermittent, and/or chronic? How long have they been there?
- **Character:** Are the lymph nodes painful? What is their approximate size? Are they mobile or fixed? Are they soft or hard? Matted or discrete? Is there any surrounding redness or red streaks present?
- **Associated symptoms:** Do you have any other symptoms of fever, chills, fatigue, night sweats, sore throat, abdominal pain, nausea/vomiting, arthralgias, or rashes?

- **Aggravating factors:** Have you had any recent infections/illnesses?
- **Relieving symptoms:** Have you tried any pharmacologic treatment, including over-the-counter (OTC) pain relief or nonpharmacologic treatment, including application of heat or cold to the affected areas?

HEALTH HISTORY

PAST MEDICAL HISTORY

- Chronic diseases (cancers, congenital disorders, autoimmune disorders, cardiovascular disease [CVD], renal diseases, HIV)
- Anemia
- Surgeries (including lymph node dissection/removal)
- Blood transfusions
- Radiation therapy
- Recent injury, trauma, or skin infection
- Recent strep throat or mononucleosis
- Allergies
- Allergic reactions
- Chronic venous insufficiency
- Tuberculosis (TB)

Medications

- Prescribed and OTC medications or supplements, including dose and frequency
- Medications that weaken the immune system (e.g., chemotherapy, tumor necrosis factor [TNF] inhibitors, and corticosteroids)

Immunizations

- **Risks for vaccine-preventable illness:** Vaccine status, risks of TB, recent tuberculin skin test (TST), recent COVID-19 vaccine

FAMILY HISTORY

- Cancer
- Infectious disease
- Immune disorders
- Anemia
- TB/positive TB reading

SOCIAL HISTORY

- Smoking history or history of tobacco use
- Intravenous (IV) drug use/drug use prescribed, not prescribed
- Recent travel out of the country
- Sleep history
- Sexual history (including risk factors for HIV exposure)
- Animal or food contact

- Exposure to cat feces
- Insect bites
- Stress and coping

REVIEW OF SYSTEMS

- **General:** Weight loss or gain, fatigue, fever, pain
- **Head, eyes, ears, nose, throat:** Headache, ear pain, nasal congestion, sinus pain, sore throat
- **Cardiovascular/respiratory:** Shortness of breath at rest or with exertion, cough, chest pain, orthopnea
- **Gastrointestinal/genitourinary:** Abdominal pain, nausea, vomiting, difficulty swallowing, black or tarry stools, dysuria, vaginal/penile discharge, dyspareunia
- **Neurologic:** Weakness, numbness, dizziness
- **Endocrine:** Changes to skin and hair, temperature intolerance
- **Hematologic:** Bruising, bleeding, jaundice, paleness
- **Skin:** Itching; rashes; lesions changing shape, size, or color; sores/wounds that are not healing
- **Psychiatric:** Depression, sadness, worry, insomnia; changes in memory, concentration, or mood

RED FLAGS IN SUBJECTIVE HISTORY

- Unintentional weight loss
- Unexplained fevers
- Night sweats
- Lymphadenopathy without known infection that is persistent, enlarging, or present in multiple locations

PHYSICAL EXAMINATION

GENERAL SURVEY

- Vital signs including temperature, pulse rate, respiratory rate, and blood pressure
- Height, weight, and body mass index as compared with previous visits (if available)
- Toxic versus nontoxic appearance

INSPECTION

- Do a complete visual inspection, including the axillae and groin (**Figure 6.1**).
- Lymph nodes and lymphatic organs should never be visible on inspection.
- Note any edema or redness, including erythematous lines along nodal tracks, lesions/rashes, or indications of trauma on the skin.
- Note any areas of localized edema in the limbs.

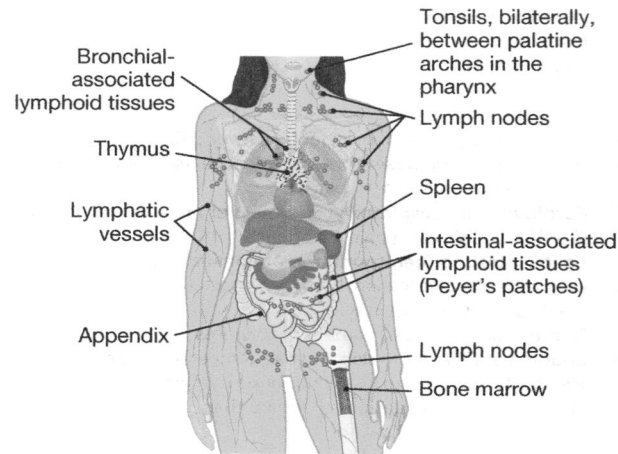

FIGURE 6.1 Lymphatic organs.

PALPATION

- The clinician's hands should be clean, dry, and warm, and the fingernails should be short.
- The clinician's fingers should be placed firmly in alignment and against one another to provide a large surface area and better coverage for detection of enlargement or abnormalities. The pads of the fingers should be used for palpation.
- Palpation should be completed using a fluid, circular motion. Soft palpation should be followed by a deeper palpation in order to feel for any hidden enlargement. Too much pressure can cause a mobile lymph node to move out of the clinician's line of palpation.
- Care should be taken to ensure the entire surface area of the lymphatic region is palpated. Remember what part of the body a particular lymph node drains so the clinician can also examine this particular area for local signs of infection or abnormality. It is important to palpate the surrounding tissues since lymph nodes are often found in chains.
- If a lymph node is palpated, the clinician should note the size, consistency, discreteness, mobility, tenderness, warmth, and border edges of the lymph node.

Head and Neck

- Ask the patient to remove all clothing from the regions of the head, neck, and upper shoulders.

- Ask the patient to tilt their head slightly down and relax the neck and shoulder muscles. Using both hands, palpate the occipital and posterior cervical lymph nodes.
- Have the patient return their neck to its upright position and ask them to raise their chin. Palpate the submental, submandibular, retropharyngeal, tonsillar, preauricular, postauricular, and anterior cervical lymph nodes (**Figure 6.2**).
- Ask the patient to move their shoulders slightly forward and palpate the supraclavicular fossa for supraclavicular lymph nodes (**Figure 6.3**). Then palpate below the clavicles to feel for any infraclavicular lymph nodes.
- Evaluate for symmetry. Clinically significant lymph nodes often present asymmetrically.

Axillae
- Make sure clothing has been removed from the area. Have the patient lay supine and raise their arm over their head. Axillary palpation can occur with the patient sitting in an upright position, but this method can be limiting (**Figures 6.4** and **6.5**).
- Use the same circular motion; ensure the entire surface has been palpated then move the hand slowly down toward the elbow until the epitrochlear notch has been located. Epitrochlear nodes are found on the medial aspect of the elbow, about 4 to 5 cm above the humeral epitrochlea. Repeat on the other side.

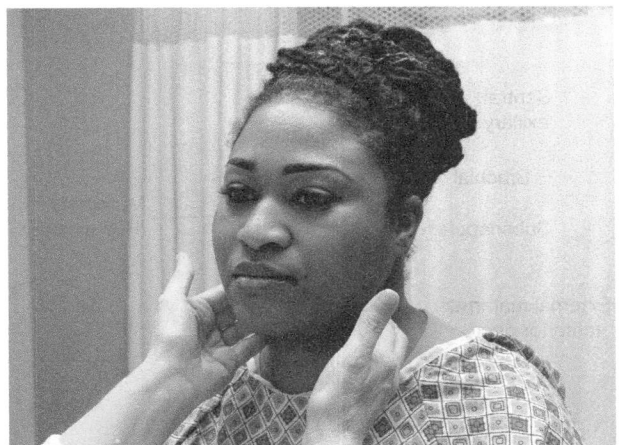

FIGURE 6.2 Proper hand placement for palpation of the anterior cervical lymph nodes.

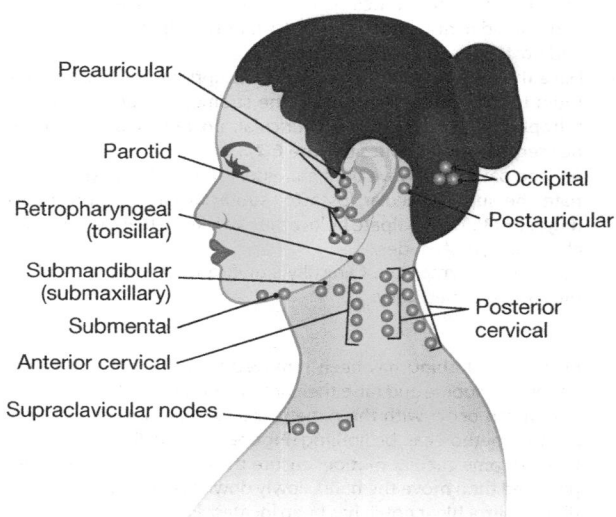

FIGURE 6.3 Lymph nodes of the head and neck.

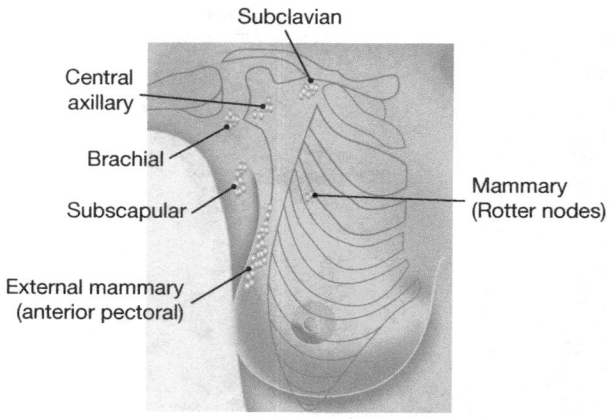

FIGURE 6.4 Axillary lymph nodes.

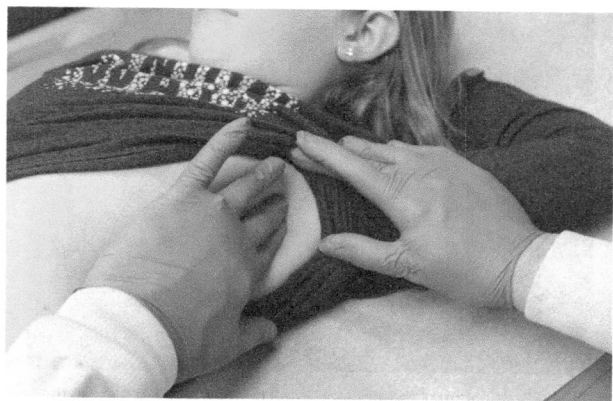

FIGURE 6.5 Palpation of the axillary lymph nodes in supine position.

Inguinal
- Have the patient lay supine. Remove all clothing from the area but maintain a modest environment for the patient by keeping them covered before and after the exam.
- Locate the iliac crest. Move the hand toward the midline, then palpate downward in a diagonal line, remaining parallel to the crease separating the upper thigh from the abdomen (**Figures 6.6** and **6.7**).
- Cover the entire region using a firm, circular motion. Repeat on the other side. With the patient already lying supine, palpate for the spleen if needed.

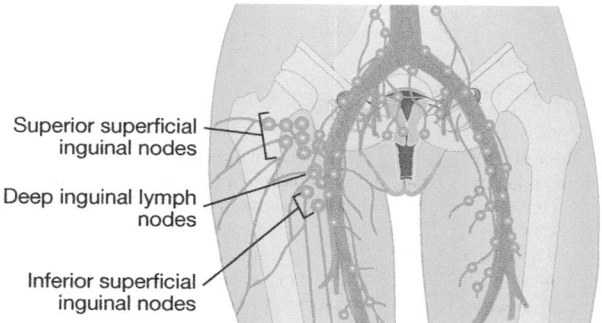

Superior superficial inguinal nodes

Deep inguinal lymph nodes

Inferior superficial inguinal nodes

FIGURE 6.6 Deep inguinal lymph nodes.

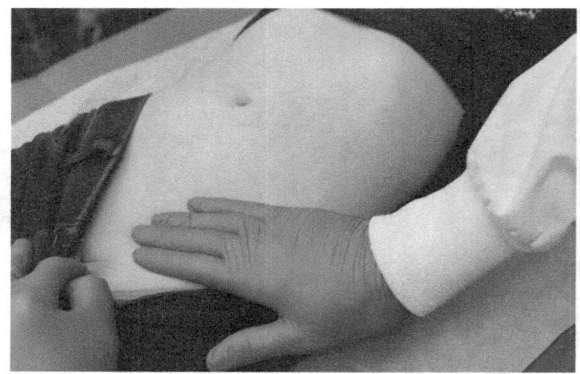

FIGURE 6.7 Palpation of the inguinal lymph nodes with the patient in the supine position.

RED FLAGS IN OBJECTIVE EXAM
Lymph nodes with the following characteristics:
- Hard
- Fixed
- Matted
- >1 cm in size
- Located in the supraclavicular, infraclavicular, iliac, popliteal, or epitrochlear regions
- Generalized
- Unilateral
- Symptoms:
  - Weight loss
  - Fever
  - Night sweats

PEDIATRIC CONSIDERATIONS
- Roughly 50% of healthy children have palpable lymph nodes at any one time that are either benign or infectious in etiology, with up to 90% of children aged 4 to 8 having palpable cervical lymph nodes. The lymphadenopathy is typically self-limiting and does not require further workup or treatment.
- Similar to adults, large and supraclavicular lymph nodes in children need further investigation in addition to the presence of systemic symptoms.

CONSIDERATIONS FOR THE OLDER ADULT

In older adults, malignant disease is the most common cause of persistent lymphadenopathy.

ABNORMAL FINDINGS

COMMON LYMPHATIC DISORDERS

Cat Scratch Disease
A bacterial infection caused by the organism *Bartonella henselae*.

History
- Scratch or bite from a cat/kitten
- Anorexia, fever, malaise, headache

Physical Examination
- Fever
- Erythema, edema, and/or purulent discharge at the site of the bite or scratch
- Persistent regional lymphadenopathy (e.g., if bite is on the arm, axillary lymphadenopathy)
- Positive *B. henselae* immunofluorescence assay (IFA) blood test

Considerations
- Disease spreads to the human when an infected cat licks a person's open wound or bites or scratches hard enough to break the surface of the skin.
- It can have serious complications if not caught early.

Human Immunodeficiency Virus/Acquired Immunodeficiency Syndrome
A virus that enters the body and invades helper T cells

History
- Varied symptoms based on disease stage; some individuals asymptomatic
- History of high-risk sexual activity (e.g., multiple partners, unprotected, prostitution)
- History of IV drug use

Physical Examination
- **Stage I—acute HIV:** Flu-like symptoms, positive HIV test
- **Stage 2—chronic HIV:** Often asymptomatic and can last up to 10 years
- **Stage 3—AIDS:**
  - Rapid weight loss; lymphadenopathy; chronic diarrhea; mouth, anus, and/or genital sores; night sweats

- Opportunistic infections (e.g., pneumonia, tuberculosis)
- Cancers (Kaposi sarcoma, cervical cancer)
- Memory loss, depression, and other neurologic disorders
- Decreasing CD4+ lymphocytes and increasing viral load levels (CD4+ count is <200 cells/mm^3)

Considerations
- It is a retrovirus, a type of virus that integrates its viral DNA into the DNA of the host cell by converting its RNA to DNA.
- HIV destroys the T cells, making it hard for the body to fight infection or infection-related cancers.

Lymphadenitis
An inflammation or infection of one or more lymph nodes

History
- Often has a history of fever and malaise
- Reports pain/tenderness in the lymph node

Physical Examination
- Often unilateral
- Lymph node enlargement, node filled with exudate
- Can have erythema or red streaking over the lymph nodes

Considerations
- It most often results from an acute streptococcal or staphylococcal infection.
- Pain and tenderness typically distinguish lymphadenitis from lymphadenopathy.

Lymphangitis
An inflammation or infection of the lymphatic vessels that commonly develops after cutaneous inoculation of microorganisms into the lymphatic vessels through a wound in the skin

History
- History of fever and malaise
- History of abrasion, wound, or coexisting infection (cellulitis) of the skin

Physical Examination
- Fever
- Enlarged lymph nodes (often in the axillae, groin, or epitrochlear regions)
- Red streaking that extends proximally from a wound or site of infection toward regional lymph nodes
- Leukocytosis

Consideration
- It most often results from an acute streptococcal or staphylococcal infection of the skin. It can have serious complications if not caught early.

Lymphatic Filariasis
A parasitic disease that is transmitted through mosquitoes, which impairs the normal function of the lymphatic system, causing edema and decreased immune function

History
- Travel to endemic areas, such as Asia, Africa, Western Pacific, Haiti, Dominican Republic, Brazil, Guyana, and parts of the Caribbean
- Can be asymptomatic
- Increased infections in the skin and lymph systems

Physical Examination
- Gross edema of an entire limb or body area (most commonly affects the legs, but can occur in the arms, breasts, vulva, or scrotum)
- Hardening and thickening of the skin in the affected extremity
- Elevated levels of antifilarial immunoglobulin (Ig) G4 in serum
- Microfilariae in a blood smear by microscopic examination

Consideration
- *Wuchereria bancrofti* is responsible for 90% of cases.

Lymphedema
Edema or enlargement due to localized lymphatic fluid retention

History
- History of congenital malformations and/or dysfunction to the lymphatic system
- History of injury, removal, or damage to the lymphatic vessels from surgery, radiation, infection, or malignancy
- History of lymph node dissection
- A feeling of heaviness, fullness, or tightness, or aching, tingling, or discomfort to the affected area
- History of recurring infections
- Noticeably tighter clothing or jewelry in the affected area
- No improvement in swelling even with diuretics
- May have improvement in swelling with elevation of the limb in the early stages but not as the condition progresses

Physical Examination
- Swelling of part or all of the arm or leg, including fingers or toes
- Restricted range of motion and decreased flexibility in nearby joints

- Changes in skin texture or appearance, such as tightness, redness, or hardening
- May or may not pit to palpation

Considerations
- **Primary lymphedema:** Congenital malformation or dysfunction of the lymphatic system
- **Secondary lymphedema:** From surgery, radiation, or malignancy

Lymphoma
A form of cancer that originates in the lymphatic system

History
- Lymphoma
- Personal history of Epstein–Barr virus (EBV)
- Fever and night sweats, fatigue
- Severe pruritus
- Chest or abdominal pain

Physical Examination
- Generalized, painless lymphadenopathy (with the exception of the inguinal region)
- Fever, unexplained weight loss

Considerations
- There are two main types, Hodgkin lymphoma and non-Hodgkin lymphoma, although many different subtypes exist.
- Tumors develop from the T cells or B cells.

Mononucleosis (or Mono)
A contagious illness caused by EBV that invades the body's B cells

History
- Most common in children and young adults
- Reports extreme fatigue that can last for months
- Throat pain often severe
- Headaches, myalgias

Physical Examination
- Fever (children may not have)
- Anterior/posterior cervical lymphadenopathy, although others can be enlarged
- White exudate on posterior pharynx and tonsillar; petechiae on the soft and hard palates
- Evanescent nonpruritic maculopapular rash (often occurs early in the illness)
- Palpebral edema
- Splenomegaly (50% of cases), hepatomegaly (10% of cases), jaundice (5% of cases)

- Elevated liver enzymes
- Positive mononucleosis spot blood test

Considerations
- It is spread through saliva.
- Children typically do not have as dramatic a presentation, so it is often missed.

PHYSICAL EXAMINATION DOCUMENTATION

Documentation should include results of inspection and palpation.

EXAMPLE OF NORMAL FINDINGS
Anterior cervical lymph nodes soft, mobile, and tender to palpation bilaterally. Size of lymph nodes estimated at 8 to 10 mm. All other lymph nodes nonpalpable, nontender.

REFERENCES

References for this chapter draw from Chapter 13, Evidence-Based Assessment of the Lymphatic System, of the textbook *Evidence-Based Physical Examination: Best Practices for Health and Well-Being Assessment (Second Edition)*. The references may be accessed in the digital version of the handbook at https://connect.springerpub.com/.

7

Evidence-Based Assessment of the Head and Neck

CLINICAL CONSIDERATIONS

- Assessment of the head and neck includes review of neurologic, musculoskeletal, and vascular systems.
- Signs and symptoms of thyroid dysfunction can be mild, nonspecific, and varied, and may include symptoms of depression and anxiety.
- Physical examination begins with a general survey, observation, and inspection of the head and neck.
- Expose the neck and clavicles to fully view the head and neck for symmetry, obvious masses, or lesions.
- Infants and children with craniofacial abnormalities may have an underlying genetic syndrome.
- More than 90% of individuals who present with a headache have a primary headache disorder and their physical exam will be normal.

SUBJECTIVE HISTORY

COMMON REASONS FOR SEEKING CARE

- Headache
- Head injury or trauma; limited mobility of the neck or jaw, neck pain
- Difficulty or pain with chewing or swallowing, sense of lump in the throat with swallowing
- Dyspnea when lying supine caused by compressive changes associated with thyroid enlargement
- Constellation of symptoms including constipation, fatigue, irritability, temperature intolerances, weight gain or loss, skin or hair changes, hoarseness or change in voice

HISTORY OF PRESENT ILLNESS

- **Onset:** When did the symptoms start? In what way did the symptoms begin? Did the symptoms occur suddenly or gradually? Was any type of prodrome or aura experienced?

- **Location:** Where is pain or discomfort located? Is pain or discomfort unilateral or bilateral; in a generalized area or at a specific location of the head, face, or neck?
- **Duration:** How long do the symptoms or episodes of having the symptoms last? Has pain or discomfort persisted since the onset? Are symptoms becoming progressively worse?
- **Characteristics:** How would you describe the pain? Is it sharp, dull, stabbing, burning, crushing, throbbing, or nauseating? Does the pain move or radiate when it occurs?
- **Aggravating factors:** What actions, activities, or body positions make the symptoms worse? Are symptoms worsened by lights or sounds?
- **Relieving factors:** What actions, activities, or body positions decrease the symptoms? If relieved, how long does the relief last?
- **Treatment:** What medications has the individual taken to help with the symptoms? Clarify the dosage and frequency of any medications.
- **Severity:** How severe are the symptoms on a scale of 0 to 10, currently and when the symptoms are at their worst? Do the symptoms limit participation in activities? Does pain force the individual to lie down, sit down, or slow down?

HEALTH HISTORY

Past Medical History
- Headaches
- Injury or trauma to the head or neck
- Recent motor vehicle accident
- Past surgical history
- Cancer, past history of radiation therapy
- HIV or other viral infections that cause damage to the immune system
- Elevated blood pressure, hypertension, heart disease
- Smoking history
- Depression, anxiety, or mental health disorder
- Osteoarthritis or rheumatoid arthritis
- Poor visual acuity, need for corrective lenses

Medications
- Prescribed and over-the-counter (OTC) medications or supplements, including dose and frequency
- Medications that weaken the immune system (e.g., chemotherapy, corticosteroids)

Allergies
- Allergies to medications, or seasonal, environmental, and/or food allergies? If yes, clarify reactions.

Immunizations
- **Risks for vaccine-preventable illnesses:** Vaccine status, including human papillomavirus (HPV) immunizations, needed or received

FAMILY HISTORY
- Migraine or recurrent headaches
- Neck or thyroid cancer
- Thyroid disorders or dysfunction
- Endocrine disorders or dysfunction
- Arthritis, inflammatory disorders
- Infectious diseases
- Immune disorders

SOCIAL HISTORY
- Use of tobacco, including cigarettes, smokeless tobacco, e-cigarettes or vaping, cigars
- Typical use of alcohol, episodes of binge drinking, alcohol misuse
- Use of prescription medications, OTC drugs, or illicit substances used for nonmedical purposes
- Environmental exposures at work or at home
- Health behaviors, including sleep and rest, coping with stress, nutrition, physical activity
- Sports participation (specifically, contact sports like football, soccer, boxing, or hockey)
- Social support system

REVIEW OF SYSTEMS
- **General:** Fever, fatigue, weight changes, appetite changes
- **Lymph:** Lymph node swelling and/or tenderness, bruising, bleeding
- **Eyes, ears, nose, throat:** Ear pain, eye drainage or redness, nasal congestion, sinus pain, sore throat
- **Neurologic:** Weakness, numbness, loss of consciousness, headache, recent fall, dizziness
- **Musculoskeletal:** Injury history, pain with movement; neck pain, stiffness, or swelling
- **Gastrointestinal:** Nausea, vomiting, constipation, abdominal pain
- **Mental health:** Sadness; insomnia; uncontrolled worry; changes in mentation, memory, or mood; current stress level and coping mechanisms; history of panic attacks
- **Endocrine (skin, hair, nails):** Changes in skin, hair, or nails; temperature intolerance; weight changes, fatigue

RED FLAGS IN SUBJECTIVE HISTORY
- Secondary headaches are those with an underlying cause (e.g., tumor, trauma, infection, or inflammation). Although less than

10% of headaches have a secondary cause, the higher likelihood of serious complications with secondary headaches warrants a comprehensive history and exam.
·   **Box 7.1** includes a summary list of symptoms (using the mnemonic SNOOP) that indicate risk for secondary headache.

PHYSICAL EXAMINATION

INSPECTION
·   Inspect the position of the head and symmetry of the cranium; note the quality and condition of the hair and scalp.
·   Inspect the face and facial expressions for symmetry; note alignment of the eyebrows, eyes, ears, nose, and mouth.
·   Inspect the skin integrity of the head, face, and neck; inspect the neck for deformities, pulsations, areas of edema, and limitations in movement.

PALPATION
·   Palpate the head for areas of edema or tenderness, including the mastoid process; test sensation of light touch on the forehead, cheeks, and chin.
·   Palpate while the individual clenches their jaw; palpate the temporomandibular joint (TMJ) with opening and closing of the mouth.
·   Palpate the submental, submandibular, retropharyngeal, tonsillar, preauricular, postauricular, and anterior and posterior cervical lymph nodes (see Chapter 6, Evidence-Based Assessment of the Lymphatic System).

BOX 7.1 Red Flags in Subjective History That Indicate Risk for Secondary Headache

S: Systemic symptoms
> Unexplained fever, weight loss, myalgia, fatigue

N: Neurologic symptoms
> Motor weakness, sensory loss, diplopia, tinnitus

O: Onset
> Sudden "split second" or "thunderclap"

O: Older age
> New onset of "migraines" in those over 50

P: Pattern change
> Progressing to daily, precipitated by Valsalva, exacerbated by postural change

- Palpate the thyroid gland to assess for nodules; enlargement begins with identifying the structures (**Figure 7.1**) and the landmarks of the neck (**Figure 7.2**).
- An anterior or posterior approach can be used for thyroid palpation (**Figure 7.3**).
- To palpate the thyroid gland using a *posterior* approach (**Figure 7.3A**), ask the patient to tip their chin slightly forward; stand behind the individual and place fingers on the patient's neck just below the cricoid cartilage. Ask the patient to swallow while keeping the fingers steady in this position; the thyroid isthmus can be felt rising under the pads of the fingers as the person swallows. To palpate the lobes of the thyroid, the clinician can (a) ask the individual to tip their chin to

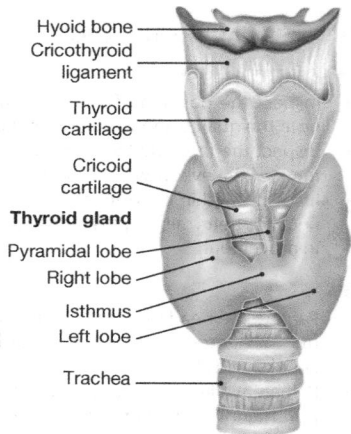

FIGURE 7.1 Midline structures of the neck within the anterior triangle.

Hyoid bone
Cricothyroid ligament
Thyroid cartilage
Cricoid cartilage
Thyroid gland
Pyramidal lobe
Right lobe
Isthmus
Left lobe
Trachea

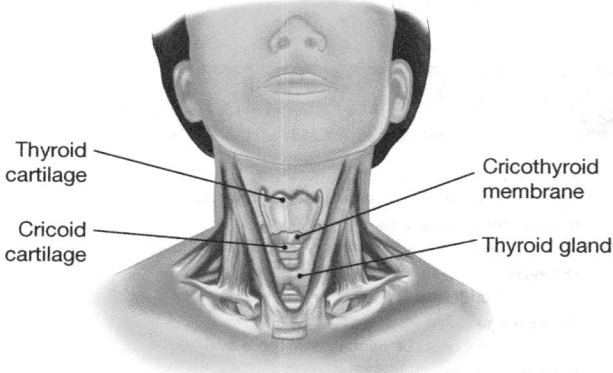

Thyroid cartilage
Cricoid cartilage
Cricothyroid membrane
Thyroid gland

FIGURE 7.2 Anatomic structures and landmarks of the neck used to assess the thyroid gland.

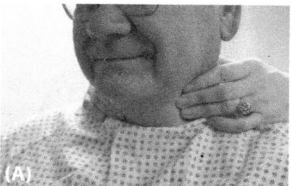 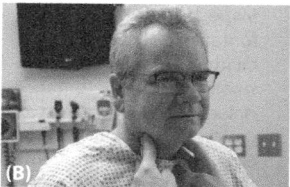

FIGURE 7.3 Palpation of the thyroid. (**A**) Posterior approach. (**B**) Anterior approach.

their chest; (b) displace the individual's trachea slightly and gently to the right with their left hand; and (c) in this position, palpate the right thyroid lobes with their right hand. Repeat this technique on the other side by displacing the trachea to the left with the right hand and palpating the left thyroid lobes.

- To use an *anterior* approach to thyroid assessment (**Figure 7.3B**), ask the patient to tip their head back slightly, and use the landmarks of the notched thyroid cartilage and the cricoid cartilage to locate the thyroid. Palpate the region below the cricoid cartilage to identify the contours of the thyroid. Simultaneously moving the sternocleidomastoid muscles further apart causes the skin to be taut over the thyroid gland and can enhance the anterior inspection and palpation techniques. To verify the location of the thyroid gland, ask the patient to swallow and note movement of the thyroid isthmus. With palpation, the thyroid gland is normally soft, without distinctly palpable nodules.

PERCUSSION AND AUSCULTATION

- Auscultation and percussion of the head and neck are not components of the routine head and neck exam for asymptomatic, healthy individuals.

PEDIATRIC CONSIDERATIONS

- Inspect the head of a newborn, infant, or child to assess size, shape, and form, including the presence of fontanels and suture ridges. An accurate head circumference measurement, using a nonstretchable measuring tape to measure above the eyebrows and ears, should be compared with the expected size on the growth chart. Inspect for symmetry or asymmetry of an infant or child's head from above and from all angles. Confirm that the line of the eyes is horizontal and that the child's ears are in alignment to confirm head symmetry.
- During the first days of life, expect that the newborn will have cranial molding. Inspect and palpate the head, noting overlapping suture ridges. A newborn's scalp is likely to be diffusely soft and swollen, a condition called *caput succedaneum*.

- Inspect and palpate the fontanels of infants and children under age 2. The small posterior fontanel is located where the two parietal bones join the occipital bone; the larger anterior fontanel is palpable where the two frontal and two parietal bones join (**Figure 7.4**). Although the posterior fontanel is often not palpable beyond 2 months of age, the anterior fontanel can be palpable up to the age of 2 years. Fontanels should be flat, not depressed or bulging, when palpated. Begin the exam while the infant is calm. Palpate the fontanels while the child is held in

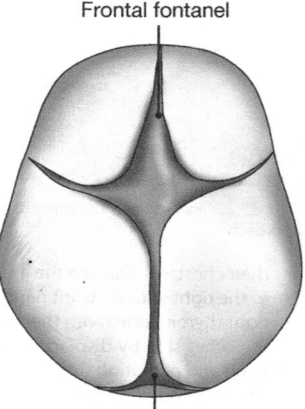

Frontal fontanel

Occipital fontanel

FIGURE 7.4 Anterior and posterior fontanels of the newborn's skull.

both supine and upright positions. Palpation of the anterior fontanel in the upright position may reveal a normal, slight pulsation. If the anterior fontanel has closed prematurely, percuss the skull near the junction of the frontal, temporal, and parietal bones to assess for Macewen's sign, an unusually resonant, "cracked-pot" sound that indicates increased intracranial pressure. Infants with an asymmetrical shape of the cranium that has resulted from positioning, a condition known as *plagiocephaly*, will have normal cranial suture lines and flat fontanels.

- Observe the infant's or child's neck control, head movement, and position. Palpate the neck for masses and/or lymphadenopathy. To assess the neck of a newborn more easily, elevate the upper back of the infant to allow the head to extend slightly. Infants and children should have full and easy range of motion of the neck. Nuchal rigidity, or resistance to flexion of the neck, is associated with meningeal irritation. Postural torticollis, twisting of the neck muscles, is relatively common in newborns related to positioning in utero; associated physical exam reveals a preference for tilting the head in one direction.

RED FLAGS IN OBJECTIVE EXAM

- The initial assessment of an individual who has sustained a head injury should include evaluation of neurologic and mental status testing. Red flags indicating severe traumatic brain injury (TBI) are listed in **Box 7.2**.

> **BOX 7.2 Red Flags in Objective Exam That Are Indications of Severe Traumatic Brain Injury**
>
> · Progressive decline in consciousness, profound confusion
> · Persistent mental status changes, incoherent speech
> · Loss of coordination, seizures
> · Pupil dilation
> · Mastoid ecchymosis (Battle sign)
> · Bruising around the orbits of the eyes (raccoon eyes)
> · Clear fluid drainage from the eyes, ears, or nose
> · In children, may include symptoms such as persistent crying, inability to be consoled, or unusual irritability

ABNORMAL FINDINGS

HEADACHE

Primary headaches are those that have no identifiable cause on exam; the diagnosis of a primary headache is made based on recognition of a pattern (which is the reason why only the history is listed in this section). Migraine with and without aura, tension-type, and cluster headaches are primary headaches. Headaches associated with COVID-19 are classified as secondary headaches, yet often present in a manner similar to primary tension-type headaches or migraines.

Migraine Headache
History
- Gradual in onset, builds in intensity
- Unilateral in most adults, bilateral in children and teens
- Lasts from 4 to 72 hours, may be recurrent
- Moderate to severe intensity, described as throbbing
- May have aura or prodrome
- Associated symptoms likely to include photophobia, phonophobia, nausea, or vomiting
- Preference for dark, quiet setting to relieve symptoms
- Triggers including stress, food, alcohol, hunger, weather, menstrual cycle, hormones, environment, and/or sleep disturbances

Tension-Type Headache
History
- Gradual onset
- Bilateral, generalized or localized
- Lasts from 1 hour to 1 week; can be infrequent, frequent, or chronic

- Described as pressure, heaviness, or band-like tightness
- No nausea or vomiting associated; may have fatigue, stress, and anxiety
- May be related to stress and tension in the neck and back
- Can be precipitated or co-occur with migraine

Cluster Headaches
History
- Quick onset, pain intense within minutes
- Unilateral, begins around the eye, temple
- Recurrent, short, painful attacks of 15 minutes to a few hours
- Describes pain as severe or very severe burning, piercing, or stabbing
- Ipsilateral lacrimation and redness of the eye, congestion, pallor, sweating, or ptosis
- Can remain active despite headache pain
- Can have abrupt onset at night; attacks occurring one to eight times daily for weeks, followed by remission

HEAD INJURY OR TRAUMA
The initial assessment of an individual who has sustained a head injury should include evaluation of neurologic and mental status testing. See **Box 7.2** for red flags indicating severe TBI.

Epidural Hematoma
History
- Experience of blunt trauma or traumatic injury of the skull
- Progressively worsening headache, vomiting
- Dizziness, drowsiness, confusion
- Typically have brief loss of consciousness after trauma, become alert, then rapidly deteriorate

Physical Examination
- Initial Glasgow Coma Scale score a predictor of outcome
- Abnormal neurologic exam
  - Pupils unequal, dilated
  - May become obtunded, have difficulty breathing
  - Risk of seizure
  - Can progress to loss of brain function and death

Considerations
- Neurosurgical emergency
- Occurs less often than subdural hematomas and usually occurs in young adults
- Occurs four times as often in males

Facial Fractures
History
- These are generally trauma-related (e.g., road traffic collisions, fights, and falls).
- The most common are injuries to the nasal bone with profuse bleeding, swelling, and bruising.

Physical Examination
- Deformity, discoloration
- Profuse swelling and/or bleeding
- Anesthesia of skin at fracture site, may be exquisitely tender to touch
- Cranial nerve abnormalities which may be associated with orbital fracture
- Broken or missing teeth with jaw fracture; trouble with chewing, eating, or speaking

Consideration
- Imaging recommendations depend on the location and extent of injury.

Skull Fractures
History
- Trauma, for example, blow to the head, falls, or high-impact motor vehicle collisions
- Pain, bruising, and/or swelling at the area of impact

Physical Examination
- Neurologic changes, including changes in the level of consciousness, vision, and balance
- Bleeding or clear fluid from the nostrils or ears
- Bruising at the trauma site, under the eyes, or behind the ears (**Figure 7.5**)

Considerations
- The type of fracture is determined by the location of the fracture and the mechanism of injury.
- Thin-slice CT has become an integral part of the diagnosis of subtle skull base fractures.
- There are four types: depressed, linear, diastatic, and basal skull fractures.

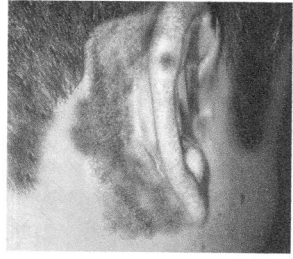

FIGURE 7.5 **Battle sign.**
Source: Image courtesy of S. Bhimji. © 2019 StatPearls Publishing LLC.

Acute, Mild Traumatic Brain Injury (Concussion)
History
- Recent motor vehicle accident, fall, occupational accident, assault, or sports injury
- Injury from direct external contact force or from acceleration/deceleration forces
- Headache, dizziness
- Emotionality, irritability
- Fatigue, drowsiness
- Difficulty concentrating

Physical Examination
- Incoordination, delayed verbal expression
- Inability to focus, blank stare, or stunned appearance
- Disorientation, slurred, and incoherent speech
- Memory deficits

Considerations
- Information from an observer or bystander can provide key information as individuals often experience posttraumatic amnesia.
- Use of a concussion assessment checklist is invaluable for needed, ongoing assessments.

PARATHYROID DISORDERS
Hypoparathyroidism
History
- Surgery of the thyroid or neck (as the most common cause is accidental removal of the parathyroid glands during surgery)
- Numbness and tingling in the fingertips, lips, and toes
- Fatigue
- Dry skin
- Muscle aches

Physical Examination
- Paresthesia in the fingertips, lips, and toes
- Muscle spasms

Consideration
- Signs and symptoms are related to the hypocalcemia that results from the decreased secretion or activity of the parathyroid hormone (PTH).

Hyperparathyroidism
History
- History of kidney stones, osteoporosis
- Abdominal pain, joint or bone pain
- Fatigue, depression symptoms

Physical Examination
- Elevated blood pressure
- Positive depression screening
- Abnormal labs and imaging

Consideration
- Enlargement of one or more of the parathyroid glands causing excess production of PTH results in hypercalcemia.

THYROID DISORDERS

Hypothyroidism

History
- Fatigue, weakness, dyspnea on exertion
- Intolerance to cold temperatures
- Weight gain
- Constipation
- Decreased hearing
- Hoarseness
- Coarse, brittle hair; dry skin
- Myalgia, arthralgia
- Difficulty concentrating
- Heavy menstrual bleeding (women)

Physical Examination
- Cognitive dysfunction, slow movement, or slow speech
- Bradycardia, diastolic hypertension
- Delayed relaxation of tendon reflexes
- Signs of carpal tunnel syndrome, paresthesia
- Periorbital edema and enlargement of the tongue
- Nonpitting edema (myxedema)
- Pleural effusion, ascites

Considerations
- Key assessments indicating hypothyroidism are related to metabolic changes that result from lack of thyroid hormone.
- Goiter is a visible, diffuse or nodular enlargement of the thyroid gland; resultant thyroid activity may result in hypothyroidism *or* hyperthyroidism (**Figure 7.6**).

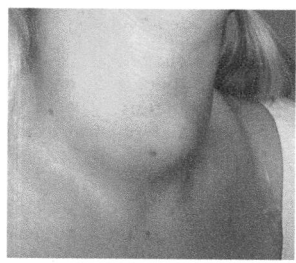

FIGURE 7.6 **Goiter.**
Source: Image courtesy of Drahreg01.

Hyperthyroidism
History
- Increased perspiration and heat intolerance
- Itching, thinning of hair
- Dysphagia due to goiter, weight loss
- Urinary frequency and nocturia
- Amenorrhea or oligomenorrhea (women)
- Anxiety, emotional lability

Physical Examination
- Hyperpigmentation
- Stare and lid lag, impairment of eye muscle function
- Proptosis or exophthalmos, periorbital edema
- Tachycardia, systolic hypertension, atrial fibrillation
- Weakness, tremor, and palpitations

Considerations
- Older adults often have isolated symptoms that warrant evaluation, including unexplained weight loss, decreased appetite, weakness, and new onset of atrial fibrillation.
- Graves disease, an autoimmune disease that causes hyperthyroidism, can precipitate thyroid eye disease, which causes upper eyelid retraction, lid lag, conjunctivitis, and bulging eyes (exophthalmos).

Thyroid Cancer
History
- Dysphagia
- Vocal cord paralysis causing voice changes or hoarseness
- History of childhood head or neck irradiation
- Family history of thyroid cancer

Physical Examination
- Palpable fixed, hard thyroid mass
- Lymphadenopathy

Considerations
- Thyroid nodules can be incidental findings during routine exams or imaging tests.
- History and physical exam have low accuracy in predicting malignancy.

PEDIATRIC CRANIOFACIAL DISORDERS
- *Cleft lip and palate* abnormalities result when the lip and/or palate do not completely form; degree varies from mild notch to severe large opening extending to the nasal cavity.
- *Craniosynostosis,* early fusion of the bones of the skull, results in increased intracranial pressure and/or skull abnormalities;

it differs from plagiocephaly, which is a flat area on the head or side of the infant's head resulting from positioning.

- *Down syndrome, trisomy 21,* is associated with craniofacial abnormalities that include flattened nasal bridge, shortened neck, small low-set ears, and slanted epicanthal folds.
- *Fetal alcohol syndrome* is associated with facial abnormalities, including smooth philtrum, thin upper lip, flat nasal bridge, short or upturned nose, and wide-set eyes.
- *Hemangioma* is an abnormal collection of blood vessels in the skin that is faint at birth, but then appears larger and darker in the first few months after birth; it is also known as *port wine stain, salmon patch,* or *strawberry hemangioma.*
- *Treacher Collins syndrome* is a genetic disorder that causes maxillary hypoplasia and auricular deformities, in addition to a smaller skull or microcephaly.
- *Turner syndrome* is a genetic disorder that affects development in females; appearance can include thickened neck, low hairline, prominent earlobes, and crowding of teeth.

PHYSICAL EXAMINATION DOCUMENTATION

Documentation should include results of inspection and palpation.

EXAMPLE OF NORMAL FINDINGS

Appears stated age, in no distress. Awake, alert, and oriented to person, place, and time. Articulates clearly, ambulates without difficulty. Skin warm, dry, intact without obvious lesions or edema; turgor with quick response. Hair with even distribution and pattern. Normocephalic, no lesions, lumps, scaling, or tenderness of the head or scalp. Face symmetric, no weakness or involuntary movements. Extraocular muscle function intact, no nystagmus. No ptosis or lid lag. Neck supple with full range of motion, symmetric, no masses, tenderness, or lymphadenopathy. Trachea midline. Thyroid nonpalpable, nontender.

EXAMPLE OF ABNORMAL FINDINGS

Appears stated age, in no distress. Awake, alert, and oriented to person, place, and time. Articulates clearly, ambulates without difficulty. Blood pressure 140/90; heart rate, temperature, and respiratory rate within normal limits. Body mass index 40. Skin dry without obvious lesions, generalized nonpitting edema of upper and lower extremities. Coarse, brittle, thinning hair. Normocephalic, no scaling, or tenderness of the head or scalp. Face symmetric, no weakness or involuntary movements. Extraocular muscle function intact, no nystagmus. No ptosis or lid lag. Generalized periorbital puffiness noted. Neck supple with full range of motion, symmetric, no tenderness or lymphadenopathy. Trachea midline. Diffuse, nodular thyroid enlargement palpable.

REFERENCES

References for this chapter draw from Chapter 14, Evidence-Based Assessment of the Head and Neck, of the textbook *Evidence-Based Physical Examination: Best Practices for Health and Well-Being Assessment (Second Edition)*. The references may be accessed in the digital version of the handbook at https://connect.springerpub.com/.

8

Evidence-Based Assessment of the Eyes

CLINICAL CONSIDERATIONS

- Changes in vision and/or eye pain may indicate systemic as well as ocular disease. Early detection and prompt referral can prevent long-term disabling effects.
- Patients who are at high risk for retinopathy benefit from vision screening with a dilated eye exam. The fundoscopic exam (direct ophthalmoscopy) in the undilated eye yields limited assessment findings. However, dilating a patient's pupils in the primary care setting has risks and challenges. Dilated exams are unsafe for small children, infants, anyone who is hyperopic, and anyone who has had previous acute angle-closure glaucoma. Consider deferring an undilated eye exam; often, patients who have had an undilated eye exam believe that they have had the exam as recommended and forgo the specialist evaluation by dilated eye exam. The consequence of failing to have recommended dilated eye exams for these populations can be significant vision loss.
- While comprehensive clinical examination of the eye is not typically performed as part of routine adult wellness exams, a thorough exam should be performed for any individual presenting with acute or chronic eye concerns, such as eye pain, eye injury, red eye, vision loss, eye discharge, double vision, dry eye, or floaters.
- Early recognition of visual disorders is especially important in children. Comprehensive assessment of the eye is a recommended routine component of pediatric wellness exams.

SUBJECTIVE HISTORY

COMMON REASONS FOR SEEKING CARE
- Eye pain
- Eye swelling and/or itching
- Eye redness and/or drainage

- Decreased visual acuity or vision loss
- Blurry vision or floaters, cloudy vision, or diplopia (double vision)
- Photophobia (painful spasm on exposure to bright light)

HISTORY OF PRESENT ILLNESS

- **Onset:** When did the symptoms start? Are the symptoms recent? Recurring? Chronic?
- **Location:** Are the symptoms unilateral or bilateral? Which part of the eye is being affected?
- **Duration:** Are the symptoms persistent or transitory? Increasing or unchanged?
- **Characteristics:** How would you describe the symptoms? Is there itching, tearing, burning, foreign body sensation, photophobia, deep pain, pain on eye movement, tenderness to touch, flashing lights in vision, or floaters? Any vision changes—for example, loss in vision, decrease in visual acuity, double vision, or blurry vision?
- **Aggravating factors:** Any recent eye injury, foreign body, or chemical substance in the eye, recent illness, stressors, sleep problems, and/or overuse of digital devices/screens?
- **Relieving factors:** What actions or activities decrease the symptoms, including flushing of the eye or application of heat or cold? If relieved, how long does the relief last?
- **Treatment:** What medications has the individual taken to help with the symptoms? Clarify the dosage and frequency of over-the-counter (OTC) and prescribed medications.
- **Severity:** How severe are the symptoms on a scale of 0 to 10?

HEALTH HISTORY

Past Medical History

- Recent injury, trauma, or infection
- Past history of eye problems, disorders, diseases, injury, surgery
- Prescription eyewear, glasses, contacts; myopia, astigmatism
- If contact wearer, current practices, including daily cleaning, sleeping/napping in contacts, change contacts as prescribed
- History of systemic disease/disorder with ocular signs and symptoms
  - **Metabolic endocrine:** Diabetes, thyroid disorders
  - **Vascular:** Hypertension, stroke, migraines, clotting disorders, sickle cell anemia
  - **Autoimmune:** Systemic lupus erythematosus (SLE), sarcoidosis, temporal (giant cell) arteritis, rheumatoid arthritis (RA), Sjögren syndrome, myasthenia gravis
  - **Inflammatory bowel disease:** Crohn's, ulcerative colitis
  - **Idiopathic disorders:** Multiple sclerosis (MS)
  - **Infective disorders:** Cytomegalovirus (CMV), HIV

○ **Neoplastic disorders:** Melanoma, pituitary adenoma, metastatic carcinoma, lymphoma
○ **Congenital disorders:** Marfan syndrome, Down syndrome, neurofibromatosis

Medications
- Prescribed and OTC medications or supplements, including dose and frequency
- Use of any eye drops, contact lens solutions, or solutions to flush or dilate the eyes

Allergies
- Allergies to medications; seasonal, environmental, and/or food allergies
- Reaction to allergens, including ocular symptoms, anaphylaxis

Preventive Care Considerations
- Diet including fruits, vegetables high in vitamin A, antioxidants
- Use of sunglasses to limit sun exposure/damage
- Regular handwashing and avoidance of touching the eye
- Health behaviors, including sleep and rest, strategies to avoid eye strain, limiting screen time

FAMILY HISTORY
- **Ocular history:** Glaucoma, cataracts, retinal detachment, blindness
- **Visual history:** Poor visual acuity, macular degeneration
- **History of diseases impacting vision:** Diabetes, hypertension, stroke, migraines, genetic disorders, clotting disorders, sickle cell anemia, ulcerative colitis, Marfan syndrome

SOCIAL HISTORY
- Use of tobacco, including cigarettes, smokeless tobacco, e-cigarettes or vaping, cigars
- Environmental exposures at work or at home
- Occupational, educational, or recreational vision requirements, use of protective eyewear
- Risk factors for HIV exposure
- Typical use of alcohol, episodes of binge drinking, alcohol misuse
- Use of prescription medications, OTC drugs, or illicit substances for nonmedical purposes

REVIEW OF SYSTEMS
- **General:** Weight loss or gain, fatigue, fever, pain
- **Head/neck:** Acute or recurrent headache, neck pain, lymphadenopathy

- **Ear, nose, throat:** Ear pain, nasal congestion, rhinorrhea, sinus pain, sore throat, and itchy ears, nose, or throat
- **Eyes:** Additional symptoms of redness, discharge, blurry vision, eye pain, vision loss
- **Cardiovascular/respiratory:** Shortness of breath at rest or with exertion, cough, chest pain, orthopnea
- **Gastrointestinal/genitourinary:** Nausea, vomiting; likelihood of pregnancy
- **Musculoskeletal:** Inflamed joints, arthritis, weakness, gait or posture defects, need for assistive devices
- **Neurologic:** Numbness, dizziness, light sensitivity, asymmetric facial movements
- **Endocrine:** Polyuria, polydipsia, polyphagia
- **Integumentary:** Itching; rashes; lesions changing shape, size, or color; nonhealing sores/wounds
- **Mental health:** Depression, sadness, worry, insomnia; changes in memory, concentration

RED FLAGS IN SUBJECTIVE HISTORY
- Acute angle-closure glaucoma is uncommon and should be treated as a medical emergency. See **Box 8.1** for a list of symptoms.

PHYSICAL EXAMINATION

Examination of the eye by the generalist clinician involves inspection in conjunction with various clinical techniques that incorporate careful observation.

INSPECTION
- Inspect the eyelids, eyelashes, conjunctivae, sclera, corneas, and irises for abnormal lesions, rashes, redness, swelling, or drainage.

BOX 8.1 Red Flags in Subjective History That Indicate Possible Acute Angle-Closure Glaucoma

- Sudden onset of severe eye pain
- Acute change in visual acuity, loss of vision
- Halos around lights, double vision, photophobia
- Eye redness
- Severe headache
- Nausea and vomiting

ASSESSMENT OF CORNEAL LIGHT REFLEX

- To perform the Hirschberg test, shine a light directly in front of the patient who is focusing on an object across the room (**Figure 8.1**). Observe where the light reflects back within the pupil of both eyes simultaneously.

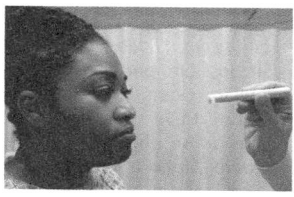

FIGURE 8.1 Hirschberg test to assess corneal light reflex.

- Corneal light reflex and observation are the primary methods for assessing eye alignment in infants. In young cooperative children, the cover test can also be used. To perform the cover test, have the child focus on an object straight ahead. Check for deviation in either eye. Cover one eye for 3 seconds (**Figure 8.2**).

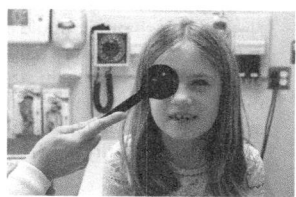

FIGURE 8.2 Pediatric binocular assessment with cover test.

The tested, uncovered eye is observed for movement out of (or back into) its original position. The untested eye is uncovered, while the tested eye is again observed for any deviation out of (or into) alignment. Repeat for the other eye.

- Asymmetric corneal light reflex indicates misalignment of the eyes (strabismus; **Figure 8.3A**); inward deviation of the eye (esotropia) resolves when the opposite eye is covered (**Figure 8.3B**).

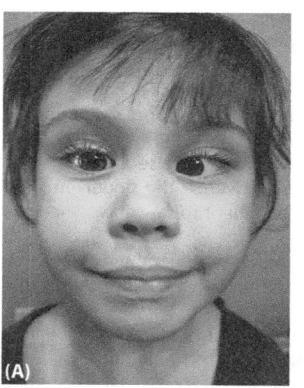
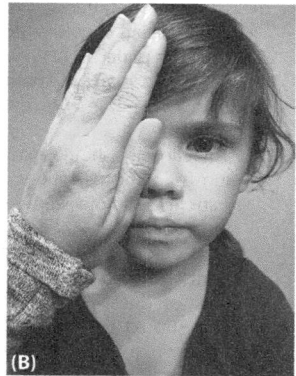

FIGURE 8.3 Esotropia. (**A**) Uncorrected. (**B**) Corrected during exam.

PUPILLARY ASSESSMENT
Pupillary Light Reflex
- If possible, perform the pupillary exam in a dimly lit room. Have the patient focus on an object across the room. Shine a light in each pupil, and note the size, position, shape, equality of the pupils, and their response to bright light (**Figure 8.4**).

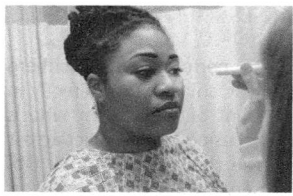

FIGURE 8.4 Assessing direct response to light.

Note that each pupil should constrict with direct illumination and will also constrict when a light is directed at the opposite pupil. Pupils should be equal in size, round, and react briskly with both direct and consensual response to light. Appropriate pupillary response requires an intact optic nerve, or cranial nerve (CN) II, and reflects the integrity of CN III, IV, and VI.

Accommodation Reflex
- Pupils should change in size when the eyes change focus on near and far objects. To assess this accommodation reflex, have the patient focus on a distant object, then focus on a penlight and slowly move the penlight toward the patient's nose. Both eyes should turn inward (convergence), and both pupils should constrict (accommodation). These functions are necessary for near and far vision.

VISUAL FIELD TESTING
- Confrontation visual field testing is used as a screening for integrity of CN II, visual field defects, scotomas (blind spots), and serious ocular disorders. The following are the steps to test visual fields by confrontation:
  - The clinician should sit (or stand) approximately 2 feet away from the patient.
  - The clinician and the patient should face one another.
  - Both cover one eye (as a mirror image) and maintain eye contact.
  - The clinician should extend an arm and raise a finger. Starting from the periphery, slowly advance the finger into the patient's field of vision. Ask the patient to say "now" when the finger becomes visible.
  - Assuming the clinician has normal peripheral vision, the patient should be able to see the finger at the same time the clinician does.
  - This should be repeated through all fields of vision. (Note that novice clinicians may incorrectly test only the right visual fields when testing the right eye, and the left visual fields when

testing the left eye. Because the visual fields of both eyes overlap, each eye should be tested independently through temporal, upper, nasal, and lower visual fields.)

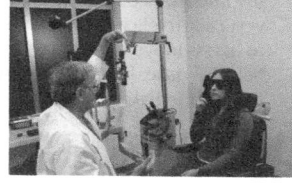

FIGURE 8.5 Simultaneous visual field testing by confrontation.

- Alternatively, the clinician can hold up a certain number of fingers peripherally, equidistant between themselves and the patient. The patient is asked to correctly identify the number of fingers. All quadrants (upper and lower, temporal, and nasal) should be tested.
- Confrontation visual field testing is highly specific but has limited sensitivity. To improve identification of any defects in central processing, the clinician may perform additional testing with both eyes open, presenting stimuli in the right and left visual fields simultaneously (**Figure 8.5**).

TESTING MOVEMENT OF THE EXTRAOCULAR MUSCLES

- Smooth and coordinated eye movement requires the use of the extraocular muscles (EOMs) of each eye that are innervated by CN III, IV, and VI. Eye movement occurs in six cardinal fields of gaze.
- To assess EOMs, the clinician stands in front of the patient and asks the patient to follow the clinician's finger with their eyes while keeping the head still and steady in a neutral position. If the clinician uses their finger to trace an "H" or a rectangular shape in front of the patient, all EOMs will be required by the patient to follow their finger smoothly (**Figure 8.6**). Note

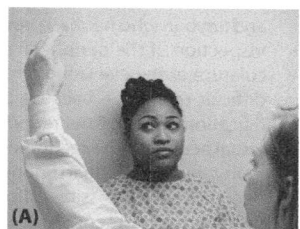

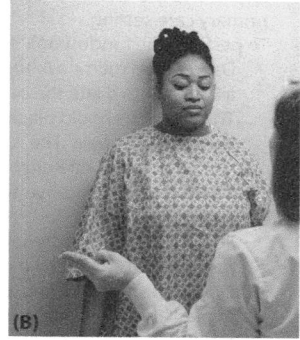

FIGURE 8.6 Assessment of extraocular muscles. (**A**) Assess upward gaze (top of the "H" on the patient's right side). (**B**) Assess downward gaze (bottom of the "H" on the patient's right side).

the importance of moving the finger far enough out laterally and vertically to elicit the full range of eye movements, and remember to assess movement across the entire "H" to assess the six cardinal fields of gaze: lateral and upward, lateral and downward, lateral, medial, medial and upward, and medial and downward.

DIRECT OPHTHALMOSCOPY

- Direct ophthalmoscopy, or fundoscopy, is used to assess concerns related to the retina, macula, optic nerve, or vasculature of the eye. Signs, symptoms, and/or history that are concerning for serious eye disease or increased intracranial or intraocular pressure should be urgently referred. A dilated fundoscopic exam (facilitated by mydriatic drops) should be performed by an ophthalmologist or optometrist for diagnostic purposes. Dilating an individual's pupils in the primary care setting is associated with risk of precipitating acute angle-closure glaucoma. Dilated exams are unsafe for small children, infants, anyone who is hyperopic, and anyone who has had previous acute angle-closure glaucoma.
- Inspection of the peripheral retina, optic nerve, macula, and vasculature of the eye using direct ophthalmoscopy is a particularly difficult technique because of the small field of view and magnification adjustments required for the individual who has poor visual acuity. As the technology for digital ocular fundus photography, including smartphone-assisted screenings, continues to become more accessible, affordable, and accurate with remote or validated assessment review, the use of retinal photographs may allow for a more reliable assessment of the undilated eye in the primary care setting.
- To perform the fundoscopic exam as effectively as possible:
  - ○ Darken the room; ask the patient to focus on an object far away to help dilate the pupil.
  - ○ The clinician should place the ophthalmoscope firmly against their own cheek. The clinician and the ophthalmoscope should move as one unit.
  - ○ Use the right hand/eye to assess the patient's right eye and vice versa.
  - ○ Look through the ophthalmoscope to determine whether it is in focus and adjust the diopter setting if needed.
  - ○ Direct the light of the ophthalmoscope into the pupil at a medial angle and watch for the red reflex, the red or reddish orange reflection of light from the fundus.
  - ○ Slowly move toward the patient while following the red reflex. If the red reflex is lost, start over. Follow the red reflex all the way in until the vasculature is seen. Follow the direction of the blood vessels in until the optic disc is visualized.

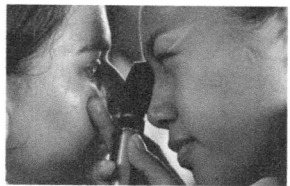

FIGURE 8.7 Ophthalmoscopy.

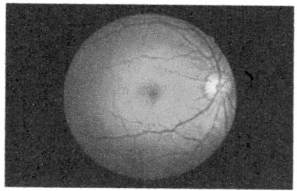

FIGURE 8.8 Normal fundal exam.

- At this point, the clinician is approximately nose-to-nose with the patient (**Figure 8.7**) and can pivot the ophthalmoscope to view the remainder of the retina, macula/fovea, and blood vessels (**Figure 8.8**).

Assessment of the Red Reflex

- Assessment of the red reflex bilaterally is a priority for infants and young children who are unable to verbalize visual disturbances. Any asymmetry in red reflex, dark spots, or leukocoria (white reflex) is abnormal and may be indicative of cataracts, retinal disease, retinoblastoma, or ocular tumor (**Figure 8.9**).

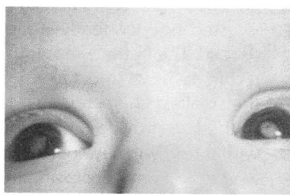

FIGURE 8.9 An infant with cataracts from congenital rubella syndrome. *Source:* Image courtesy of Centers for Disease Control and Prevention.

- These abnormalities have been identified through lack of "red eye" in photographs. To best assess the red reflex in clinical practice, use an ophthalmoscope to visualize the pupil. Look through the ophthalmoscope while shining the light into the pupil. This technique works best in a dimly lit room with a calm, awake infant or young child. The clinician may need to view at different angles to elicit the reflex.

MEASUREMENT OF VISUAL ACUITY

- Visual acuity is not assessed on a routine basis as a component of physical exams in most cases, except for children; however, assessing visual acuity can provide useful data when patients present with clinical concerns as acute change in visual acuity may be a worrisome sign.
- Snellen visual acuity charts are widely used. They have been modified over the years for different languages and include numbers and pictures for children and others who cannot read the letters.

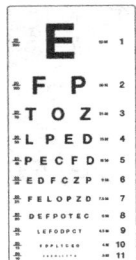 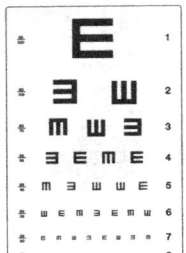 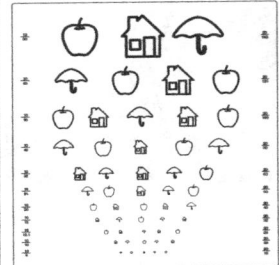

FIGURE 8.10 Snellen visual acuity chart.

- When testing visual acuity with a Snellen chart (**Figure 8.10**), the patient should stand at a 20-foot distance from the chart. Each eye is tested independently—one eye is covered, while the other is used to read. The patient should be allowed to wear glasses; document results as "best corrected vision." Ask the patient to read the line with the smallest characters that they can see. The numbers at the end of the line provide an indication of the patient's acuity compared with those who have normal vision. The larger the denominator, the worse the acuity. For example, 20/200 indicates that the patient can see at 20 feet what an individual with normal vision can see at 200 feet. If the patient is unable to read any of the lines on the chart, an estimate of what they are capable of seeing should be assessed (e.g., ability to count fingers, detect motion, or perceive light).

PEDIATRIC CONSIDERATIONS

- At each routine wellness visit, the following assessments should be performed on all children from newborn to 3 years of age:
  - Vision assessment, including visual fixation, tracking, visual interest, and attentiveness
  - Inspection of the eyes, including the lids, eyelashes, conjunctiva, corneas, sclera, irises, and pupils
  - Assessment of corneal light reflex and movement of the eyes (EOMs)
  - Pupillary function, including reaction to light, accommodation, and convergence
  - Red reflex (may appear gray or cream-colored in infants with darker pigmented skin)
- For children aged 3 years and older, age-appropriate visual acuity screening and fundoscopy should be included as components of the pediatric eye exam. Clinicians should complete these screening exams when children are able to be cooperative, and not when they are experiencing illness or fatigue.

PREGNANCY CONSIDERATIONS

Numerous physiologic effects occur within the body during pregnancy, and the eye is no exception. Normal physiologic changes include the following:

- Decrease in corneal sensitivity
- Slight increase in corneal thickness
- Changes in corneal curvature
- Contact lens intolerance as a result of a change in corneal curvature, increased corneal thickness/edema, or an altered tear film
- Decreased or transient loss of accommodation

CONSIDERATIONS FOR THE OLDER ADULT

Age-related changes include the following:

- Eyelid laxity and deepening of the lines of expression
- Changes in corneal curvature and decreased corneal luster
- Increased resistance to the outflow of aqueous humor in the trabecular network
- Hardening (nuclear sclerosis) of the lens
- Less collagen, which causes liquefaction of the vitreous humor
- Decline in visual function, including function of the lens, resulting in presbyopia (farsightedness)
- Decreased contrast sensitivity resulting in reduced depth perception
- Increased susceptibility to age-related diseases (e.g., macular degeneration)

RED FLAGS IN OBJECTIVE EXAM

- Timing is everything. Do not hesitate to refer patients to ophthalmology for abnormal findings associated with ocular assessment and vision.
- Red flags indicating serious neurologic or ocular disorders are listed in **Box 8.2**.

BOX 8.2 Red Flags in Objective Exam That Are Indications of Serious Neurologic or Ocular Disorders

- Intense eye redness of conjunctiva, sclera, lens, cornea
- Severe, purulent discharge from eye(s)
- Lens opacities, hazy cornea
- Loss of vision, visual field defects, change in visual acuity
- Pupil dilation or pupils unequal in size or shape
- Slow or absent pupil reaction to light
- Papilledema
- Periorbital or orbital erythema, edema, and tenderness
- Ptosis, painful or limited extraocular movements

ABNORMAL FINDINGS

The abnormal findings and differential diagnoses listed in this section are in alphabetical order, not in order of prevalence. The list is not exhaustive.

CATARACTS

History
- Cloudy, blurry vision
- Poor night vision, halos around lights
- Typically slow progression of symptoms, over years
- Risk factors including diabetes, smoking, alcohol use, and prolonged exposure to UV sunlight

Physical Examination
- Cloudy changes to the lens of the eye
- Missing or irregular red reflex (often leads to the discovery of cataracts in children)

Considerations
- The incidence increases with age.
- Pediatric cataracts are either present at birth (congenital) or develop in early childhood.

CONJUNCTIVITIS

History
- Burning, itching, foreign body sensation, and/or eye drainage
- Increased risk among contact lens wearers

Physical Examination
- Common signs include injection or redness and swelling of the conjunctiva, and eye drainage.

Considerations
- The etiology of conjunctivitis needs to be differentiated to ensure appropriate treatment.
  - Chemical irritants and fungal organisms can infect the eye and lead to conjunctivitis.
  - The incidence of conjunctivitis in patients with COVID-19 is being studied to determine exposure and transmission risks.
  - The three most common causes or types of conjunctivitis are viral, bacterial, and allergic.

Allergic Conjunctivitis
History
- Itchy eyes, intense itching of the eyelids
- Watery or clear mucoid drainage
- Co-occurring extraocular allergy symptoms, rhinorrhea

Physical Examination
- Reddened sclera from injected conjunctivae
- May have edema and erythema of the eyelids, loss of lashes (**Figure 8.11**)
- May have hypertrophy of conjunctiva resembling "cobblestones"
- Associated signs of allergies, including rhinitis, allergic shiners

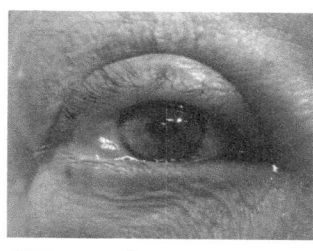

FIGURE 8.11 Allergic conjunctivitis.
Source: Image courtesy of James Heilman, MD.

Considerations
- Caused by reaction to allergens such as pollen, ragweed, dust mites, molds, pet dander, medicines, or cosmetics
- Not contagious, occurs more commonly in people with other allergic conditions like asthma or eczema

Bacterial Conjunctivitis
History
- Significant crusting and matting of eyelashes from mucopurulent drainage, especially after waking
- May be unilateral, although commonly spreads to both eyes
- Comorbid otitis media common in children

Physical Examination
- Scleral erythema, injected conjunctivae
- Purulent eye discharge (**Figure 8.12**), may have lid swelling

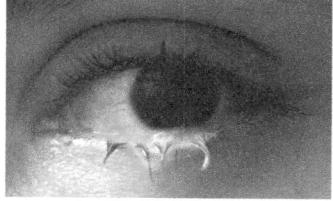

FIGURE 8.12 Bacterial conjunctivitis.
Source: Image courtesy of Tanalai.

Considerations
- Referred to as *pink eye*, highly contagious
- More common in children than adults
- If present in newborn, gonorrhea or chlamydia may be causal agent; treatment needed to prevent sepsis and vision loss

Viral Conjunctivitis
History
- Usually occurs concomitantly with symptoms of upper respiratory infection
- Symptoms often beginning in one eye, but can be in both

Physical Examination
- Reddened sclera and watery drainage (**Figure 8.13**)

Considerations
- The most common viral cause is adenoviruses.
- Conjunctivitis caused by viruses like measles or herpes simplex virus present with additional extraocular, cutaneous lesions consistent with the causative agent.

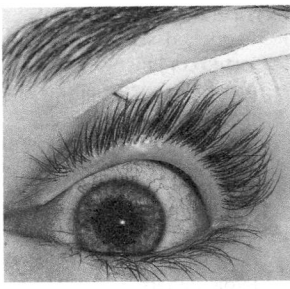

FIGURE 8.13 Viral conjunctivitis.
Source: Image courtesy of Joyhill09.

CORNEAL ABRASION

History
- Injury to the eye caused by foreign body, contact lens, trauma
- Excruciating eye pain that precludes normal daily activities
- Inability to open the affected eye due to foreign body sensation

Physical Examination
- Fluorescein staining reveals abrasion on the surface of the cornea.
- If a foreign body is suspected, the clinician may perform a lid eversion, "flipping" the lid inside out to inspect for a retained foreign body.

Consideration
- Penetrating trauma (ruptured globe) should be ruled out with a penlight exam by evaluating eye structures and pupil function; assess for clear drainage of aqueous humor.

DACRYOSTENOSIS

History
- Newborn with excess tearing
- A congenital lacrimal duct obstruction that typically resolves spontaneously by 6 to 12 months of age; gentle massage may help relieve the blockage

Physical Examination
- Persistent clear eye discharge without reddened sclera

Considerations
- It can be acquired in other age groups after injury or surgery.
- Dacryocystitis, an infection of the nasolacrimal duct system, is a rare complication of dacryostenosis; key signs and symptoms include erythema, swelling, warmth, and tenderness of the nasolacrimal sac, and/or purulent eye drainage.

DIPLOPIA

- Causes of diplopia (double vision) depend primarily on whether the diplopia is monocular or binocular. Binocular diplopia is present when both eyes are open and absent when one eye is closed. Monocular diplopia persists even when one eye is closed.
- Monocular diplopia is suggestive of local unilateral eye disease or refractive error. Causes of monocular diplopia include cataracts; high astigmatism error; keratoconus, a collagen vascular condition causing a very steep cornea; and displacement or subluxation of the lens, highly associated with Marfan syndrome.
- Binocular diplopia results from ocular misalignment. Sudden development should be evaluated urgently to rule out neurologic disorders, vascular pathologies, or mass/lesion etiologies. Common causes include strabismus; palsy of CN III, IV, or VI; myasthenia gravis or Graves disease; and trauma to the eye muscles.

GLAUCOMA

Acute Angle-Closure Glaucoma

Optic neuropathy characterized by unequal or elevated intraocular pressure (IOP) from insufficient drainage or excessive production of aqueous humor; can lead to vision loss if untreated

History

- Dramatic onset of symptoms (see **Box 8.1** for red flags)

Physical Examination

- Severely elevated and/or asymmetric IOPs
- Conjunctival injection
- Fixed or sluggish, dilated pupil (**Figure 8.14**)

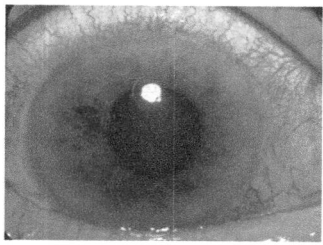

Considerations

- Causes sudden and severe damage to the optic nerve
- Should be treated as a medical emergency!

FIGURE 8.14 Acute angle-closure glaucoma.
Source: Image courtesy of Jonathan Trobe, MD.

Open-Angle Glaucoma

Glaucoma is optic neuropathy characterized by unequal or elevated IOP from insufficient drainage or excessive production of aqueous humor; can lead to vision loss if untreated

History

- Patchy blind spots in the peripheral or central vision
- Tunnel vision in advanced stages
- Risk factors including family history, ethnicity, and age over 65

Physical Examination
- Asymmetric IOPs
- May have retinal hemorrhages

Considerations
- Known as the *silent blinder* because it is often asymptomatic

MACULAR DEGENERATION

History
- Patients over 50 years of age most at risk
- Increased difficulty adapting to low-light levels, increased blurriness of printed words
- Difficulty recognizing faces

Physical Examination
- Reduced central vision in one or both eyes
- May have focal areas of retinal pigment loss and lesions on fundoscopic exam

Consideration
- An Amsler grid can be used to detect vision changes associated with macular degenerations (**Figure 8.15**).

OPTIC NEURITIS AND RETROBULBAR NEURITIS
This is an inflammatory condition of the optic nerve.

History
- Sudden onset of unilateral visual loss, unilateral orbital pain
- Occurs most often in ages 18 to 45 years
- Loss of color vision in the affected eye

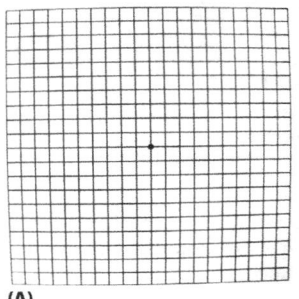
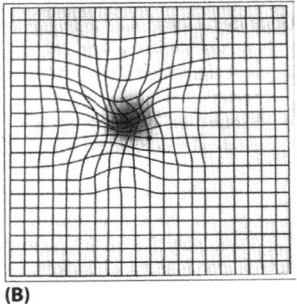

(A)   **(B)**

FIGURE 8.15 Amsler grid. (**A**) Amsler grid used to detect changes in vision. (**B**) Distorted Amsler grid.
Source: Part A image courtesy of Rosmarie Voegtli. Part B image courtesy of National Institutes of Health and National Eye Institute.

Physical Examination
- Absent or diminished pupillary response
- Visual field defects (central or peripheral)
- May have papilledema, flame-shaped hemorrhages, and vitreous cells on fundoscopy

Consideration
- Causes include MS, infective organisms (including viruses), granulomatous inflammatory conditions, tuberculosis, syphilis, sarcoidosis, and autoimmune disorders.

ORBITAL AND PERIORBITAL CELLULITIS
Periorbital cellulitis is an infection of the anterior portion of the upper and/or lower eyelid(s). Orbital cellulitis is an infection of the tissue in the orbit (eye socket).

History
- With either type of cellulitis, history includes eye pain with eyelid swelling and erythema.
- Orbital cellulitis generally presents with more severe clinical features, such as pain with eye movements, impaired eye movement, and proptosis (forward displacement of the globe).

Physical Examination
- Both conditions cause eyelid swelling and erythema surrounding the eye (**Figure 8.16**).

Considerations
- The most common cause of periorbital cellulitis is infection secondary to local skin trauma.
- The most common causes of orbital cellulitis are acute sinusitis, ophthalmic surgery, and orbital trauma.

PINGUECULUM
Benign growth of the conjunctiva

History
- Chronic dry eyes
- Recurrent exposure to wind, dust, and UV light or sunlight

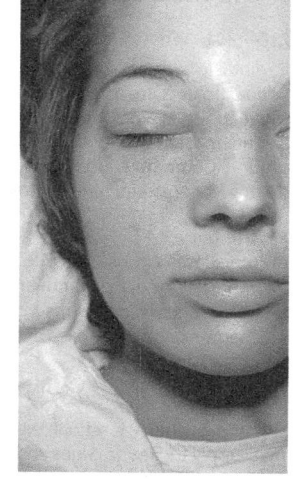

FIGURE 8.16 Orbital cellulitis.
Source: Image courtesy of Centers for Disease Control and Prevention/Dr. Thomas F. Sellers, Emory University.

Physical Examination
- Growth appears as a yellow bump on the inner canthus of the conjunctiva (**Figure 8.17**).

Consideration
- Can progress to pterygium

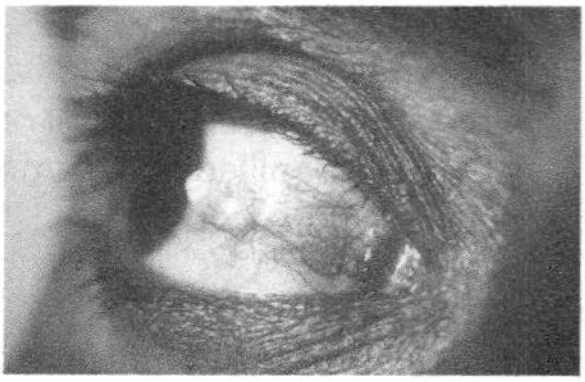

PTERYGIUM
Benign growth of the conjunctiva

FIGURE 8.17 Pinguecula.
Source: Image courtesy of Centers for Disease Control and Prevention.

History
- Chronic dry eyes
- Recurrent exposure to wind, dust, and UV light or sunlight

Physical Examination
- Growth of fleshy tissue that often arises from the pinguecula (**Figure 8.18**)

Consideration
- Can potentially obstruct vision by causing an astigmatic distortion of the cornea

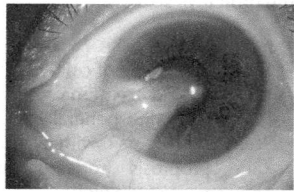

FIGURE 8.18 Pterygium.
Source: Image courtesy of Jmvaras.

RETINAL ABNORMALITIES
Retinal Floaters
Retinal floaters are a condition in which specks, black spots, or threads "float about" in a person's vision. These floaters move as the eyes move and are most noticeable to people when looking at a plain, bright background. Common causes are age-related. However, more serious conditions like posterior vitreous detachment can be an underlying cause.

Retinal Tears
In some cases of posterior vitreous detachment, the vitreous can pull away hard enough to tear the retina. A torn retina may result in a torn retinal vessel, which results in blood leaking into the vitreous (vitreous hemorrhage). Any case of floaters should be evaluated for retinal tear by a specialist.

Retinal Detachment
This occurs when the retinal cells separate from the layer of blood vessels that supply the retina. Signs and symptoms include acute onset of floaters, flashes of light (photopsia), blurred vision, and impaired peripheral vision. Any acute visual changes are concerning for a serious condition and should be evaluated urgently by an ophthalmologist. Infants and young children who present with suspicion of abusive head trauma should be evaluated emergently for retinal tears, hemorrhage, or detachment.

RETINOPATHY

Diabetic Retinopathy

A condition in which damage to the retina causes visual impairment

History

- Floaters, blurry vision, poor night vision, impaired color vision, and blank/dark areas in the field of vision
- Both eyes typically affected
- Occurs more often in patients with chronic diabetes (>5 years) and history of uncontrolled blood sugar (hemoglobin A1c [HbA1c] significantly above 7.0)

Physical Examination

- Defects in visual acuity, visual fields
- Chronically elevated blood sugar levels
- May have microaneurysms, retinal hemorrhages, cotton-wool spots, and macular edema on fundoscopic exam (**Figure 8.19**)

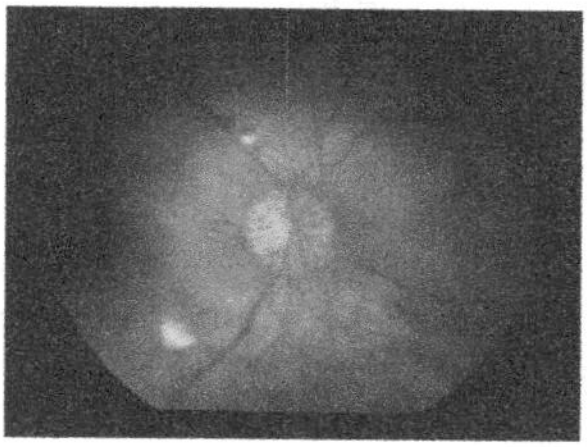

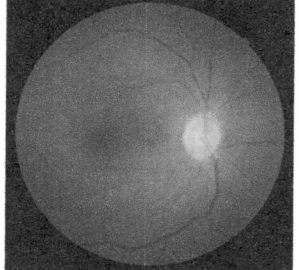

FIGURE 8.19 Proliferative diabetic retinopathy.
Source: Image courtesy of National Institute of Health and the National Eye Institute.

Considerations

- Diabetic retinopathy occurs primarily in two forms: proliferative and nonproliferative, which refer to whether there is growth of abnormal blood vessels on the retina.
- It causes vision loss, glaucoma, retinal detachment, and blindness.

Hypertensive Retinopathy

History

- Floaters, blurry vision
- Occurs more often in patients with chronically elevated blood pressure, those with a genetic predisposition, or younger patients with secondary hypertension

Physical Examination

- Chronic uncontrolled hypertension
- Can have arteriolar constriction, arteriovenous crossing or nicking, retinal hemorrhages, and blurred disc margins on fundoscopic exam (**Figure 8.20**).

FIGURE 8.20 Hypertensive retinopathy.
Source: Image courtesy of Frank Wood.

Consideration
- Visual changes can occur with advanced disease; less common to cause blindness.

Retinopathy of Prematurity
History
- It occurs in a small percentage of premature infants born less than 31 weeks' gestation.
- Infants at risk are those who require intensive respiratory support, such as oxygen therapy.

Physical Examination
- Digital retinal imaging is a useful tool to screen and document retinal changes.

Consideration
- The condition is thought to be a result of disorganized growth of retinal blood vessels, which can cause retinal scarring and detachment. Oxygen toxicity and hypoxia may also contribute to the development of retinopathy of prematurity.

SCLERITIS AND EPISCLERITIS

Scleritis
Scleritis is the inflammation of the sclera or choroid of the eye.

History
- Severe "boring" or penetrating pain, watery discharge, extreme photophobia

Physical Examination
- Exquisite tenderness to palpation
- Severe inflammation, injection of the sclera
- Decreased visual acuity

Considerations
- It is associated with SLE, RA, ankylosing spondylitis, inflammatory bowel disease, and infectious diseases.
- Scleritis can be anterior or posterior, diffuse, focal, nodular, or necrotizing.

Episcleritis
Episcleritis is localized inflammation of the episcleral tissues (outer covering of the sclera). Unlike scleritis, this condition is self-limiting and benign with mild discomfort.

History
- Red eye without discharge of drainage

Physical Examination
- May note a discrete, elevated area of inflamed episcleral tissue (nodular type) or an area of diffuse, vascular congestion in the absence of an obvious nodule (simple type)

Considerations
- Typically involves only one sector or area of the episclera
- Resolves over a few weeks

STRABISMUS
Strabismus is a misalignment of the eyes that is often congenital and occurs with various degrees of severity. The misalignment occurs because of an imbalance in EOM function.

History
- More common in children than adults
- Particularly more common in children with neurologic disorders like cerebral palsy

Physical Examination
- There is asymmetric corneal light reflex and the cover test is abnormal; the axis of misalignment can occur in one of several directions. As one eye fixates, the other eye may deviate inward (esotropia), outward (exotropia), upward (hypertropia), or downward (hypotropia).

Considerations
- Pseudostrabismus describes a condition in which the eyes appear to be misaligned when in fact they are not. If patients or young children have undeveloped facial features or a variation in the slant of palpebral fissures, symmetric corneal light reflex confirms pseudostrabismus not strabismus.
- Strabismus can lead to amblyopia (reduced vision) or blindness, as the child's developing brain prioritizes vision in the aligned eye and disregards the visual stimulus in the deviated eye, adversely affecting visual development. Persistent loss of visual stimulation in the affected eye eventually leads to amblyopia. Early intervention and treatment is crucial.
- Acute onset of strabismus in an older adult can be indicative of a more serious condition, for example, a CN VI or CN III palsy, and should be considered a medical emergency.

STY (HORDEOLUM)
An acute pustular infection of the eyelid margin

History
- Redness of the eyelid, tearing
- No changes in vision

Physical Examination
- Red, tender papule/pustule on the eyelid margin (**Figure 8.21**)
- Can present externally at the area of an eyelash follicle or tear gland, or internally just under the conjunctival side of the eyelid

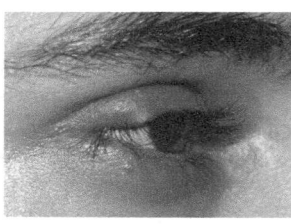

FIGURE 8.21 Sty of the upper eyelid.

Considerations
- A sty, or hordeolum, may evolve into a chronic inflammatory lesion (chalazion), which presents as a firm, rubbery nodule within the eyelid.
- When an individual presents with eyelid redness but not tearing, the condition is more likely blepharitis, inflammation of the eyelids, which can be caused by an infection or a systemic illness, such as seborrheic dermatitis, rosacea, or dry eye syndromes.

SUBCONJUNCTIVAL HEMORRHAGE

Demarcated area of ruptured blood vessels just beneath the surface of the eye

History
- Asymptomatic; no itching, drainage, pain, or discomfort

Physical Examination
- Distinct collection of blood within the sclera (**Figure 8.22**)
- Differs from more generalized hyperemia associated with acute conjunctivitis

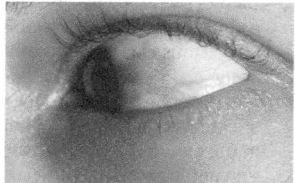

FIGURE 8.22 Subconjunctival hemorrhage.
Source: Image courtesy of Daniel Flather.

Considerations
- Can be caused by traumatic injury to the head or eye, but may also occur with Valsalva-associated coughing, straining, or vomiting; from anticoagulant therapy; or with contact lens insertions or removal
- Diagnosed by clinical appearance; further evaluation needed if the patient presents with a history of head trauma

UVEITIS

An inflammatory condition of the uveal tract

History

- Usually appears suddenly, with nonspecific symptoms of eye pain, redness, severe photophobia, and diminished vision

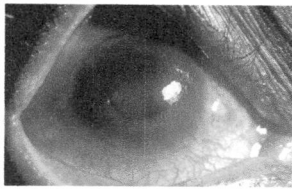

FIGURE 8.23 Acute anterior uveitis.
*Source: Community Eye Health Journal,
18(53), March 2005. www.cehjournal.org.*

Physical Examination

- Reduced visual acuity
- Deep hyperemia extending beyond the conjunctiva (**Figure 8.23**)
- Varied physical findings depending on the portion of the uveal tract affected, either anterior chamber (iritis), ciliary body, posterior chamber (retinitis), or dissemination throughout

Consideration

- Cause varies depending on the etiology of the inflammation. Infectious causes include herpes; CMV; toxoplasmosis; syphilis; tuberculosis; and West Nile, Ebola, and Zika viruses. Systemic or immune conditions include spondyloarthritis, sarcoidosis, juvenile idiopathic arthritis, psoriatic arthritis, inflammatory bowel disease, MS, Vogt–Koyanagi–Harada syndrome, Behçet syndrome, Sjögren syndrome, and SLE.

PHYSICAL EXAMINATION DOCUMENTATION

Documentation should include results of inspection and special tests.

EXAMPLE OF NORMAL FINDINGS

Visual fields full by confrontation, extraocular muscles intact, no nystagmus. No ptosis, lid lag, discharge, or crusting. Corneal light reflex symmetric, no strabismus. Conjunctiva clear, sclera white, no lesions or redness; pupils equal, round, and react to light and accommodation (PERRLA). Optic discs with sharp margins on digital fundoscopy; retinal background with even color without hemorrhages or exudate.

EXAMPLE OF NORMAL FINDINGS FOR PEDIATRIC WELLNESS EXAM

Visual acuity 20/20 with use of Snellen tumbling E chart for each eye and both eyes. Extraocular muscles intact, smooth, with no nystagmus, ptosis, or lid lag. Corneal light reflex symmetric; no strabismus as indicated by cover test. Conjunctiva clear, sclera white, no lesions, redness, or discharge noted. Pupils equal, round, and react to light and accommodation (PERRLA). Red reflex equal bilaterally.

REFERENCES

References for this chapter draw from Chapter 15, Evidence-Based Assessment of the Eyes, of the textbook *Evidence-Based Physical Examination: Best Practices for Health and Well-Being Assessment (Second Edition)*. The references may be accessed in the digital version of the handbook at https://connect.springerpub.com/.

9

Evidence-Based Assessment of the Ears, Nose, and Throat

CLINICAL CONSIDERATIONS

- To visualize the tympanic membrane (TM) in an adult, pull the helix up and back. In children under the age of 3, the angle of the ear canal is less acute, so the clinician will need to pull back and down on the posterior helix to see the TM.
- Pneumatic otoscopy is recommended to evaluate for effusion in the middle ear and can be very helpful when evaluating children.
- When evaluating a patient with hearing loss, use tuning forks to confirm diagnosis.
- If a patient presents with otalgia with a normal exam, consider other pathology, such as temporomandibular joint (TMJ) disorders, cervical pain, dental abscess, and cancer of the oropharynx and larynx.
- Rhinoscopy is a commonly overlooked part of the ear, nose, and throat exam. It should be completed in any patient who presents with an ear/nose/throat concern.
- When performing an oral exam, have the patient remove their dentures to ensure all of the oral mucosa is evaluated.
- If the clinician cannot get a good view of the posterior pharynx because the patient is guarding, have the patient pant in and out or yawn. This will elevate the soft palate, while relaxing the tongue.
- It is important for the clinician to be able to identify red flags in both the history and the physical examinations of the ear, nose, and throat (**Boxes 9.1** and **9.2**).

SUBJECTIVE HISTORY

COMMON REASONS FOR SEEKING CARE
- Otalgia
- Nasal congestion/rhinitis
- Sore throat

HISTORY OF PRESENT ILLNESS
- **Onset:** When did the symptoms start? What was the individual doing when they became symptomatic? Did this occur suddenly, or has it been developing gradually?

BOX 9.1 Red Flags in Subjective History

- History of sudden or rapidly progressive hearing loss
- Unilateral hearing loss of sudden or recent onset
- History of pain, active drainage, or bleeding from an ear
- Acute, chronic, or recurrent episodes of dizziness
- Evidence of congenital or traumatic deformity of the ear
- Unilateral or pulsatile tinnitus

- **Location:** Does the symptom have associated pain or discomfort? If so, where is the discomfort located? Which ear is affected? Is the nasal discharge one side or both?
- **Duration:** How long do the symptoms last? Over what period of time has the ear/nose/throat symptom developed? Have the symptoms been occurring for days/months/years?
- **Characteristics:** Is the pain aching, burning, sharp, dull, or throbbing? What color is the nasal/ear exudate?
- **Associated symptoms:** Have there been any fevers, chills, or night sweats? Any eye drainage or itching, ear drainage, hearing loss, tinnitus, anosmia, enlarged lymph nodes, coughing, postnasal drip, or sinus pain or pressure? Is there any pus on the back of the throat?
- **Aggravating factors:** What actions, activities, or body positions make the symptoms worse? Does it hurt to swallow? Does laying on the ear or swimming make the pain worse? Has exposure to smells, dust, pollen, smoking, or activities caused an increase in symptoms?
- **Relieving factors:** What actions, activities, or body positions decrease the symptoms? If relieved, how long does the relief last?
- **Treatment:** What medications has the individual taken to help with the symptoms? Have nasal corticosteroids or allergy medications or injections ever been tried? Clarify the dosage and frequency of any medications. Are there any pain or cold/sinus medications being used for the symptoms?
- **Severity:** How severe are the symptoms on a scale of 0 to 10? Do the symptoms affect the patient's quality of life? Are the symptoms worsening?

HEALTH HISTORY

Past Medical History

- History of ears, nose, and throat (ENT) illnesses throughout their life span
- Premature birth history, low birth weight, or birth complications such as severe asphyxia or low Apgar scores

- Previous diagnoses of asthma, sleep-disordered breathing, cystic fibrosis (CF), migraine, stroke, ciliary dyskinesia, autoimmune disorders, anemia, hematologic disorders, gastroesophageal reflux disease (GERD), Parkinson
- Previous ED visits or hospital stays for ear/nose/throat or respiratory problems
- Previous head and neck procedure(s) or surgery, including myringotomy with tympanostomy tubal placement
- History of trauma to the nose
- History of eczema or asthma
- Viral diseases such as Epstein–Barr virus (EBV), meningitis, or recent viral upper respiratory infection
- History of frequent ear infections as a child/adult, sudden hearing loss, eardrum rupture, deviated or perforated septum, recurrent sinus infections, nasal polyps, conjunctivitis, vitamin deficiencies, lichen planus, frequent strep throat/ tonsillitis, tonsilliths, sexually transmitted infections
- Anatomic malformation of the head or neck, craniofacial abnormalities (e.g., cleft palate)
- History of allergy testing and results
- Exposure to radiation
- Frequency of routine dental exams and cleanings
- Comorbidities or risk factors related to ear/nose/throat disease
- Recent exposure to individual with flu, flu-like symptoms, or COVID-19 symptoms
- Known or suspected pulmonary, cardiac, liver, or renal disease
- History of malignancy
- Recent surgery, hospitalization, or immobility
- Pregnancy status, noting the likelihood of pregnancy or if currently or recently pregnant
- Use of hearing aids, date of last adjustment

Medications
- Prescribed or over-the-counter (OTC) medications or supplements, including dose and frequency, nonsteroidal anti-inflammatory drugs (NSAIDs), antibiotic use (aminoglycosides), oxymetazoline, anticoagulants (prescribed and OTC), chemotherapy, steroids (including oral steroid inhalers), bisphosphonates, hormones, OTC saline rinses or saline irrigations, recent antibiotic use

Allergies
- Allergies to medications, or seasonal, environmental, and/or food allergies? If yes to being allergic to any substance or environmental trigger, clarify reaction:
  - Swelling of tongue, lips, face?
  - Dyspnea, wheezing, dizziness?

Immunizations
- **Risks for vaccine-preventable illnesses:** Vaccine status; date of last COVID-19, influenza, human papillomavirus (HPV), and tetanus vaccinations

Pediatric Considerations
- Sniffing or tripod position (may indicate epiglottis in children)
- Number of ear infections in the past 6 months
- Family members or school contacts with illness
- Concern for a possible foreign body (in the ear, nose, or throat)

FAMILY HISTORY
- Hearing loss, especially in childhood
- Head and neck cancers
- Allergic rhinitis (AR)
- Asthma
- Eczema
- Sinus disease
- Bleeding disorders
- Ciliary dyskinesia
- Autoimmune disorders
- Genetic malformations
- HIV
- Laryngeal disorders
- Thyroid disorders
- Perinatal viral infections such as cytomegalovirus (CMV), HPV, rubella, herpes, toxoplasmosis, or syphilis

SOCIAL HISTORY
- Tobacco use, including chewing tobacco, snuff, e-cigarettes, cigarettes, and cigars; pack-years (or equivalent), secondary exposure, quitting history and attempts, current desire to quit
- Alcohol use, including frequency, quantity, and type
- Illicit drug use, especially intranasal use
- Use of headphones, gun use, attendance at loud music concerts, playing in a band
- Occupation:
  - Operation of heavy machinery, exposure to loud noises
  - Exposure to wood dust, chemicals, asbestos, nickel
  - Teachers, speakers, singers, or professionals who use their voice often
- Recreation, such as frequent swimming
- Use of paan (betel quid)
- High-risk sexual behavior or exposure to HPV

REVIEW OF SYSTEMS
- **General:** Fatigue, fevers, unintended weight loss, weakness
- **Eyes:** Eye pain, double vision, blurry vision

BOX 9.2 Red Flags in Objective Exam

- Suspected foreign body in the ear or nose
- Blood discharge from the ear
- Uncontrolled or frequent episodes of epistaxis
- Persistent hoarseness, voice changes, or sore throat
- Difficulty breathing or shortness of breath
- Tripod positioning with drooling, stridor, dyspnea, and tachypnea
- Persistent sore or ulcer in the nose or mouth that does not resolve
- Red or white patches on the gums, tongue, or tonsils that do not resolve or worsen over time
- Head or neck mass
- Ear, nose, and throat symptoms associated with unintentional weight loss or other systemic symptoms

- **Ears, nose, throat:** Dental pain or caries, trismus, change in voice, hoarseness, odynophagia, sinus pain/pressure, bloody noses
- **Lymphatics:** Lymphadenopathy
- **Cardiovascular:** Chest pain, palpitations
- **Respiratory:** Shortness of breath, cough, wheezing
- **Gastrointestinal:** Abdominal pain, gastroesophageal reflux, diarrhea, constipation, blood in stool
- **Neurologic:** Headaches, facial palsies, dizziness, numbness
- **Skin:** Rashes, ulcers, sores, lumps

PHYSICAL EXAMINATION

GENERAL SURVEY AND VITAL SIGNS
- Rate, rhythm, depth, and effort of breathing
- Posture and position
- Vital signs including temperature, pulse rate, respiratory rate, and blood pressure

INSPECTION OF THE EAR
- Inspect the outer ear. Look for erythema, edema, tissue deformity, lesions, or masses.
- Use an otoscope to see the ear canal and TM. The clinician should place the otoscope in their dominant hand and place the nondominant hand on the helix, then pull up and back for an adult or pull back and down for a child (**Figures 9.1 and 9.2**).

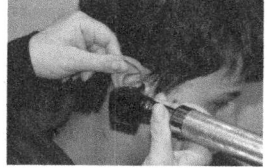

FIGURE 9.1 Adult ear exam technique.

- The otoscope can be held several different ways based on the preference and comfort of the clinician. One way is to put the handle between the thumb and the fingers, wrapping the hand around the handle, with the handle pointing toward the floor. This works well when examining adult patients and you do not expect much movement of the head.

- Pneumatic otoscopy is recommended for evaluation of effusion in the middle ear. Pneumatic otoscopy is a method of examining the middle ear by using an otoscope with an attached rubber bulb to change the pressure in the ear canal (**Figure 9.3**). Changing the pressure in the ear helps the clinician determine whether the TM moves. If the middle ear is well aerated, the TM will move from the pressure exerted with the rubber bulb. If an ear has an effusion, the TM cannot move because fluid is pushing against it.

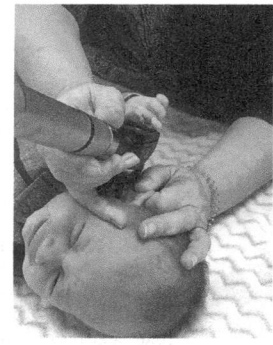

FIGURE 9.2 Infant ear exam technique.

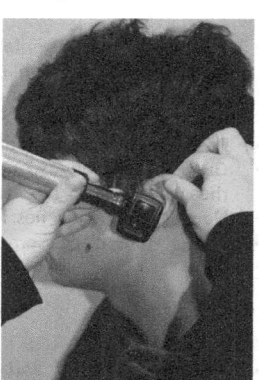

FIGURE 9.3 Pneumatic otoscopy.

PALPATION OF THE EAR

- Palpating the tragus and mastoid, or pulling up on the pinna, can provide information as to whether there is an ongoing, infective process as these maneuvers will generally produce pain if inflamed.

ASSESSING AUDITORY ACUITY

- The patient will be asked to occlude one ear canal. If the patient cannot do this, the clinician can press on the tragus, occluding the ear canal. The clinician should stand behind the patient or cover their mouth to ensure that the patient does not read the clinician's lips.

- Standing about 1 to 2 feet away, the clinician should exhale fully and whisper softly three words or numbers toward the unoccluded ear. The words or numbers should be equally accented syllables like "baseball" or "99." If the patient repeats them back correctly, the hearing is considered normal. If the patient does not respond correctly, repeat using three different words or numbers. The patient is considered to pass if they repeat three out of six answers correctly.

Finger Rub Test

- Standing in front of the patient, the clinician should hold their hands to the side of the patient's head. Gently rub the fingers on one side together, asking whether the patient hears the sound. Repeat on the other side.
- Wait for the patient's response. Repeat again with both hands, asking whether the patient hears them equally on both sides.

ASSESSING AIR AND BONE CONDUCTION

The tuning fork exam should be used in addition to the physical exam when evaluating hearing. This provides valuable information and can assist in distinguishing diagnoses that are consistent with a conductive or sensorineural hearing loss. The following are screening tests and do not replace formal audiometry.

Weber Screening Test

- In a quiet room, lightly hit the fork to start a light vibration. The clinician can do this by hitting the tuning fork on their knuckles/elbow or stroking the forks between their fingers. Once vibration is felt, lightly place the 512-Hz tuning fork on the patient's scalp at midline

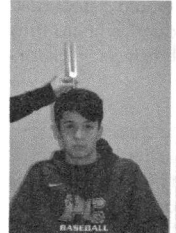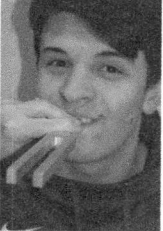

FIGURE 9.4 Weber exam techniques.

(**Figure 9.4**). Ask the patient whether they hear the tone louder in the left ear, the right ear, or if it is equally loud in both ears. The exam is considered normal if the sound is heard equally in each ear.
- In unilateral conductive hearing loss, the sound lateralizes to the affected ear (it will be heard louder in the affected ear). In unilateral sensorineural hearing loss, the sound lateralizes away from the affected ear (it will be heard louder in the normal ear). If nothing is heard, try again or move the turning fork onto the upper front teeth. This cannot be done if the patient is edentulous or has false teeth.

Rinne Test

- Place a lightly vibrating 512-Hz tuning fork on the mastoid bone behind the ear (**Figure 9.5A**). Ask the patient to cover the opposite ear with their hand. When the patient can no longer hear the sound,

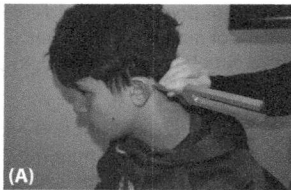
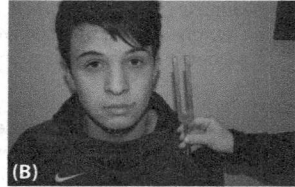

FIGURE 9.5 Conducting the Rinne test. (**A**) Assessing bone conduction.
(**B**) Assessing air conduction.

move the vibrating tuning fork in front of the same ear canal. Avoid
touching the ear. The "U" portion of the tuning fork should face forward in order to maximize the sound for the patient. The patient
should report when they can no longer hear the vibratory sound.
- A normal test is when the patient continues to hear the vibratory
sound for twice the amount of time when the tuning fork is held
next to their ear (**Figure 9.5B**) than when it was placed on their
mastoid bone. This indicates that air conduction (AC) is greater
than bone conduction (BC), signifying a normal test.
- The Rinne test would detect unilateral conductive hearing loss if
the vibratory sound is heard through the bone as long or longer
than through the air (AC < BC or AC = BC).

AUDIOMETRY
Testing Recommendations
- Tympanometry should be done in a patient with suspected otitis
media. This can be available in some medical offices or performed
by a licensed audiologist.
- In patients with a concern for hearing loss, an audiogram by a licensed audiologist is recommended.
- Any abnormal tuning fork exam findings should prompt a referral
for an audiologic evaluation.

PEDIATRIC CONSIDERATIONS
- In children under the age of 3, the angle of the ear canal is less acute,
so the clinician will need to pull back and down on the posterior helix. This allows for proper placement of the speculum into the external ear canal. A parent or assistant can help stabilize the head for you.
- It may be difficult to see the posterior pharynx in an infant. It is
best visualized when the infant is crying. If you cannot get good
visualization, listen to the quality of the infant crying as this can
indicate if there is any obstruction or restriction of the airway.

INSPECTION OF THE NOSE AND SINUSES
- Inspect the outside of the nose. Look for shape, deformity, lesions, asymmetry, and deviation. Assess the nares as the patient

breathes in and out of the nostrils. To
assess for nasal obstruction, press on
one naris at a time, asking the patient
to breathe in and out, assessing airflow
through the nasal vestibules.
- Palpate the sinuses to evaluate for tenderness. Palpate the frontal sinuses,
which are located under the eyebrows,
without pressing on the eyes. Palpate
the maxillary sinuses, which are located
approximately 1 cm lateral to the nasal
bridge bilaterally.
- Inspect the inside of the nose with an
otoscope and the largest ear speculum
available. Have the patient tilt the head

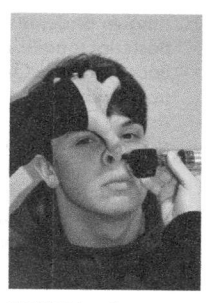

FIGURE 9.6 Otoscope
technique for anterior
rhinoscopy.

back and press the nasal tip up to open the nasal vestibule. Grab-
bing the otoscope between the thumb and index finger, brace the
otoscope using the clinician's fifth digit against the patient's cheek
(**Figure 9.6**). This will stabilize the scope and prevent sudden jerking movements in the nose.
- Look posteriorly and superiorly to visualize the anterior septum,
anterior inferior turbinate, and possibly the middle turbinate.
Evaluate the septum for deviation, lesions, perforation, bleeding,
and/or crusting. Assess the nasal cavity and mucosa for color, lesions, drainage, ulcerations, and polyps. Assess the turbinates for
color, size, polyps, lesions, and ulcerations.

INSPECTION OF THE MOUTH AND POSTERIOR PHARYNX
Lips
- Inspect the oral cavity, starting with the lips. Ensure the lips are
symmetrical at the oral commissure. Asymmetry can indicate
stroke or facial nerve palsies.
- Assess the lips for color, lesions, and closure. Nonhealing lesions
on the lip can indicate cancer.

Mouth
- Inspect the mouth with a light source and tongue depressor.
- Inspect the gingiva and dentition for caries, abscesses, periodontal disease, and lesions. Note the condition of the teeth and provide education on oral hygiene if poorly maintained.
- Look at the floor of the mouth under the tongue for pooling of
saliva or ulcerations, which could indicate cancer.

Tongue
- Inspect the buccal mucosa, dorsal tongue, ventral tongue, floor of
the mouth, retromolar trigone, hard palate, and soft palate. Use
the tongue blade to help pull back the buccal mucosa, lift the

tongue, or depress the tongue to get good visualization of the posterior tongue, lateral sides of the tongue, ventral tongue, and floor of mouth. Check for masses, ulcerations, and discolorations (red or white patches).

- Ask the patient to stick out the tongue and move it from side to side, assessing for fasciculation, symmetry, and function of cranial nerve (CN) XII. In infants and young children, have the patient sit on a parent's or adult's lap. The parent/adult should hold the head stable while the clinician examines the mouth with a tongue blade and light source. Inspect the frenulum of the tongue.

Posterior Pharynx

- Inspect the posterior pharynx by asking the patient to say "ahh" (**Figure 9.7**). Watch the soft palate elevate. This examines the function of CN X.
- Assess the uvula for deviation. Deviation can indicate peritonsillar abscess or CN X paralysis.
- Inspect the posterior pharynx, tonsillar pillars, retromolar trigone, soft palate, and uvula.

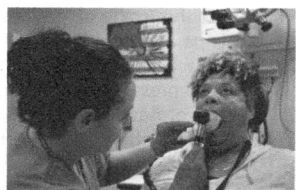

FIGURE 9.7 Inspection of the oral cavity and posterior pharynx.

- Inspect the tonsils for symmetry, size, crypts, exudates, white spots (tonsilliths), and/or masses.

PALPATION OF THE MOUTH AND JAW

- With gloved hands, ask the patient to stick out their tongue. Move it side to side, assessing for color, lesions, asymmetries, rough texture/smooth texture, and/or white/red patches (**Figure 9.8**).
- Next palpate the entire tongue—lateral surfaces, dorsal surface, ventral surface, and floor of the mouth (**Figure**

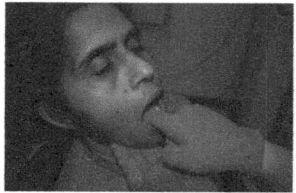

FIGURE 9.8 Palpation during the oral examination.

9.9). If there is asymmetry of the tonsils or a concern for a sore throat in a patient who is a tobacco user, palpate the tonsils and the base of the tongue. Oral or tonsillar lesions can cause referred pain to the ear.

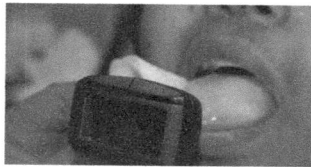
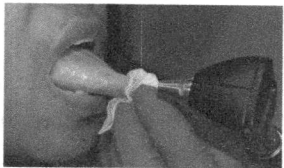

FIGURE 9.9 Inspection and palpation of the tongue.

TEMPORAL MANDIBULAR JOINT

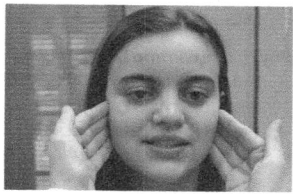

FIGURE 9.10 Assessing the temporal mandibular joint.

- Palpate and examine the TMJ. Assess the patient opening and closing the mouth and palpate the TMJ joint with adduction and abduction of the jaw (**Figure 9.10**). Patients with TMJ arthritis may have pain that radiates to the ear, causing ear pain.
- The clinician can also feel for crepitus or shifting of the joint when affected patients open their mouth.

PEDIATRIC CONSIDERATIONS

- Otitis media with effusion (OME) can cause significant hearing problems in children, resulting in speech and learning delays. Clinicians should assess children between the ages of 2 and 12 who exhibit speech or learning problems.
- Subtle symptoms of poor balance, behavioral problems, school performance issues, or speech delay may also point to an underlying hearing problem. It is important to rule out OME in these children as management can improve hearing outcomes.
- An additional consideration in the pediatric population is the heightened activity of the tonsil and adenoid tissue from ages 4 to 10. The most common bacterial infection that affects this area is group A beta-hemolytic *Streptococcus* (GABHS), which causes tonsillitis.
- The Paradise criteria for tonsil infection include a sore throat plus at least one of the following features: temperature over 38.3°C (100.9°F), adenopathy, tonsil exudate, or a positive culture for GABHS.

ABNORMAL FINDINGS

EAR

Otitis Media
An infection or inflammation that involves the middle ear

History
- Otalgia (typically unilateral)
- Reported fever, may have additional symptoms of upper respiratory infection concurrent or prior to symptoms
- Difficulty hearing typically described as muffled hearing

Physical Examination
- Bulging, erythematous TM (**Figure 9.11**); posterior to TM, purulent fluid noted inside the middle ear
- Weber lateralization to the affected ear
- No movement of TM with pneumatic otoscopy or autoinsufflation

Consideration
- Otitis media can be purulent and symptomatic with otalgia and fever, or there can be serous or mucoid fluid behind the TM that may or may not cause hearing impairment and rarely other associated symptoms.

Otitis Media With Effusion
Fluid accumulates behind an intact TM.

History
- Hearing loss often described as muffled hearing
- Aural fullness/pressure
- May report vertigo or tinnitus
- Often following an upper respiratory infection or with seasonal allergies

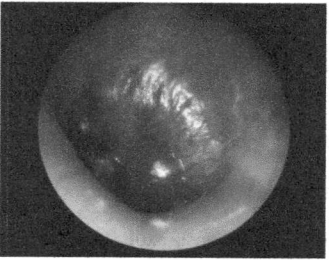

FIGURE 9.11 Otitis media.
Source: Image courtesy of B. Welleschik.

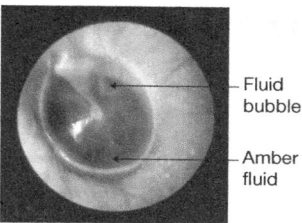

FIGURE 9.12 Otitis media with effusion.
Source: Image courtesy of Michael Hawke, MD.

Physical Examination
- Amber fluid and bubbles are seen behind the TM (**Figure 9.12**).
- Weber test lateralizes to the affected ear.
- Audiogram will reveal conductive or mixed hearing loss of the affected ear.

Considerations
- OME may occur spontaneously due to poor eustachian tube function or as an inflammatory response following an acute otitis media (AOM).
- Between 60% and 70% of OME will resolve spontaneously within 3 months.

Cholesteatoma
A condition in which squamous epithelium becomes entrapped either behind the ossicles or within the crevices of the temporal bone and causes bony erosion, hearing loss, and TM perforations

History
- Difficulty hearing
- History of chronic ear infections and/or eustachian tube dysfunction
- Chronic otorrhea
- May experience vertigo and tinnitus

Physical Examination
- Debris accumulates most often in the upper ear above the malleus (pars flaccida); debris can resemble white skin and/or may be mixed with cerumen.
- Bony erosion is seen in the upper ear canal (scutum erosion; **Figure 9.13**).

Considerations
- Cholesteatoma is due to long-term eustachian tube dysfunction and/or repeated middle ear infections, resulting in severe retraction of the TM around these osseous structures.

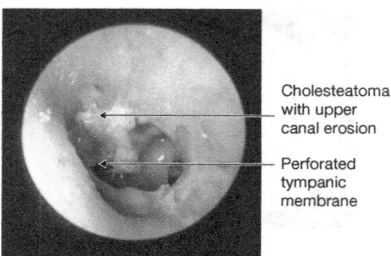

Cholesteatoma with upper canal erosion

Perforated tympanic membrane

FIGURE 9.13 Cholesteatoma with upper canal erosion.
Source: Image courtesy of Michael Hawke, MD.

- If cholesteatomas are left untreated, they can cause hearing loss, infections, dizziness, and injury to the facial nerves.

Eustachian Tube Dysfunction
An ear condition that occurs when there is negative pressure in the middle ear and the TM is pulled into the middle ear cavity

History
- Difficulty hearing usually described as muffled hearing
- Difficulty popping or equalizing pressure in the ear
- Otalgia
- Tinnitus
- Aural fullness in the affected ear
- History of frequent ear infections

Physical Examination
- TM is sucked into the middle ear space, creating a pocket.
- Weber lateralizes to the affected ear.

Consideration
- Blockage of the eustachian tube isolates the middle ear space from the outside environment, creating a negative pressure that pulls the TM inward, causing pressure, pain, and accumulation of fluid.

Hearing Loss
Hearing loss can have multiple causes and presentations. See **Table 9.1** and **Figure 9.14**.

Tinnitus
Typically described as ringing in the ears but can be any type of sound one hears that is not external.

TABLE 9.1 Causes of Hearing Loss With Expected Exam Findings

Causes of Hearing Loss	Assessment Noted on Exam
Conductive hearing loss	
Cerumen	Yellow, orange, brown waxy substance in the ear canal blocking visualization of the TM
Otitis media with effusion (most common in children)	Usually painless with amber fluid behind the TM; usually can see air bubbles; immobility of the TM with pneumatic otoscopy
Acute otitis media	On inspection, bulging, erythematous TM with purulent material behind the TM
TM perforation	Hole in the TM with view into the middle ear
Otosclerosis	Not visible on exam but will demonstrate conductive hearing loss
Otitis externa	Erythema, edema, and exudate within the ear canal; can have white, yellow debris or purulent drainage
Ear canal mass/middle ear mass (glomus tumor, osteomas)	White, hard round masses within the ear canal (osteomas) or red pulsating mass within the middle ear that may extend through the TM
Tympanosclerosis	Scarring on the TM; usually white in color
Cholesteatoma	White skin debris or hard cerumen that usually occurs in the pars flaccida
Causes of sensorineural hearing loss[a]	
Presbycusis	This is a gradual, symmetric, high-frequency, permanent hearing loss that occurs over the age of 60.
Noise exposure	Exposure to loud noise, typically over 85 decibels; the louder the sound, the shorter amount of time it takes to cause hearing loss.
Hereditary	In infants, this can affect between 1 and 3 children per 1,000; newborn hearing screening can detect this hearing loss.

(continued)

TABLE 9.1 Causes of Hearing Loss With Expected Exam Findings *(continued)*

Causes of Hearing Loss	Assessment Noted on Exam
Ototoxicity	Certain drugs are known to cause ototoxic effects in the cochlea: aminoglycoside antibiotics, platinum-based chemotherapeutic medications, loop diuretics, and salicylates/NSAIDs.
Sudden idiopathic hearing loss	This is considered a medical emergency and needs to be identified early in order to preserve hearing. Physical exam reveals normal ear exam and Weber lateralizes away from the affected ear. Immediate referral to otolaryngologist is indicated.
Autoimmune hearing loss	This is very rare; symptoms include fluctuating hearing loss and possibly vertigo.
Ménierè disease	This is an inner ear disorder believed to be caused by too much endolymph inside the cochlea.
Vestibular schwannoma	This is rare, affecting 1 to 2 per 100,000 people, and is a slow-growing, benign tumor. Physical exam findings reveal normal otoscopy. If the tumor is large, the patient may have facial paresis due to compression of CN VII (facial nerve).
Infections (meningitis, viral labyrinthitis)	In meningitis, the patient may have severe headache, fevers, cranial nerve palsies, and decreased hearing. In viral labyrinthitis, some patients may have precipitating viral upper respiratory infection causing vertigo, as well as decreased or sudden hearing loss.

[a]In all of these situations, otoscopy is normal. Weber would lateralize away from the affected ear. Air conduction should be louder than bone conduction.
CN, cranial nerve; NSAIDS, nonsteroidal anti-inflammatory drugs; TM, tympanic membrane.

History
- Subjective sound reported as hissing, ringing, buzzing, humming, or chirping in one or both ears; can be reported as pulsatile (sound like heartbeat is in the ear); heard constantly or intermittently
- Can occur in one or both ears
- Causes interference with concentration and hearing
- Can lead to decreased quality of life

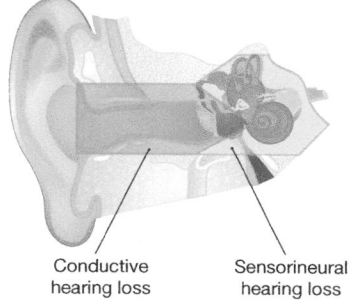

FIGURE 9.14 Conductive and sensorineural hearing loss. Conductive hearing loss occurs when sound waves do not reach the inner ear. Sensorineural hearing loss occurs when sound waves are not correctly processed.

Conductive hearing loss

Sensorineural hearing loss

Physical Examination
- Otoscopic exam is typically normal.
- Audiogram typically shows hearing loss.

Consideration
- Tinnitus is a subjective perception of sound that originates in the brain and not an outside source.

Malignant Otitis Externa
The sequela of a severe outer ear infection, mostly from *Pseudomonas aeruginosa* or *Staphylococcus aureus*

History
- Otalgia, otorrhea
- Change in hearing
- Immunocompromised status or uncontrolled diabetes
- Granulation at the bony cartilaginous junction of the ear canal

Physical Examination
- Pain with manipulation of the auricle
- Culture from otorrhea positive for *P. aeruginosa*
- Facial weakness in severe cases
- Osteomyelitis noted on CT temporal bone or gallium scan

Consideration
- The infection begins as an external otitis media and progresses into an osteomyelitis of the temporal bone.

NOSE
Allergic Rhinitis
An inflammatory immunoglobulin E (IgE)-mediated disease triggered by exposure to allergens

History
- Sneezing, nasal congestion
- Itchy eyes, nose, or throat
- Nasal congestion

Physical Examination
- Postnasal drip
- Clear, watery, bilateral rhinorrhea
- Pale, boggy nasal mucosa
- Swelling of turbinates
- Puffiness/darkening around the eyes or "allergic shiners"
- Posterior pharynx cobblestoning
- Nasal polyps (occasional)

Consideration
- AR can also be associated with other conditions such as atopic dermatitis, eczema, asthma, sleep-disordered breathing, conjunctivitis, rhinosinusitis, and otitis media.

Nonallergic Rhinitis
An inflammation of the nasal tissues with an etiology that is not immune-related and most often due to a virus or irritant; results in nasal congestion, rhinitis, and sneezing

History
- Environmental triggers (e.g., pollen, grass)
- Postnasal drip
- Congestion, sneezing
- Lack of nasal itching the *key difference between this and AR*

Physical Examination
- Edematous turbinates
- Rhinorrhea (clear)
- Allergy testing negative for IgE

Consideration
- Usually viruses or environmental irritants will trigger it, but it can be triggered by medications or pregnancy.

Sinusitis
An inflammation of the paranasal sinus cavities (**Figure 9.15**) due to a virus, bacteria, fungus, or an allergic reaction

History
- **Bacterial sinusitis:** Symptoms persist over 10 days or worsen after an initial improvement.
- **Viral sinusitis:** Symptoms peak at day 3 and gradually decline within 10 to 14 days.
- **Acute sinusitis:** Symptoms last <4 weeks in duration.

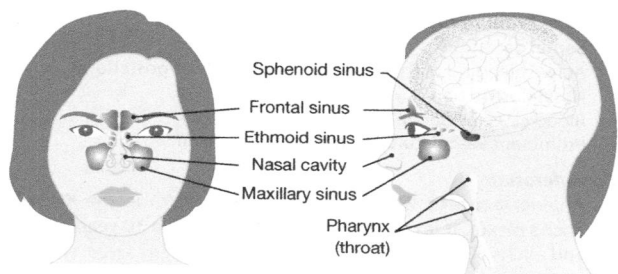

FIGURE 9.15 Paranasal sinuses.

- **Chronic sinusitis:** Symptoms persist >12 weeks.
- The three core symptoms are purulent nasal drainage, facial pain/pressure, and nasal obstruction/congestion.
- Additional symptoms include cough, headache, maxillary dental pain, aural fullness, sinus tenderness, and anosmia.

Physical Examination
- Purulent nasal drainage
- Edematous, erythematous nasal mucosa
- Injected throat, with purulent mucus in the posterior pharynx
- Possible head and neck lymphadenopathy
- Occasional anatomic findings such as deviated septum, turbinate hypertrophy, nasal mass, and/or nasal polyps (more likely found in chronic sinusitis)

Consideration
- Sinusitis can be acute or chronic in nature. With chronic sinusitis, there can be a history of allergic rhinitis and allergies.

Epistaxis
Bleeding from the nose caused by a ruptured blood vessel

History
- Reported digital trauma
- Use of certain medications (e.g., warfarin)
- Dry environment
- History of elevated blood pressure, hypertension, vascular malformations, or coagulopathies
- History of or current upper respiratory infection and/or allergic rhinitis
- Reported trauma to the nose or face
- Use of inhaled illicit drugs (e.g., cocaine)
- Alcoholism
- History of nasal cannula use

Physical Examination
- Septal deviation
- Active bleeding of the nose either anteriorly or posteriorly
- Nasal obstruction
- Blood clots inside the nose
- Prominent vasculature on the anterior septum

Consideration
- Anterior epistaxis is most common (90%–95%) in the Kiesselbach's plexus. It is common among children 2 to 10 years of age and adults 50 to 80 years of age.

Nasal Polyp
Mucus-filled lobular lesion that occurs within the nose and paranasal sinuses (**Figure 9.16**)

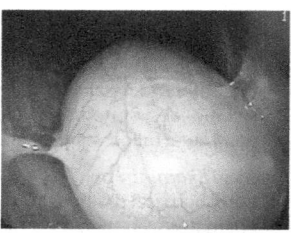

History
- Nasal congestion, postnasal drip, rhinorrhea
- Will likely have allergy symptoms such as itchy watery eyes, itchy nose, and sneezing
- May have a history of chronic sinus infections due to the obstruction
- History of CF, allergic fungal sinusitis, and aspirin allergy

FIGURE 9.16 Nasal polyp in the left nares between the inferior turbinate and the septum.

Physical Examination
- Nasal obstruction
- Boggy pale, enlarged turbinate(s)
- Round, symmetric, pale grape-like mass

Consideration
- Nasal polyps can occur in response to a foreign body in the nose.

Septal Perforation
Refers to a hole within the septum of the nose

History
- History of cocaine use
- Epistaxis
- Crusting

Physical Examination
- May be entirely asymptomatic
- A whistling noise when breathing through the nose

- Malodorous smell in the nose
- Hole in the septum (can be tiny or involve the majority of the septum)
- Saddle nose deformity

Consideration
- Septal perforation can be a result of trauma to the nose, post-surgical trauma, or due to an iatrogenic cause.

THROAT
Acute Pharyngitis
Edema, odynophagia, and/or scratchiness in the pharynx typically due to a viral or bacterial infection

History
- Sudden-onset sore throat; often accompanied by rhinorrhea, cough, fever, fatigue, malaise, and/or myalgia
- Odynophagia
- Absence of a cough (typical of streptococcal pharyngitis)
- History of exposure to strep throat

Physical Examination
- Anterior and posterior cervical lymphadenopathy
- Fever
- Tonsillar hypertrophy
- White exudate on tonsils
- Palatal petechiae (**Figure 9.17**)
- Erythematous rash that blanches with a sandpaper quality (scarlet fever or scarlatina)

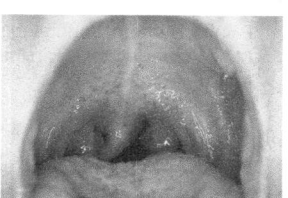

FIGURE 9.17 **Strep pharyngitis.**
Source: Centers for Disease Control and Prevention/Heinz F. Eichenwald, MD.

Consideration
- Bacterial (or streptococcal) pharyngitis needs to be treated with antibiotics to prevent complications including rheumatic fever and glomerulonephritis.

Angioedema
Swelling of the deeper layers of the skin in response to an allergen, commonly affecting the eyes, cheeks, and lips

History
- History of medications known to cause reactions (e.g., angiotensin-converting enzyme [ACE] inhibitors, antibiotics)
- History of allergies (e.g., certain foods, latex, insect venom)
- Can be a hereditary disorder

Physical Examination

- Sudden swelling of the face, lips, and/or tongue, but can occur in any part of the body
- Swelling of the airway
- Sudden, severe shortness of breath or trouble breathing
- Voice changes
- Stridor
- May have other allergic reaction symptoms such as pruritus or rash
- Edema of the lips, around the eyes; may cause edema of the oral mucosa and tongue

Consideration

- If not treated, severe cases can be life-threatening due to risk of airway compromise.

Aphthous Ulcer

Small, painful lesions that occur inside the lips or on the tongue, buccal or palatal mucosa, and floor of the mouth; frequently referred to as cold sores

History

- Painful, burning, or tingling sensation at the site of the ulcer
- More common during an immunocompromised state
- May report a fever
- Lasts about 1 to 2 weeks

Physical Examination

- Shallow ulcer with white or yellow center surrounded by erythema (**Figure 9.18**)
- Can occur on ventral tongue, gingiva, or buccal mucosa

Consideration

- Typically self-resolves without treatment

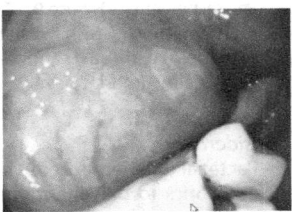

FIGURE 9.18 Aphthous ulcer.

Herpangina

A contagious illness most often caused by the coxsackie group A viruses

History

- Typically found in young children (ages 3–10)
- More frequent in the summer and fall months
- Reported high fever
- Reported fussiness or refusing to eat in young children

- Headache, anorexia, sore throat
- Odynophagia

Physical Examination
- High fever
- Ulcerative lesions in the mouth and throat; similar lesions on the feet, hands, and buttocks
- Vomiting

Consideration
- Herpangina is most commonly spread through contact with respiratory secretions or via the fecal–oral route. It is similar to hand, foot, and mouth disease; see Chapter 5, Evidence-Based Assessment of the Skin, Hair, and Nails.

Leukoplakia
Thin white lesion on the mucosal surface anywhere within the oral cavity; usually not painful and does not brush or rub off

History
- History of heavy smoking or chewing tobacco, heavy alcohol use
- Often asymptomatic
- Nonpainful, nontender

Physical Examination
- White, thick patches on the mucosa and/or tongue
- Can be thickened or hardened patches
- Can be seen along with raised, red lesions
- Does not rub off

Consideration
- It can be a premalignant lesion in some cases and is diagnosed with a biopsy.

Oral Candidiasis
A white lesion due to a fungal infection involving the mucosal surfaces, commonly referred to as thrush

History
- Often seen in infants and older adults
- Immunocompromised status
- Use of an inhaled steroid
- Wears dentures
- History of diabetes, HIV, or cancer
- Reports soreness or pain around the area, difficulty eating or swallowing
- Reduced feeding (infants)
- Loss of taste

Physical Examination
- White lesion that will leave an erythematous base when scraped off
- Generally has a flaky-type appearance involving several areas
- Patches typically found on the tongue or inner cheek
- Can spread to the roof of the mouth, gingiva, tonsils, or posterior pharynx (**Figure 9.19**)

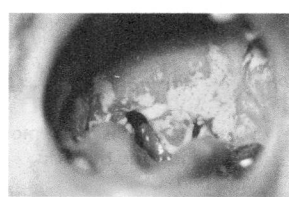

FIGURE 9.19 Oral candidiasis.
Source: Centers for Disease Control and Prevention.

Consideration
- It can be spread from the infant to the mother during breastfeeding.

Nasal/Oral Cancers
Malignancy in the nasal/oral cavities, typically due to a squamous cell carcinoma

History
- History of HPV
- History of smoking or chewing tobacco, heavy alcohol use
- Poor oral hygiene
- Pain
- Dysphagia
- Odynophagia
- Hoarseness
- Unilateral otalgia, nasal obstruction, rhinorrhea, sinus infections, epistaxis, or orbital symptoms

Physical Examination
- Unintentional weight loss
- Neck mass
- Red or white patch or ulcer on the lips, tongue, cheeks, floor of the mouth, hard and soft palate, sinuses, and pharynx (throat) that does not resolve
- Tender to palpation
- May be firm and/or fixed on palpation
- Loose teeth
- Adenopathy

Consideration
- There are many kinds of head and neck cancers but many of them have the same risk factors, specifically tobacco and heavy alcohol use.

PHYSICAL EXAMINATION DOCUMENTATION

Documentation should include results of inspection and palpation.

EXAMPLE OF NORMAL FINDINGS

Conjunctiva clear without erythema or drainage bilaterally. Pupils equal, round, and reactive to light and accommodation. Vision 20/20 on Snellen chart. No frontal or maxillary sinus tenderness on palpation. No tragus or pinna tenderness bilaterally. Tympanic membranes pearly gray and translucent with no bulging or retraction bilateral. Cone of light visible at 5 o'clock in right ear and 7 o'clock in left ear. Nasal turbinates nonedematous and nonerythematous bilaterally without drainage. Dentition intact with no caries. Oral membranes moist and pink. Posterior pharynx nonerythematous. Tonsils 1+ without exudate. No occipital, preauricular, postauricular, posterior cervical, anterior cervical, submandibular, submental, or supraclavicular lymphadenopathy.

EXAMPLE OF ABNORMAL FINDINGS

No tragus or pinna tenderness bilaterally. Right tympanic membrane (TM) pearly gray and translucent with no bulging or retraction. Left TM with clear fluid, no movement of TM with insufflation. Nasal turbinates edematous with clear drainage bilaterally. Posterior pharynx erythematous with cobblestoning and clear drainage. Tonsils 1+ without exudate. No occipital, preauricular, postauricular, posterior cervical, submandibular, submental, or supraclavicular lymphadenopathy. Several shotty anterior cervical lymph nodes palpable.

REFERENCES

References for this chapter draw from Chapter 16, Evidence-Based Assessment of the Ears, Nose, and Throat, of the textbook *Evidence-Based Physical Examination: Best Practices for Health and Well-Being Assessment (Second Edition)*. The references may be accessed in the digital version of the handbook at https://connect .springerpub.com/.

10

Evidence-Based Assessment of the Neurologic System

CLINICAL CONSIDERATIONS

- Develop a routine for the neurologic examination. Perform the examination the same way each time to ensure no portion of the examination is missed or forgotten.
- Several neurologic conditions do not present with neurologic deficits.
- Older adults may present with altered levels of cognition, not associated with or occurring as part of a neurologic disease.
- Depression screening is important in older adults to determine whether changes in cognition are related to depression or as part of a neurologic disorder.

SUBJECTIVE HISTORY

COMMON REASONS FOR SEEKING CARE
- Headaches
- Dizziness/vertigo
- Weakness

HISTORY OF PRESENT ILLNESS
- **Onset:** When did the symptoms start? What was the individual doing when they became symptomatic? Did this occur suddenly, or has it been developing gradually?
- **Location:** Does the symptom have associated pain or discomfort? If so, where is the discomfort located? Is the headache on one side or both? Is the weakness localized to one area of the body or is it generalized?
- **Duration:** How long do the symptoms last? Over what period of time has the neurologic symptom developed? Do the symptoms come and go or are they always present?
- **Characteristics:** Is the headache aching, pulsating, sharp, shooting? Would you describe the headache as a thunderclap, abrupt-onset headache? Did the headache wake you from sleep? Would you describe the dizziness as lightheadedness, disequilibrium, or like the room is spinning?

- **Associated symptoms:** Do you experience any nausea, vomiting, vision changes, confusion, weakness, or aura with the headache? Does the weakness worsen with effort? Does the weakness include sensory loss?
- **Aggravating factors:** What actions, activities, or body positions make the symptoms worse? Is the headache exacerbated by light, sound, noise, or smell? Can you identify any triggers (e.g., dehydration, certain foods, alcohol, fatigue, stress) for the headache? Is the dizziness worse with movement or going from sitting to standing? Is the weakness worse with movement or when completing certain activities? If so, what activities?
- **Relieving factors:** What actions, activities, or body positions decrease the symptoms? If relieved, how long does the relief last? Does the headache improve with sleep or going into a dark room? Does the weakness improve with rest?
- **Treatment:** What medications has the individual taken currently or in the past to help with the symptoms? Clarify the dosage and frequency of any medications.
- **Temporal:** Are the symptoms worse at a certain time of day? Do you wake up in the morning with a headache?
- **Severity:** How severe are the symptoms on a scale of 0 to 10? Do the symptoms limit participation in activities or daily activities? Are the symptoms worsening?

HEALTH HISTORY
Past Medical History
- History of trauma, such as concussion/brain injury, spinal cord injury or localized injury, central nervous system insult, seizures, birth trauma, and stroke
- Premature birth history or neurologic disease diagnosed during childhood
- Previous diagnoses of meningitis, encephalitis, lead poisoning, and poliomyelitis
- Previous ED visits or hospital stays for neurologic problems
- Previous or current history of neurologic disorders, neuro/brain surgeries, or any residual effects
- History of migraines or headaches
- History of deformities, congenital anomalies, genetic syndromes, and developmental delays in children
- Hand, eye, and foot dominance
- Recent illness or tick bite

Comorbidities or Risk Factors Related to Neurologic Diseases
- History of cardiovascular (CV) or circulatory problems, such as hypertension, aneurysm, peripheral vascular disease, and stroke
- History of diabetes or endocrine disorders
- Known or suspected respiratory, cardiac, or renal disease
- History of malignancy
- History of autoimmune disorders
- Recent surgery, hospitalization, or immobility
- Pregnancy status, noting the likelihood of pregnancy or if currently or recently pregnant
- Recent or past infection with *Campylobacter jejuni*, Epstein–Barr virus (EBV), cytomegalovirus (CMV), Lyme disease, or COVID-19

Medications
- Prescribed medications, including the dose, frequency, and the last time blood levels were checked (if applicable)
- Over-the-counter (OTC) medications or supplements, including the dose and frequency
- Any new medications that have been recently started or had the dosage adjusted
- Any medication-induced tardive dyskinesia

Allergies
- Allergies to medications, or seasonal, environmental, and/or food allergies? If yes to being allergic to any substance or environmental trigger, clarify reactions.

Immunizations
- **Risks for vaccine-preventable illnesses:** Vaccine status; date of last influenza, meningococcal, *Haemophilus influenzae* type B, pneumococcal, tetanus, and polio
- History of Guillain–Barre syndrome following vaccine

Pediatric Considerations
- **Gestation:** Mother's health during pregnancy? Exposures or illnesses during pregnancy? Fetal abnormalities identified during the prenatal stage? Substance use during pregnancy?
- **Birth history:** Delivery eventful or uneventful, vaginal or Cesarean section, prolonged or abrupt? Prolapsed cord, malpositioned placenta, premature rupture of membranes, or abruptio placentae? Any respiratory distress after birth? Any apneic episodes? Did the child require oxygen, pulse oximetry monitoring, or support for breathing as an infant? Apgar scores at birth?
- **Growth and development history:** Meeting developmental milestones (motor, adaptive, language, and personal–social behavior)? Has there been any regression of developmental

milestones? Suboptimal growth or poor weight gain (based on pediatric growth charts)? Academic performance?

- **Eating and nutritional history:** How has the child been eating? Is the infant breast- or bottle-fed? Has the child's eating pattern changed?

FAMILY HISTORY

- Neurologic disorders, such as amyotrophic lateral sclerosis (ALS), arteriovenous malformation (AVM), brain tumors, headaches (migraine, cluster), Alzheimer, Creutzfeldt–Jakob, Huntington, Parkinson, multiple sclerosis (MS), stroke, cerebral palsy (CP), epilepsy, trigeminal neuralgia, dementia, neurofibromatosis, muscular dystrophy
- Metabolic disorder, thyroid disease, hypertension, diabetes
- Developmental delays, learning disorders, intellectual disability, attention deficit hyperactivity disorder (ADHD)
- Addiction (and/or use of alcohol or drugs during pregnancy)
- Family patterns of dexterity and dominance

SOCIAL HISTORY

Environmental Exposures

- Current and past occupations
- Exposure to pollutants, neurotoxins, insecticides, herbicides, fungicides, other harmful chemicals and/or irritants in the work environment
- Low-level chronic exposure to hazardous substances at work or at home

Lifestyle Behaviors (Including Substance Use)

- Typical use, type, amount of alcohol consumed
- Use of prescription medications or illicit substances for nonmedical purposes
- Use of OTC drugs for reasons other than health-related
- Use of tobacco, including cigarettes, smokeless tobacco, e-cigarettes or vaping, cigars
- Caffeine use (amount, frequency of intake)
- Hygiene, activities of daily living, finances, communication, shopping, ability to fulfill work expectations
- Social support system
- Use of cane or assistive device

REVIEW OF SYSTEMS

- **General:** Fever, chills, sleeplessness, fatigue, dizziness, unintentional weight loss
- **Head, eyes, ears, nose, throat:** Visual disturbances/visual difficulty, tearing or redness of the eyes

- **Cardiovascular/respiratory:** Respiratory irregularities, bruits, thrills
- **Gastrointestinal/genitourinary:** Nausea, vomiting, urinary frequency, hesitancy, urgency, incontinence
- **Neurologic:** Weakness, numbness/tingling, change in sensation, loss of consciousness, headaches, falls, dizziness, tremor, sensory disturbances, changes in balance or coordination, confusion
- **Musculoskeletal:** Headache, backache, nuchal rigidity, unsteadiness when standing/walking, myalgias, arthralgias
- **Mental health:** Depression; anxiety; changes in mentation, memory, or mood

PHYSICAL EXAMINATION

GENERAL SURVEY
- Assess/compare vital signs with past measurements to identify possible disease/predisease markers.
- Height, weight, and body mass index (BMI) calculation should be completed and compared with previous visits to identify signs of chronic disease or weight loss.
- Note the patient's demeanor, speech, presence of a resting tremor, affect, and ability to articulate and communicate.

INSPECTION
- Observe the patient's gait, balance, and coordination. Listen to the patient's response to questions, which provides information regarding the patient's ability to follow directions. Important to note for older adults as depression is more common in older adults and those with chronic diseases, including neurologic disorders such as dementia, MS, and Parkinson.
- Inspection of the face includes attention to symmetry, shape, features, facial expression, symmetry of the eyebrows, eyes, ears, nose, and mouth, as well as position of the nasolabial folds, and inspecting for facial muscle atrophy and tremors (see Chapter 7, Evidence-Based Assessment of the Head and Neck).

MENTAL STATUS EXAMINATION
- Refer to the mental status exam in Chapter 16, Evidence-Based Assessment of Mental Health Including Substance Use Disorders.

CRANIAL NERVES
Olfactory (I)
- This should be tested when the patient is unable to discriminate odors. Ensure the patient's nares are clear. Ask the patient to occlude one naris at a time and close their eyes while you hold an

open vial or other distinguishable aroma (e.g., alcohol pad) under their nose. Ask the patient to breathe deeply. Use a different aroma to test the other side. Repeat two to three times with two to three different odors. Patients are expected to perceive an odor on each side and identify it.

Optic (II)
- Test distant and near vison.
- Test visual fields by confrontation and extinction.
- Test each eye separately and both eyes together. In patients with partial vision loss, testing of both eyes can reveal a visual field deficit, whereas testing with one eye will miss this finding. See Chapter 8, Evidence-Based Assessment of the Eyes for specifics about assessment of vision, including when ophthalmoscopic exam is warranted.

Oculomotor, Trochlear, and Abducens (III, IV, VI)
- These are tested with movement of the eyes through the six cardinal points of gaze.
- Visualizations of pupil size, shape, response to light, accommodation, and opening of the upper eyelids are described in Chapter 8, Evidence-Based Assessment of the Eyes.

Trigeminal (V)
- Its primary function is to provide sensory and motor innervation to the face.
- **Motor function:** Observe the face for muscle atrophy, deviation of the jaw to one side, and muscle twitching. Ask the patient to clench their teeth tightly as the muscles over the jaw are palpated, evaluating tone (**Figure 10.1**). Facial tone should be symmetric, without tremor.

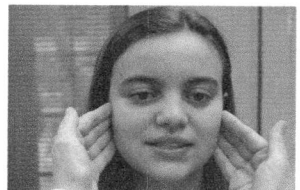

FIGURE 10.1 Motor function assessment of the trigeminal nerve.

- **Sensory function:** The three trigeminal nerve divisions are evaluated for sharp, dull, and light touch sensations. Have the patient close their eyes, then touch each side of their face at the scalp, cheek, and chin alternately using the sharp and smooth edges of a broken tongue blade or paper clip. Ask the patient to report whether each sensation is sharp or dull. Stroke the face in the same six areas with a cotton wisp, asking the patient to report sensation. Discrimination of all stimuli is expected over all facial areas (**Figure 10.2**).

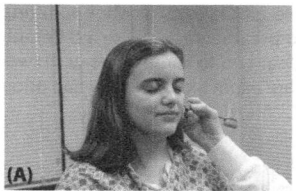 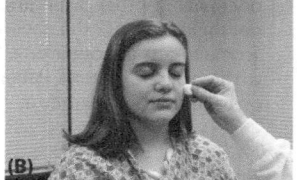

FIGURE 10.2 Evaluation of sensation in the trigeminal nerve divisions using
(A) a dull edge and **(B)** a cotton ball.

Facial (VII)

- The facial nerve has both sensory and motor functions. It controls
  facial movements, taste, and movement of the lacrimal, submaxil-
  lary, and submandibular glands.
- Ask the patient to form specific facial expressions to test for facial
  symmetry **(Figure 10.3)**.

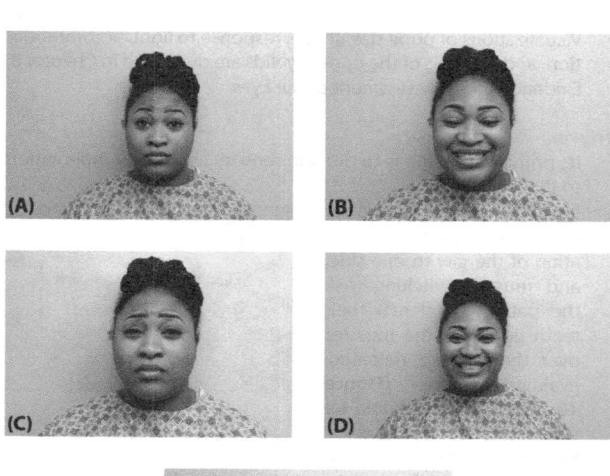

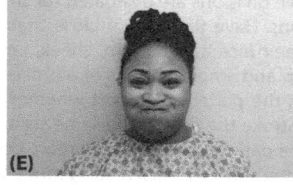

FIGURE 10.3 Facial nerve testing. Among other expressions, the patient **(A)**
raises their eyebrows, **(B)** squeezes their eyes shut, **(C)** frowns, **(D)** smiles, and **(E)**
puffs out their cheeks.

- Observe for tics, unusual facial movements, and asymmetry. Drooping of one side of the mouth, a flattened nasolabial fold, and/or sagging of the lower eyelid are signs of muscle weakness.

Vestibulocochlear (VIII)

- This cranial nerve (CN) is responsible for hearing and maintaining body balance.
- Assess hearing with the whispered voice test. Ask the patient to repeat numbers whispered into one ear while blocking or rubbing your fingers next to the opposite ear. An audiometry examination

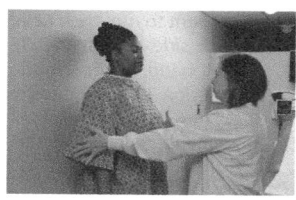

FIGURE 10.4 Romberg test.

can also be completed if a more thorough examination is necessary.
- The Romberg test assesses vestibular function (position sense; **Figure 10.4**).

Glossopharyngeal (IX) and Vagus (X)

- Test the ability to identify sour and bitter tastes on the posterior third of each side of the tongue, gag reflex, ability to swallow, inspection of the palate and uvula, and speech sounds.
- Observe for difficulty swallowing; assess for guttural speech or hoarse voice sounds.
- Sensory function of taste may be completed during the CN VII evaluation.
- Glossopharyngeal nerve function is simultaneously tested during the evaluation of the vagus nerve for nasopharyngeal sensation (gag reflex) and the motor function of swallowing.
- Gag reflex is initiated by touching the patient's posterior pharyngeal wall with an applicator while observing for upward movement of the palate and contraction of the pharyngeal muscles. Uvula should remain midline; drooping or absence of an arch on either side of the palate is abnormal.
- Motor function is evaluated with inspection of the soft palate for symmetry. Have the patient say "ah" and observe the movement of the soft palate. If there is damage to the vagus or glossopharyngeal nerve, the palate does not rise and the uvula will deviate from midline. Have the patient sip and swallow water. The patient should be able to swallow easily.

Spinal Accessory (XI)

- Evaluate the size, shape, and strength of the trapezius and sternocleidomastoid (SCM) muscles.
- To test the trapezius muscle, stand behind the patient and observe for atrophy or flickering movement of the skin (a symptom of disease of the nervous system). Place a hand on each

shoulder and ask the patient to shrug upward; observe the strength and contraction of the muscles (**Figure 10.5**).

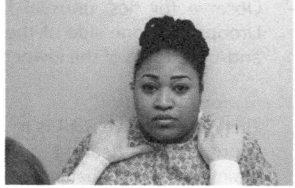

FIGURE 10.5 Testing the trapezius muscle.

- To test the SCM muscle, ask the patient to turn their head to each side against the clinician's hand, observing the contraction of the opposite SCM muscle and force of movement against the hand.

Hypoglossal (XII)

- This CN innervates all but one of the muscles of the tongue.
- Inspect the patient's tongue while at rest on the floor of the mouth and while protruded from the mouth, observing for size and shape. Have the patient move their tongue in and out of the mouth, side to side, and curled upward and downward.

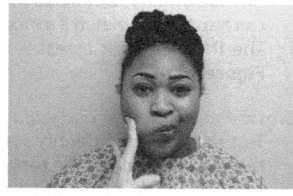

FIGURE 10.6 Testing muscle strength of the tongue.

- Test muscle strength by asking the patient to push the tongue against the cheek as the clinician applies resistance with an index finger or hand (**Figure 10.6**).
- Assess lingual speech sounds (l, t, d, n) by listening to the patient's speech (**Box 10.1**).

BOX 10.1 Mnemonic for Cranial Nerves

Olfactory	**O**n
Optic	**O**ld
Oculomotor	**O**lympus
Trochlear	**T**owering
Trigeminal	**T**ops
Abducens	**A**
Facial	**F**inn
Acoustic	**A**nd
Glossopharyngeal	**G**erman
Vagus nerve	**V**iewed
Spinal	**S**ome
Hypoglossal	**H**ops

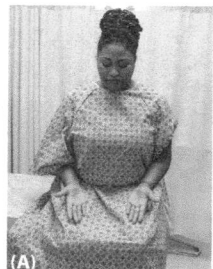 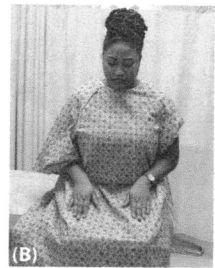

FIGURE 10.7 Testing rapid rhythmic alternative movements. The patient alternately places their palms up (**A**) and down (**B**).

PROPRIOCEPTION AND CEREBELLAR FUNCTION

Coordination and Fine Motor Skills

Observe the patient's body position during movement and at rest. Look for involuntary movements (tics or tremors), muscle bulk, muscle strength, muscle tone, and the patient's coordination. Abnormal position may be due to mono- or hemiparesis from a stroke.

Rapid Rhythmic Alternative Movements

- Ask the seated patient to pat their knees with both hands, alternately turning the palms up and down and gradually increasing the speed of movements (**Figure 10.7**).
- Alternatively, ask the patient to touch the thumb to each finger on the same hand from the little finger and back. One hand is tested at a

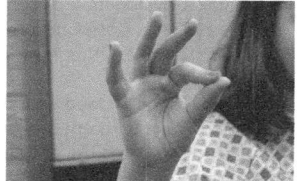

FIGURE 10.8 Testing rapid rhythmic alternating movements.

time, gradually increasing the speed (**Figure 10.8**). The clinician should model the movements for the patient before having the patient complete them. The patient should be able to accomplish these movements smoothly and rhythmically. Stiff, slow, or jerky clonic movements are abnormal.

Accuracy of Movements

- **Finger-to-nose test:** This tests the accuracy of the patient's movements (**Figure 10.9**). The clinician moves their finger position several times during the test, which is then repeated on the other hand.
- **Heel-to-shin test:** This is an alternative method to test accuracy of movement. The test can be performed with the patient sitting

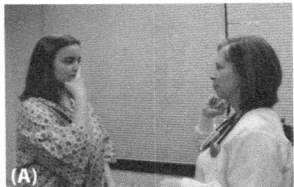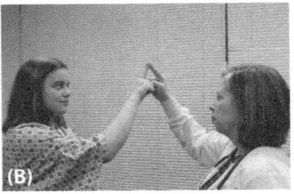

FIGURE 10.9 Finger-to-nose test. (**A**) Ask the patient to touch their nose, then (**B**) ask the patient to touch the clinician's finger. The maneuvers (**A** and **B**) are repeated several times after the clinician moves their finger position.

or supine (**Figure 10.10**). The patient should be able to move their heel up and down the shin in a straight line without deviating to the side.

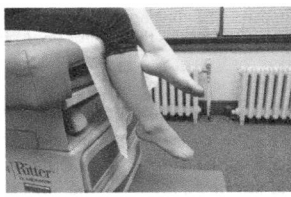

FIGURE 10.10 Heel-to-shin test.

Balance

- Complete the Romberg test (see Vestibulocochlear [VIII] section). Loss of balance is a positive sign, indicating cerebellar ataxia/dysfunction or sensory loss. If the patient staggers or loses balance, postpone other tests of cerebellar function that require balance. Other methods to evaluate balance include the following:
  ○ Have patient stand with their feet slightly apart and push the shoulders with enough effort to throw them off balance (be ready to catch the patient if needed). The patient should be able to quickly recover balance.
  ○ Ask the patient to close their eyes, hold their arms at the sides of the body, and stand on one foot, repeating the test on the opposite foot. Slight swaying is normal; the patient should be able to maintain balance on each foot for 5 seconds.
  ○ With eyes open, have the patient hop in place on one foot and then the other (tests proximal and distal muscle strength). The patient should be able to hop on one foot for 5 seconds without loss of balance. Observe for instability or need to continually touch the floor with the opposite foot or a tendency to fall. Difficulty hopping may be related to weakness, lack of position sense, or cerebellar dysfunction.

Gait

- Have the patient walk across the room or down the hall and turn and come back, observing posture, balance, swinging of the arms, and intact movement.

- The patient should then walk heel to toe in a straight line (tandem walking), walk on their toes, and then on their heels (**Figure 10.11**). Last, have the patient do a knee bend.

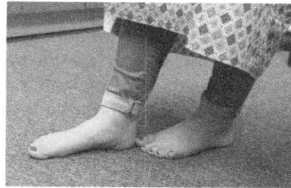

FIGURE 10.11 Assessment of gait using tandem walking.

- These tests assess for gait abnormalities that increase fall risk. An uncoordinated gait with reeling and instability is ataxic, which is seen in cerebellar disease, loss of position sense, and intoxication. Tandem walking may reveal ataxia, distal leg weakness, and is a sensitive test for corticospinal tract damage. See **Table 10.1** for abnormal gait pattern characteristics.
- **Pronator drift testing:** Muscular strength, coordination, and good position sense are tested (**Figure 10.12**).

TABLE 10.1 Corticospinal, Basal Ganglia, and Cerebellar Motor Pathways

Pathway	Function
Corticospinal (pyramidal) tract	Mediation of voluntary movement, inhibition of muscle tone, coordination of complicated movements
Basal ganglia system	Controls muscle tone and body movements, including automatically performing a learned behavior
Cerebellar system	Coordinates muscle activity, sustains equilibrium, and maintains posture

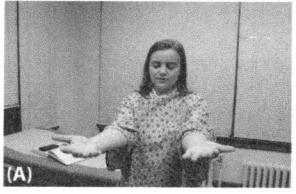
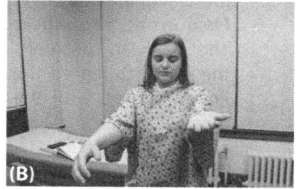

FIGURE 10.12 Testing for pronator drift. (**A**) The patient stands with their eyes closed and arms straight forward with the palms up. (**B**) Arms drifting sideward or upward after a brisk tap indicate a positive test.

Muscle Strength

- Normal muscle strength varies, so the normal standard should allow for factors such as age. The patient's dominant side is usually stronger than the nondominant side; differences may be hard to detect.
- Test muscle strength by asking the patient to actively resist the clinician's movement:
  - **Biceps and brachioradialis at the elbow flexion and extension:** The patient pulls and pushes against the clinician's hand.
  - **Extension at the wrist:** The patient makes a fist and resists as the clinician presses down.
  - **Grip strength:** The clinician asks the patient to squeeze two of their fingers as hard as possible and not let them go. Weak grip is seen in cervical radiculopathy, ulnar peripheral nerve disease, carpal tunnel syndrome, arthritis, and epicondylitis.
  - **Finger abduction:** The patient's hand is positioned down with the fingers spread. The patient tries to prevent the clinician from forcing the fingers together (**Figure 10.13**). Weak finger abduction occurs in ulnar nerve disorders.
  - **Thumb opposition:** The patient touches the top of the little finger to the tip of the thumb. The clinician then attempts to break them apart.
  - **Muscle strength of the trunk:** This is determined by flexion, extension, rotation, and lateral bending.
  - **Flexion at the hip:** The clinician places their hand on the patient's midthigh and asks them to raise the leg against their hand.
  - **Adduction at the hips:** The clinician puts their hands on the inside of the patient's knees and asks the patient to bring both legs together.
  - **Abduction at the hips:** The clinician puts their hands on the outside of the patient's knees and asks the patient to spread both legs against their hands.
  - **Extension at the knee:** The clinician supports the knee in flexion and asks the patient to straighten the leg against their hand. Expect a forceful response as the quadriceps are the strongest muscles in the body.
  - **Flexion at the knee:** The clinician positions the patient's leg so the knee is flexed with the foot resting on the bed. The clinician tells the patient to keep the foot down as they try to straighten the leg.
  - **Foot dorsiflexion and plantar flexion at the**

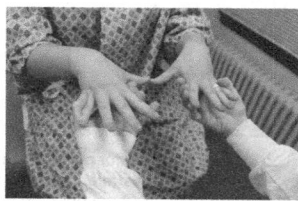

FIGURE 10.13 Finger abduction test.

ankle: The clinician asks the patient to pull up and push down against their hand. Heel and toe walk assesses foot dorsiflexion/plantar flexion.

REFLEXES

Superficial Reflexes

- **Plantar reflex:** Using the end of a reflex hammer, stroke the lateral side of the foot from heel to ball, then across the foot to the medial side with the result of plantar flexion of the toes. This is a normal sign.
- **Abdominal reflex:** With the patient supine, stroke the four abdominal quadrants with the end of a reflex hammer. Stroking downward and away from the umbilicus elicits the lower abdominal reflexes, which respond with a slight movement of the umbilicus toward the area of stimulation. Reflex response should be equal and bilateral.

Deep Tendon Reflexes

- Biceps, brachioradialis, triceps, patellar, and Achilles reflexes are deep tendon reflexes (DTRs).
- The patient should be in a seated position. Test each reflex and compare it with the other side of the body. The reflex response should be symmetric, visible, and palpable. DTRs are obtained by positioning a limb with a slightly stretched tendon and quickly tapping the tendon to be tested with a percussion hammer. The expected response is a sudden contraction of the muscle. If the tendon response is absent, consider a neuropathy. Consider an upper motor neuron disorder with hyperactive reflexes. If DTRs are symmetrically diminished or absent, use a technique of isometric contraction of other muscles which might increase reflex activity. Each reflex is scored as 0 to 4+ (**Table 10.2**).
- **Biceps reflex:** With the patient's arm bent at a 45° angle at the elbow, palpate the biceps tendon and place your thumb over the tendon and your fingers under the elbow. Strike your thumb with

TABLE 10.2 Deep Tendon Reflex Grading

Grade 0	No response
Grade 1+	Sluggish or diminished response
Grade 2+	Active or expected response (normal)
Grade 3+	Brisk/slightly hyperactive
Grade 4+	Brisk/hyperactive

the reflex hammer to elicit contraction of the biceps muscle, causing flexion of the elbow (**Figure 10.14**).

- **Brachioradialis reflex:** With the patient's arm bent at a 45° angle at the elbow, rest the patient's arm on yours. The patient's hand should be slightly pronated. The clinician directly strikes the brachioradial tendon 1 to 2 inches above the wrist with the reflex hammer (**Figure 10.15**). A normal response is forearm pronation and elbow flexion.

- **Triceps reflex:** With the patient's arm flexed at a 90° angle, support the patient's arm just above the antecubital fossa and palpate the antecubital fossa. Then directly strike the triceps tendon with a reflex hammer just above the elbow (**Figure 10.16**). A normal response is extension of the elbow.

- **Patellar reflex:** With the patient's knee flexed to a 90° angle, support the patient's upper leg with your hand to allow the patient's lower leg to hang. Strike the patellar tendon just below the patella (**Figure 10.17**). A normal response is extension of the lower leg.

- **Achilles reflex:** With the patient sitting and the knee flexed to a 90° angle, keeping the ankle in a neutral position, hold the patient's foot in your hand. Strike the Achilles tendon at the level of the ankle malleoli. A normal response is plantar flexion of the foot.

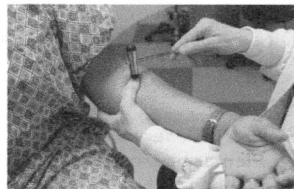

FIGURE 10.14 Biceps reflex test.

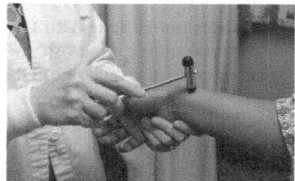

FIGURE 10.15 Brachioradialis test.

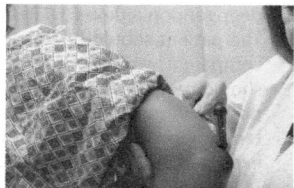

FIGURE 10.16 Triceps reflex test.

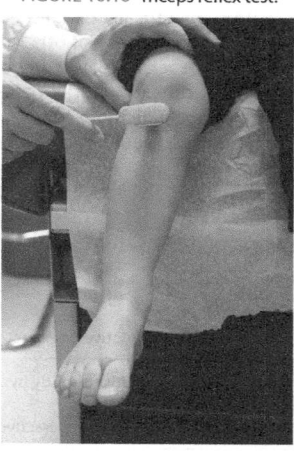

FIGURE 10.17 Patellar reflex test.

Primitive Reflex Testing in Infancy

- **Moro reflex:** Supporting the infant's head, body, and legs, the clinician suddenly lowers the body, causing the arms to abduct and extend, followed by relaxed flexion, during which the legs should flex.
- **Stepping reflex:** The clinician holds the infant under the arms, allowing one of the infant's feet to touch the surface of the examination table. The clinician observes for flexion of the hip and knee. The foot should touch the table while the other foot steps forward.
- **Palmar reflex grasp:** The clinician places a finger in the infant's hand, pressing against the palmar surface of the hand. The infant flexes all fingers to grasp the clinician's finger. A positive grasp reflex that lasts longer than 2 months indicates central nervous system damage.
- **Plantar reflex grasp:** The clinician touches the sole of the infant's foot at the base of the toes, causing the toes to curl.

SENSORY FUNCTION

- Evaluation requires testing of several kinds of sensations—for example, pain and temperature (spinothalamic tracts), position and vibration (posterior columns), light touch (spinothalamic tracts and posterior columns), and discriminative sensations that depend on pain, temperature, position, vibration, and light touch (the cortex).
- Evaluate sensation by asking the patient to identify stimuli on the hands, distal arms, abdomen, feet, and legs. Each sensation procedure is tested with the patient's eyes closed. Contralateral areas of the body are tested, and the patient is asked to compare sensations side to side. Normal findings include minimal differences side to side, correct description of sensations (hot, cold, sharp, dull), recognition of the side of the body tested, location of sensation, and recognition if proximal or distal to the site previously tested.
- When testing, the clinician focuses on the areas that have numbness, pain, motor, or reflex abnormalities. Compare symmetric areas on two sides of the body, including the arms, legs, and trunk. With pain, temperature, and touch sensation, compare distal with proximal areas of the extremities.
- Test the fingers and toes first for vibration and sensation. If tests are normal, the clinician can assume the more proximal areas are normal. Evaluation of light touch and superficial pain can be done together.
- **Monofilament testing:** Testing with a 5.07 monofilament should be done on several sites of the foot for all patients with diabetic and peripheral neuropathy. With the patient's eyes closed, the clinician places the monofilament on several sites of the plantar surface of each foot and one side of the dorsal surface of the foot

in a random pattern (**Figure 10.18**). The clinician applies pressure for 1.5 seconds to each site without repeating a test site. The correct amount of pressure is applied when the filament bends. Testing is positive if the patient cannot feel the monofilament.

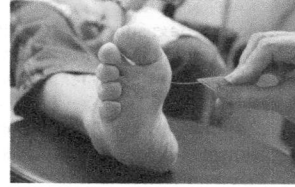

FIGURE 10.18 Monofilament test.

Primary Sensory Functions

- **Light touch:** Lightly touch the skin with a cotton wisp and ask the patient to respond when and where the sensation is felt.

- **Superficial pain:** Alternate the sharp and smooth edges of a broken tongue blade, Wartenberg wheel, or paper clip on the skin (**Figure 10.19**). Ask the patient to identify each sensation as sharp or dull and where the sensation is felt.

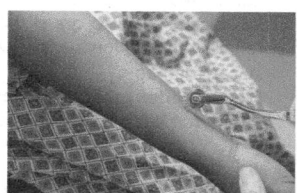

FIGURE 10.19 Testing superficial pain with a Wartenberg wheel.

- **Temperature:** Testing skin temperature is omitted if pain sensation is normal. If there are sensory deficits, use test tubes filled with hot and cold water. Ask the patient to identify whether the sensation is hot or cold and where the sensation is felt.

- **Vibration:** Place the stem of a low-pitched tuning fork (128 Hz) against a bony prominence at the toe or finger joint; ask the patient to identify when/where the buzzing sensation is felt (**Figure 10.20**).

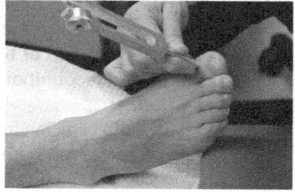

FIGURE 10.20 Testing vibration with a low-pitched tuning fork.

- **Proprioception joint position sense:** Assess the patient's ability to sense the position of their joint. This should be completed on the great toe of each foot and a finger on each hand (**Figure 10.21**). Hold the joint by the lateral aspect in the neutral position. Move the finger/toe up and down; ask the patient to identify whether the joint is forward, backward, or in the neutral position. If they cannot, it is considered an abnormal finding.

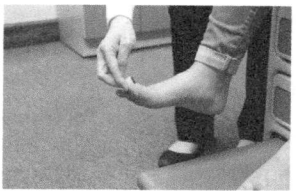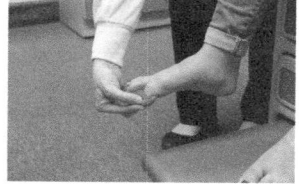

FIGURE 10.21 Testing proprioception joint position sense.

SPECIAL TESTS

Cortical Sensory Function

- Discriminatory sensory function tests assess the patient's ability to interpret sensation. Patients with lesions in the sensory cortex or posterior spinal cord would be unable to complete these tests. The patient's eyes should be closed during testing.
- **Stereognosis:** This tests the patient's ability to identify a familiar object by touch. Place a key or coin in the patient's hand; ability to identify the object is a normal response.
- **Two-point discrimination:** Using two ends of a paper clip, alternate touching the patient's skin at various locations with one or two points of the paper clip (**Figure 10.22**). The patient's ability to identify one- or two-point touch is a normal response.
- **Extinction phenomenon:** Simultaneously touch two areas on each side of the body (such as the cheek or hand) with the broken end of a tongue blade. The patient should be able to discriminate the number of touches and where they are felt bilaterally.
- **Graphesthesia:** With the blunt end of an applicator, draw a number or shape on the palm of the patient's hand. Repeat the test using a different figure on the other hand. The patient should be able to identify the shape or number.
- Other special tests are used when the clinician suspects meningeal irritation, which can occur with meningitis or subarachnoid hemorrhage:
    - **Brudzinski sign:** The clinician should not use this test if there is injury or fracture of the cervical vertebrae or cervical cord (**Figure 10.23**).

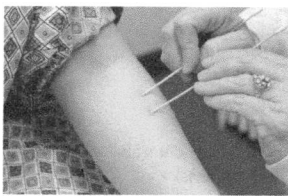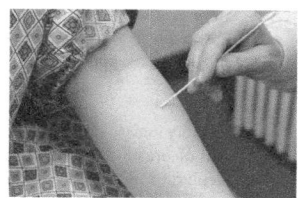

FIGURE 10.22 Two-point discrimination test.

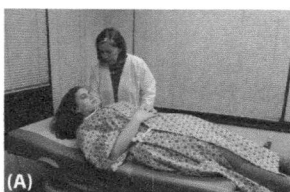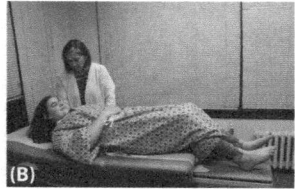

FIGURE 10.23 Brudzinski sign test. (**A**) The clinician flexes the patient's neck forward. (**B**) Test is positive when the patient bends their hips and knees in response to neck flexion.

- ○ **Kernig sign:** With the patient lying flat, flex their leg at the hip and knee, then slowly extend the leg and straighten the knee. Normally, the patient should feel some discomfort behind the knee with extension. A positive test reveals pain with knee extension.

RED FLAGS IN ASSESSMENT
- Subjective and objective findings that indicate significant neurologic disorders or impairment are summarized in **Box 10.2**.

BOX 10.2 Red Flags in History and Physical Exam

- · History of cancer or immunosuppression
- · History of trauma, fall, or loss of consciousness
- · History of previous stroke or transient ischemic attack
- · Family history of a progressive neurologic disorder
- · Reported progressive neurologic dysfunction
- · Face drooping
- · Sudden numbness or weakness of the face, arm, or leg, especially unilateral
- · Sudden confusion, trouble speaking, or issues understanding speech
- · Sudden trouble seeing in one or both eyes, abrupt vision loss, or double vision
- · Sudden trouble walking, dizziness, or loss of balance/coordination
- · Sudden severe headache
- · Abrupt onset of motor and sensory deficits
- · Seizure; status epilepticus
- · Paralysis
- · Syncope
- · Memory loss
- · Loss of already attained cognitive or developmental abilities
- · Meningitis triad (fever, headache, neck stiffness)

ABNORMAL FINDINGS

BELL'S PALSY

Bell's palsy is a condition characterized by sudden, temporary weakness or paralysis of the facial muscles on one side of the face. The exact cause of Bell's palsy is unknown but believed to be linked to viral infections and genetic or autoimmune disorders, which cause inflammation of the facial nerve.

History
- History of herpes simplex type 1 or Lyme disease
- Symptoms that typically develop abruptly (within hours), with maximum characteristics in 3 days
- Reported facial pain, pain around the ear
- Abnormal taste

Physical Examination
- Unilateral facial weakness and drooping, drooling
- Unilateral eyelid weakness, absence of a corneal reflex, reduced tearing

Considerations
- It is believed to be the result of swelling and inflammation of the facial nerve due to reactivation of an existing (dormant) viral infection. Impaired immunity from stress, sleep deprivation, physical trauma, minor illness, or autoimmune syndromes are the most likely triggers.
- Other conditions that cause facial paralysis (e.g., brain tumor, stroke, myasthenia gravis, Lyme disease) should be ruled out first.
- The patient usually recovers within 3 weeks.

CEREBRAL PALSY

CP is a group of permanent movement disorders that appear in early childhood and affect body movement and muscle coordination. It is defined as a nonprogressive motor disorder secondary to damage to the developing brain, which can occur before, during, or after birth.

History
- History of preterm birth, low birth weight, low Apgar score, neonatal encephalopathy, neonatal sepsis, meningitis
- History of maternal conditions, infections, Rh incompatibility
- Poor nutrition
- Reported sleep disruption

Physical Examination
- In infancy, abnormal muscle tone, abnormal motor development, and feeding difficulties
- Difficulty with speech, language, and communication
- Difficulty eating, drinking, and swallowing

- Pain associated with musculoskeletal disorders, including hip dislocation, nonspecific back pain, increased muscle tone (dystonia, spasticity), muscle fatigue, headache, nonspecific abdominal pain, dental pain, dysmenorrhea
- Mental health disorders, including depression, anxiety disorder, antisocial behavior, learning disabilities, ADHD
- Vision and hearing Impairment
- Vomiting, regurgitation, reflux
- Constipation
- Epilepsy

Considerations
- Symptoms of CP differ in type and severity from one person to the next and may even change in an individual over time.
- Symptoms depend on which parts of the brain have been affected.

EPILEPSY

Epilepsy is a neurologic disorder characterized by recurrent, unprovoked seizures. Seizures are episodes of abnormal electrical activity in the brain that can cause a variety of symptoms, including muscle contractions, loss of consciousness, and changes in sensation, behavior, or mood. Seizures occur secondary to brief, strong surges of abnormal and disorganized activity, which may affect all or part of the brain.

History
- History of perinatal anoxia, congenital brain malformation, genetic disorders, infectious disease, and traumatic brain injury is possible.
- Seizures are often triggered by sleep deprivation, dehydration, stress, alcohol, and/or drug use.
- It commonly interferes with school, work, and driving.
- Children may experience physical complications from seizures and are at greater risk for negative self-image, anxiety, depression, and learning disabilities.

Physical Examination
- Jerking movement of one or more extremities
- Nystagmus
- Abrupt movement of the head to one side or the other
- Moans or cries
- Fearful or sad emotions
- Humming or buzzing noises
- Tongue biting
- Intense or unpleasant smells or tastes
- Tingling in one area or side of the body
- Flashing lights in a portion of the visual fields

Consideration
- Status epilepticus is considered a medical emergency due to an increased chance of death.

HEMORRHAGIC STROKE
Bleeding directly into the brain tissue, caused by leakage from intra-cerebral arteries

History
- Trauma history
- History of hypertension, previous stroke, coagulopathies, or anti-coagulant therapy
- Reported nausea, vomiting, headache
- Advanced age
- History of alcohol abuse and/or cocaine use

Physical Examination
- Altered level of consciousness
- Seizures
- Weakness or paralysis of an extremity, half of the body, or all extremities
- Facial droop
- Monocular or binocular blindness, blurred vision
- Dysarthria and trouble understanding speech
- Vertigo or ataxia
- Aphasia
- Subarachnoid symptoms such as sudden onset of severe head-ache, signs of meningitis (nuchal rigidity), photophobia and eye pain, nausea and vomiting, and syncope

Considerations
- It is less common than ischemic stroke and is associated with a higher mortality rate.
- Patients may have neurologic deficits similar to ischemic stroke, but are more likely to have headache, altered mental status, seizures, nausea and vomiting, and/or pronounced hypertension.

INTRACRANIAL TUMOR
Intracranial tumor is an abnormal growth in the cranial cavity that may be benign or due to malignancy. Brain tumors include glioblas-tomas, meningioma, and pituitary tumors.

History
- Persistent headaches that wake the patient from sleep
- Appetite loss
- Nausea and vomiting

Physical Examination
- Ringing and hearing loss in one ear
- Reduced visual acuity, loss of vision
- Changes in behavior and personality
- Children may exhibit irritability, lethargy, cranial nerve palsies, weight loss
- Seizures
- Confusion
- Papilledema
- Aphasia
- Nystagmus
- Ataxia
- Unilateral weakness

Consideration
- Brain CT scan or MRI is needed to confirm diagnosis.

ISCHEMIC STROKE
Ischemic stroke is an embolus from atrial fibrillation or atherosclerotic disease that causes a sudden loss of blood circulation to the brain.

History
- History of smoking or excessive alcohol use
- History of oral contraceptive use or pregnancy in young women
- History of atrial fibrillation
- History of high cholesterol, hypertension, atherosclerosis, cancer, blood clots, and/or diabetes
- History of hematologic disorders (e.g., factor V Leiden, prothrombin gene mutation, sickle cell anemia)
- Hypercoagulable states
- History of transient ischemic attack (TIA)
- Recent travel

Physical Examination
- Sudden severe headache with no known cause
- Abrupt onset of hemiparesis or monoparesis
- Visual field deficits
- Facial droop
- Ataxia
- Nystagmus
- Aphasia (expressive and receptive)
- Sudden numbness or weakness of the face, arm, or leg
- Abrupt decrease in level of consciousness

Considerations
- If ischemic stroke is not treated promptly, it can lead to brain damage or death; signs and symptoms need to be identified immediately to prevent morbidity and mortality.

- Tissue plasminogen activator given within 4.5 hours of the start of symptoms is most effective at breaking up the clot.

MENINGITIS

Meningitis is inflammation of the meninges of the brain or spinal cord caused by bacterial, viral, or fungal organism colonization in the upper respiratory tract.

History

- Symptoms develop over several hours or 1 to 2 days.
- Patient has a history of exposure to a patient with a similar illness.
- Classic triad for bacterial meningitis is fever, headache, and neck stiffness; however, patients may present with only one or two of these symptoms.

Physical Examination

- Neck stiffness
- Lethargy, sleepiness
- Nausea, vomiting
- Photophobia
- Confusion, irritability
- Delirium
- Seizures
- Coma
- Altered mental status
- Nuchal rigidity
- Increased blood pressure with bradycardia
- Positive Brudzinski and Kernig signs
- Petechial and purpura rash with meningococcal meningitis
- Bulging fontanel, paradoxical irritability (quiet when lying flat, crying when held), high-pitched cry, hypotonia in infants

Considerations

- It is important to identify the causative agent in cases of meningitis.
- Bacterial meningitis (a medical emergency) must be the first and foremost consideration in the differential diagnosis of patients with headache, neck stiffness, fever, and altered mental status.

MULTIPLE SCLEROSIS

MS is a chronic autoimmune disease that affects the central nervous system. It is characterized by damage to the myelin sheath, which is the protective covering around the nerve fibers in the brain and spinal cord. The damage interferes with the normal transmission of nerve signals and can cause a wide range of symptoms, including muscle weakness, difficulty with coordination and balance, and problems with vision, speech, and bladder control.

History

- Onset typically between 20 to 40 years of age; occurs more often in women
- Reports fatigue, heat intolerance, depression, localized weakness, decreased attention span and concentration, and memory loss
- History of vision problems (double vision, loss of vision)
- Reports bowel, bladder, and sexual dysfunction
- Constipation

Physical Examination

- Localized weakness
- Paresthesia
- Muscle cramping due to spasticity
- Dysarthria, nystagmus, and intention tremor
- Lhermitte's sign (an electric shock-like sensation that occurs with flexion of the neck and goes down the spine, often going into the limbs)
- Trigeminal neuralgia
- Irregular twitching of the facial nerves
- Focal sensory disturbances (decreasing proprioception and vibration)
- Hyperreactive reflexes
- Increased muscle tone or stiffness in the extremities
- In optic neuritis, unilateral loss of visual acuity and pain

Considerations

- Signs and symptoms depend on where the nerves are demyelinated.
- The four types of MS are relapsing-remitting, secondary progressive, primary progressive, and progressive relapsing. The type of MS provides information about the general course of the disease and responsiveness of the disease to treatment.

MYASTHENIA GRAVIS

Myasthenia gravis is a common autoimmune disease that affects neuromuscular junction transmission.

History

- Patient has personal or family history of autoimmune diseases.
- Symptoms can worsen with stress, illness, and fatigue.

Physical Examination

- Weakness that worsens with activity
- Difficulty swallowing or speaking
- Drooping eyelids
- Double vision; ocular symptoms most common
- Fatigue or weakness, facial weakness when puffing out cheeks

- Difficulty walking
- Hypophonia
- Respiratory compromise or failure
- Skeletal muscle weakness
- Positive serum antibodies

Considerations
- The etiology of the disease is unknown.
- Diagnosis is based on history and physical exam findings and confirmed by electrodiagnostic testing and positive serum antibodies directed at proteins in the neuromuscular junction.

PARKINSON DISEASE
Parkinson disease is a slowly progressive neurodegenerative disorder affecting movement, muscle control, and balance, caused by destruction and loss of dopaminergic neurons.

History
- Reports early signs and symptoms which may be subtle and difficult to detect or missed secondary to slow disease progression
- Older adults (older than 60 years of age are at the greatest risk of acquiring)
- Affects men more than women
- Menopause in women
- History of head trauma
- Working with environmental toxins including pesticides and herbicides
- Carrying the alpha-synuclein gene
- Reports numbness, tingling, and muscle soreness, as well as difficulty swallowing

Physical Examination
- Nonmotor symptoms can sometimes be seen prior to motor symptoms.
- Symptoms also include constipation, depression, cognitive dysfunction, dementia, and psychosis.
- Motor symptoms considered cardinal signs of Parkinson disease include rest tremors; slowness of movement, freezing, or unable to continue movements; rigidity; and postural instability.
- Motor symptoms include pill-rolling movement of the fingers bilaterally; head tremors; drooling; stooped posture; short steps, shuffling gait, or accelerating gait to maintain posture; slow slurred speech; and softened voice.

Consideration
- Diagnosis is based on signs/symptoms, patient history, physical exam, and neurologic assessment.

PERIPHERAL NEUROPATHY

Peripheral neuropathy is the most common type of neuropathy which is caused by nerve lesions or tissue nerve damage that produces hyperexcitability of the primary sensory neurons and cells in the dorsal root ganglia.

History
- Reports numbness, tingling, shooting, burning, or electric-shock sensations; occurs in the feet or hands
- All sensation painful
- Gradual onset of symptoms; symptoms worsen at night
- History of diabetes
- History of alcohol abuse
- History of nutritional disorders
- Neurotoxic chemotherapy

Physical Examination
- Reduced touch sensation
- Reduced sensation in the feet with monofilament examination
- Diminished posterior tibial or dorsalis pedis pulses
- Distal muscle weakness; cannot stand on toes or heels
- Skin ulcerations that the patient is unable to feel (most often on the extremities)

Consideration
- Due to lack of feeling and pain, patients are at high risk for skin ulcerations. They should be advised to always wear shoes and do skin checks every day.

TRIGEMINAL NEURALGIA

Trigeminal neuralgia causes recurrent paroxysmal sharp pain radiating into one or more branches of the trigeminal nerve.

History
- More common in older adults (greater than age 50); affects women more often than men
- Reports unilateral burning, stabbing, electric shock, excruciating facial pain in the chin or cheek
- Reports pain episodes which may occur several times a day to several times/month
- Increased pain with chewing, swallowing, talking, brushing teeth, cold exposure
- Intermittent pain-free periods
- Inflammation of the maxillofacial region
- Inflammation of the ear, nose, throat
- Recent dental work
- History of MS

Physical Examination
- Patient may have normal neurologic assessment.
- Patient has slight sensory impairment in painful regions.
- Pain occurs in one or more divisions of the trigeminal nerve.

Consideration
- Other causes of trigeminal neuralgia include pressure of a tumor on the nerve or MS. Development of trigeminal neuralgia in a young adult suggests the possibility of MS.

PHYSICAL EXAMINATION DOCUMENTATION

EXAMPLE OF NORMAL FINDINGS
Patient alert and oriented ×3. Affect, behavior, speech, and communication appropriate. Patient Health Questionnaire-9 score of 6. Recent and remote memory intact. Cranial nerves I to XII intact. Pain, light touch, and vibratory sense intact. Two-point discrimination intact. Biceps, brachioradialis, triceps, patellar, and Achilles deep tendon reflexes (DTRs) 2+ bilateral. Good muscle tone. Strength 5/5 upper and lower extremities (deltoid, biceps, triceps, quadriceps. and hamstrings). Finger-to-nose and heel-to-shin testing normal bilateral. Rapid alternating movements even, equal, and coordinated. Romberg test negative. Gait smooth and coordinated with a steady base. Coordination intact as measured by heel walk and toe walk.

EXAMPLE OF CRANIAL NERVE DOCUMENTATION
(I) Able to accurately identify three scents. (II, III, IV, VI) Visual acuity (uncorrected) left eye 20/20, right eye 20/20; visual fields intact; pupils equal, round, and react to light and accommodation (PERRLA); movement of extraocular muscles (EOMs) intact without ptosis. (V) Facial sensation normal, equal bilateral to sharp, dull, and light touch stimuli; corneal reflex present; facial tone symmetrical, without tremor. (VII) Facial muscle strength normal and equal bilaterally. (VIII) Whisper test negative bilaterally. (IX, X) Palate and uvula elevate symmetrically with intact gag reflex, uvula midline without deviation; voice normal. (XI) Shoulder shrug 5/5 bilateral. (XII) Tongue protrudes midline and moves symmetrically.

REFERENCES
References for this chapter draw from Chapter 17, Evidence-Based Assessment of the Nervous System, of the textbook *Evidence-Based Physical Examination: Best Practices for Health and Well-Being Assessment (Second Edition)*. The references may be accessed in the digital version of the handbook at https://connect.springerpub.com/.

11

Evidence-Based Assessment of the Musculoskeletal System

CLINICAL CONSIDERATIONS

- History questions for the patient who presents with chronic musculoskeletal (MSK) problems include assessing for fever, weakness, inability to bear weight, stiffness, and/or swelling.
- History questions for the patient who presents with acute MSK injury include asking about the mechanism of injury and subsequent limitation in movement and activity.
- To be both systematic and thorough when completing a physical exam related to injury or pain in a joint, remember to begin with inspection, then palpate and assess strength; proceed to assess range of motion (ROM) and use special tests to note joint stability if there are no obvious deformities or point tenderness.
- In the MSK exam, a solid knowledge of the bony landmarks and underlying anatomy, along with precise palpation, is invaluable. Tenderness over a particular bony or soft tissue landmark can help determine potential differential diagnoses.

SUBJECTIVE HISTORY

COMMON REASONS FOR SEEKING CARE

- Joint pain (shoulder, elbow, wrist, hand, hip, knee, ankle, or foot pain)
- Spine pain (neck or back pain)

HISTORY OF PRESENT ILLNESS

- **Onset:** When did the symptoms start? What was the patient doing when they became symptomatic? Did this occur suddenly, or has it been developing gradually?
- **Location:** Does the symptom have associated pain or discomfort? If so, where is the discomfort located? Can you please point to the exact location of the pain or discomfort? Does the pain radiate anywhere? Are any other parts of the body affected?
- **Duration:** How long do the symptoms last? Over what period of time has the pain or symptom developed? Does the pain come and go or is it constantly present?

- **Characteristics:** How would you describe the pain—aching, burning, sharp, shooting, or deep? Is there any obvious deformity?
- **Associated symptoms:** Is there ever a click or pop associated with movement? Do you experience any other symptoms with it like weakness, stiffness, numbness, or tingling? Is there ever any instability or inability to bear weight? Are there any systemic symptoms (e.g., fever, unintended weight loss)? Are there any urinary symptoms (loss of bowel or bladder)?
- **Aggravating factors:** Was there a known injury? If so, what happened? What actions, activities, or body positions make the symptoms worse? Clarify the level of activity that causes symptom exacerbation. Is it worse at night or during the day? Is the back pain worse with bowel movements or the Valsalva maneuver?
- **Relieving factors:** What actions, activities, or body positions decrease the symptoms? Have limb elevation, ice, or heat been tried? If relieved, how long does the relief last?
- **Treatment:** What medications has been taken to help with the symptoms? Clarify the dosage and frequency of any medications. Have steroid injections been used in the past? Have any alternative treatments been tried like chiropractic care or acupuncture?
- **Severity:** How severe are the symptoms on a scale of 0 to 10? Do the symptoms limit participation in activities? Are there associated symptoms? Are the symptoms worsening?

HEALTH HISTORY

Past Medical History

- History of MSK conditions throughout the life span
- Chronic diseases (including cancers, diabetes, autoimmune disorders, osteoporosis, renal diseases, thyroid disorders)
- Osteoarthritis
- Anemia
- Surgeries
- Radiation therapy
- Recent or past injury, trauma, or car accidents
- History of physical or occupational therapy
- Anorexia/bulimia/eating disorders

Medications

- Prescribed medications (dose/frequency), including statins, steroids, antacids, antidepressants, Depo-Provera, thyroid replacement therapy, cancer chemotherapy drugs, bisphosphonates, estrogen
- Over-the-counter (OTC) medications or supplements (dose/frequency), including nonsteroidal anti-inflammatory drugs (NSAIDs), acetaminophen, glucosamine, calcium, vitamin D
- Cortisone injections

Pediatric/Adolescent Considerations
- Birth history
  - Delivery eventful or uneventful, vaginal or Cesarean section, prolonged or abrupt? Any nerve or bony injuries? Any interventions required during delivery or after birth?
  - Fetal abnormalities identified during the prenatal stage?
- Growth and development history
  - Meeting developmental milestones? Motor skills appropriate for age?
  - Suboptimal growth or poor weight gain (based on pediatric growth charts)?
- Eating and nutritional history
  - How has the child been eating? Specifically for the infant: Is the infant breast- or bottle-fed? Have the child's eating patterns changed?
  - Balanced diet? Energy expenditure related to calorie intake?
- Sports participation
  - Is the injury affecting the child/adolescent's ability to play and/or function at school?
  - Sports participation (what sports, training, frequency of participation, history of injuries)
  - History of concussions? Broken bones?

FAMILY HISTORY
- Congenital diseases (including myopathies)
- Autoimmune disease (including rheumatoid arthritis)
- Gout
- Paget disease of the bone
- Osteogenesis imperfecta
- Osteopenia/osteoporosis
- Muscular dystrophy

SOCIAL HISTORY
- **Level of physical activity:** Typical exercise routines, including type of activity, frequency, warm-up/cooldown routines, stretching programs, recent changes, increases or decreases and reasoning for this change; sports participation (e.g., type, frequency of training, cross-training)
- **Occupation:** Amount of movement during a typical workday and any repetitive motions that could put the patient at risk
- **Activities of daily living (ADL):** Patient able to dress themselves independently, brush their hair, put on their own socks; patient strong enough to walk stairs, carry loads, and reach overhead
- Smoking status
- Alcohol consumption
- Recreational or illicit drug use (type, frequency, amount)
- Diet, looking for possible nutritional deficiencies including calcium and vitamin D intake

REVIEW OF SYSTEMS

- **General:** Fever, weight loss, weight gain, fatigue, malaise
- **Head, eyes, ears nose, throat:** Conjunctivitis, vision changes
- **Cardiovascular:** Chest pain
- **Respiratory:** Shortness of breath
- **Gastrointestinal/genitourinary:** Dysuria, vaginal/penile discharge, erectile dysfunction
- **Neurologic:** Weakness, numbness, loss of sensation, balance concerns, cranial nerve deficits
- **Musculoskeletal:** Recent falls, decreased ROM, dropping things, decreased grip strength, changes in handwriting or fine motor movements, difficulty with completing ADL, multiple or diffuse joint pain, early morning stiffness, past injury or medical evaluation to affected area
- **Hematologic:** Anemia, bone pain
- **Skin:** Color, rash, erythema
- **Mental health:** Body image concerns, depression, anxiety, body dysmorphia, orthorexia, eating disorders

PHYSICAL EXAMINATION

Completing the physical exam of the MSK system includes having an appreciation for the techniques of the exam—(a) inspection; (b) palpation, including muscle strength; (c) assessment of ROM; and (d) use of special tests—as well as an understanding of how these techniques are used together to assess the integrity of the MSK system.

- Clinicians should be aware of red flags in the history and physical examination that would prompt additional work-up or emergency evaluation (**Box 11.1**).

BOX 11.1 Red Flags in History and Physical Exam

- History of cancer
- Associated neurologic deficits
- Saddle anesthesia
- Loss of bowel or bladder control
- Paralysis
- Weakness (especially unilateral with an acute onset or progressive)
- Gross deformity
- Associated unintended weight loss
- Point tenderness
- Extreme pain or pain that reoccurs over time
- Absence of pulses

GENERAL SURVEY

- Vital signs, including temperature, pulse rate, respiratory rate, and blood pressure
- Posture and position
- Gross deformities

INSPECTION

- Observe the patient throughout the exam. Observe their gait as they walk through the office, their posture, and their ability to do things, like remove their shirt. Note whether they are able to get out of a chair using only their legs or if they need their arms. If they need their arms, note whether they favor one arm versus the other.
- Observing their handwriting and asking about changes in handwriting can provide an early clue to a number of MSK or neurologic disorders.
- Identify any deformity, asymmetry, hypertrophy, or atrophy, along with any skin changes, including bleeding, bruising, swelling, and previous scars.
- Observe the anterior, posterior, lateral, and medial aspects of the joint and compare the affected joint with the joint on the opposite side of the body for symmetry.

PALPATION

- The palpation portion of the exam should include ROM and strength testing, followed by joint-specific special tests. The exam may or may not need an evaluation of deep tendon reflexes.
- After completing this portion of the exam, imaging and interventions should be considered based on current, evidence-based guidelines.

MUSCLE STRENGTH

- See Chapter 10, Evidence-Based Assessment of the Neurologic System, for information on completing this exam.
- See **Table 11.1** for the muscle strength scale.

RANGE OF MOTION AND SPECIAL TESTS

- ROM is the full movement potential of a joint; it should be completed during every MSK visit.
- Most joints will have a contralateral joint in which to compare motion and angles.
- See **Box 11.2** for a definition of different types of movements.

Head

- Have the patient open and close their mouth, move their jaw from side to side, and protract/retract their jaw. Palpate the temporomandibular joint (TMJ) during these movements; inquire about tenderness. With the patient's mouth open, place fingers below the zygomatic bone, anterior to the condyle. When the patient closes their mouth, the fingertip should fall into the depression

TABLE 11.1 Muscle Strength Testing	
Grade	Level of Function
0	No movement
1	Trace movement
2	Full passive range of motion
3	Full range of motion against gravity, no resistance
4	Full range of motion with resistance, although weak
5	Full range of motion, full strength

BOX 11.2 Types of Movements

Flexion: A movement that decreases the angle between two body parts

Extension: A movement that increases the angle between two body parts; opposite of flexion

Rotation: A movement in a circular motion around an axis

Abduction: A movement away from the midline, spreading the fingers or toes

Adduction: A movement toward or across the midline of the body, bringing the fingers or toes together

Inversion: Turning of the foot to angle the bottom of the foot toward the midline

Eversion: Turning the bottom of the foot away from the midline

Supination: Rotation of the radius that returns the bones to their parallel positions and moves the palm to the anterior-facing (supinated) position

Pronation: Body movement that moves the forearm from the supinated (anatomic) position to the pronated (palm backward) position

Circumduction: Movement of the limb, hand, or fingers in a circular pattern, using the sequential combination of flexion, adduction, extension, and abduction motions

Source: From Betts, J. G., Young, K. A., Wise, J. A., Johnson, E., Poe, B., Kruse, D. H., Korol, O., Johnson, J. E., Womble, M., & DeSaix, P. (Eds.). (2013). *Anatomy and physiology.* OpenStax. http://cnx.org/contents/14fb4ad7-39a1-4eee-ab6e-3ef2482e3e22@8.24.

anterior to the tragus as the patient opens their mouth. Feel for any clicking, popping, or catching.

- When the patient is opening and closing their mouth, the movement should be smooth and the mandible should not have left- or right-sided deviation. When opened, there should be enough room for three fingers between the incisors.

- Examine the tone of the major muscles of mastication, the temporalis, and masseter. Have the patient clench their jaw as you palpate for symmetric firmness of the muscles in contraction.

Cervical Spine

- When inspecting, look for deformities or asymmetries. Note the patient's posture; inspect for increased or decreased cervical lordosis or excessive thoracic kyphosis. Note their head position and whether they hold their head to one side or the other.

- Watch their movements. Do they have fluid, coordinated movements? Or do they appear stiff, slow, or uncontrolled?

- Palpate each spinal process. The spine has several landmarks that can assist in palpation, including the mastoid process, individual spinous processes (C7 is usually the most prominent), and facet joints, which lie approximately 1 inch lateral to each spinous process (**Figure 11.1**). These joints are not always palpable. Tenderness over the midline of the cervical spine when palpating the spinal processes could be indicative of a spinous process fracture.

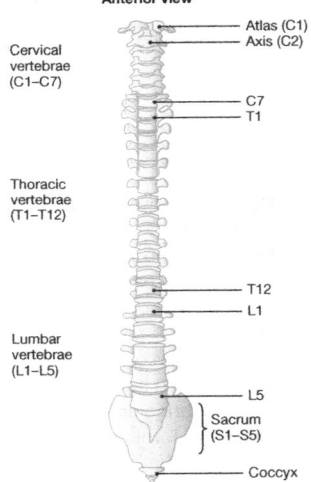

Anterior view

Cervical vertebrae (C1–C7) — Atlas (C1), Axis (C2), C7

Thoracic vertebrae (T1–T12) — T1, T12, L1

Lumbar vertebrae (L1–L5) — L5

Sacrum (S1–S5)

Coccyx

FIGURE 11.1 Spinal column.

- Palpate the soft tissue, including the paraspinal musculature, sternocleidomastoid muscle, and trapezius muscle.

- Do not test cervical ROM if unstable spine injury is suspected. Cervical ROM should include flexion, extension, lateral rotation to the left and right, and lateral bending to the left and right. The majority of flexion/extension occurs between the occiput and C1, with the majority of rotation occurring between C1 and C2.

- The following are the normal ROM values for the cervical spine: flexion, 45°; extension, 55°; lateral rotation, 70°; lateral bending, 40°.

- A proper cervical spine exam includes dermatome and myotome exams of the upper extremities, along with reflex testing of the biceps (C5), brachioradialis (C6), and triceps (C7; see **Figure 11.2** and **Table 11.2**).

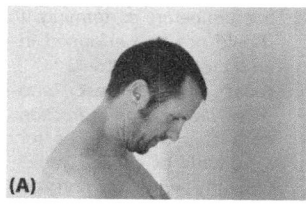

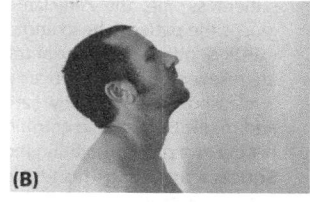

FIGURE 11.2 Range of motion of the cervical spine. (**A**) Cervical flexion. (**B**) Cervical extension.

Special Tests of the Cervical Spine

- **Spurling test:** This test identifies whether a nerve root is being compressed due to intervertebral disc pathology. Passively extend and rotate the patient's neck to the affected side. Slowly start applying axial pressure by pressing down on the top of the patient's head (**Figure 11.3**). The Spurling test is positive when radicular symptoms or pain is increased or reproduced on the ipsilateral shoulder or arm. Be sure to rule out cervical instability, vertebral artery injury, and vertebral

TABLE 11.2 Dermatomes and Myotomes of the Upper Extremity

Nerve	Dermatome	Myotome	Associated Reflex
C5	Lateral upper arm	Deltoid	Biceps
C6	Radial side of the forearm to the thumb and index finger	Biceps, wrist extensors	Brachioradialis
C7	Middle finger	Triceps, wrist flexors, and finger extensors	Triceps
C8	Ulnar forearm to the fourth and fifth digits	Finger flexors and interossei muscles	None
T1	Ulnar side of elbow	Interossei muscles	None

fracture before performing. It should not be performed in an acute trauma setting.

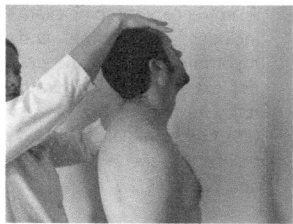

FIGURE 11.3 Spurling test.

- **Axial traction test** (*also called the traction-distraction test*)**:** This test assesses for symptoms of cervical radiculopathy with traction on the cervical spine. With the patient supine, the clinician grasps the patient's head and exerts gentle but firm axial traction; in a positive test, symptoms are relieved by the maneuver and return or increase once traction is released. The test has low sensitivity but relatively high specificity and might be useful in combination with other findings from the history and physical examination.

- **Squeeze arm test:** This test is used to distinguish patients with symptoms from shoulder pathology versus cervical nerve root compression. Placing the hand on the middle third of the upper arm with the fingers over the biceps and the thumb on the triceps, the clinician squeezes several times and has the patient rate their level of pain from 0 to 10. The clinician then palpates or squeezes two shoulder sites—the acromioclavicular (AC) joint area and the subacromial shoulder area—and has the patient again rate the level of pain. In a positive test, pain with compression of the arm is three or more points higher compared with the other sites. The concept of the test is that where there is nerve root compression there is pain involving the affected nerves in the arm that can be elicited by the squeezing maneuver.

Thoracic/Lumbar Spine

- Inspect the spine, looking for increased lumbar lordosis, kyphosis, and side curvature of the spine (scoliosis).
- Spinal curvature is best examined by having the patient flex forward while observing the spinous processes, which should form a straight line. There are two natural lordoses; when viewed from the side, the spine should form an "S"-shaped curve. The skin should be inspected for any abnormalities, including hairy patches, café-au-lait spots, or doughy lipomata. These findings could be indicative of underlying neurologic pathology.
- Observe the iliac crests, gluteal folds, posterior superior iliac spine (PSIS), and the anterior superior iliac spine (ASIS) while the patient is standing. Note any differences in height between the left and right sides.
- While the patient is supine, measure from the ASIS to the medial malleolus to check for true leg length discrepancies. Compare with the apparent leg length discrepancies as measured from the

umbilicus to the medial malleolus to evaluate for possible pelvic obliquity.

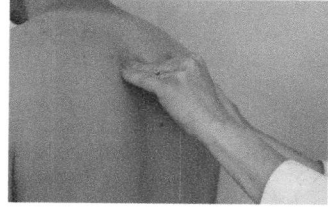

FIGURE 11.4 Palpation of the spinal processes.

- Palpation of the lumbar and thoracic spines (**Figure 11.4**) should include each of the spinous processes, iliac crests (approximately at L4 to L5 interspace), bilateral ASIS, greater trochanters, ischial tuberosities, and bilateral PSIS. The umbilicus often lies near the L3 to L4 interspace. Look for any step-off deformities. The transition from one spinous process to the neighboring ones should be smooth, with a slight divot between each.
- Normal values for the lumbar spine ROM are noted in **Figure 11.5**.
- **Table 11.3** includes a listing of dermatomes originating from the spine that affect the lower extremities.

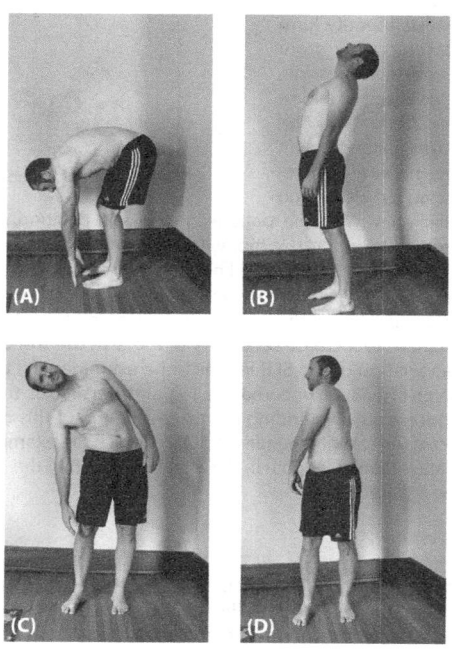

FIGURE 11.5 Range of motion of the spinal column. (**A**) Flexion: 40°–60°. (**B**) Extension: 20°–35°. (**C**) Lateral bending: 15°–20°. (**D**) Lateral rotation: 5°–20°.

TABLE 11.3 Dermatomes and Myotomes of the Lower Extremity

Nerve	Dermatome	Myotome	Associated Reflex
L4	Medial leg and medial foot	Anterior tibialis	Patella tendon
L5	Lateral leg and dorsum of the foot	Extensor hallucis longus	None
S1	Lateral foot	Peroneus longus and brevis	Achilles tendon

Special Tests of the Lumbar Spine

- **Straight leg raise (SLR) and Lasègue's test**: These tests identify lumbar radiculopathy from nerve root compression, often the result of a lumbar disc herniation. The maneuver places tension on the nerve root, reproducing or worsening

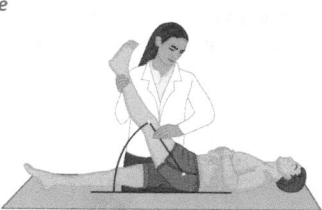

FIGURE 11.6 Straight leg raise.

radicular pain. With the patient in a supine position, passively lift the leg, flexing at the hip, with the knee in full extension; if needed, place a hand on the knee to ensure full knee extension (**Figure 11.6**). The test is positive if the maneuver causes radicular pain in the leg below the knee on the ipsilateral side at 30° to 70° of elevation. To increase sensitivity of the test, use the **Lasègue's test**, a variation of the SLR in which the examiner lifts the leg to the point of pain, lowers the leg 10°, and dorsiflexes the foot to reproduce a positive finding. Another variation of this maneuver is the crossed straight leg raise (CSLR) in which the examiner looks for sciatic or radicular pain in the affected leg when the contralateral leg is raised.

Upper Extremities
Shoulder

- When inspecting the shoulder, evaluate the patient's arm swing. Does it appear equal or does the motion seem limited in one side? Movements should be smooth and coordinated. Use the contralateral side for comparison, not just during inspection but also when testing ROM, strength, and special tests.

- Look for any muscle atrophy (indicative of a nerve palsy or extreme deconditioning), deformity (fracture or dislocation), winging scapula, Popeye deformity, discoloration, or scars.
- Palpate the following bony landmarks (**Figure 11.7**): scapula (including the coracoid process, acromion process, spine of the scapula, superior and inferior angles of the scapula, and the medial/lateral borders of the scapula), clavicle (including the sternal end, the acromial end, and the entire shaft), and humerus (including the deltoid tuberosity, the greater tuberosity [lateral], the bicipital groove, and the lesser tuberosity [medial]).
- Palpate the sternoclavicular joint, AC joint, sternoclavicular ligament, and AC ligament.
- Palpate the following areas of soft tissue: insertion point of the rotator cuff muscles at greater tuberosity; axilla borders; serratus anterior muscles; pectoralis major muscles; upper, middle, and lower trapezius; deltoid (anterior, middle posterior bellies); sternocleidomastoid; biceps insertion and belly; and latissimus dorsi muscles.
- When palpating musculature, feel for tenderness and tone; compare muscles with the contralateral side.
- **Apley's scratch test:** Ask the patient to abduct and externally rotate their arms, then reach behind their back and touch the contralateral scapula. Have the patient abduct and internally rotate their arm, then ask the patient to reach behind their back and reach as far up their back as possible. Note the extent of reach on each side and compare the range bilaterally.
- To test active horizontal adduction, have the patient abduct their arms to 90°, flex the elbow to 90°, then reach across the front of their body and touch the contralateral AC joint.

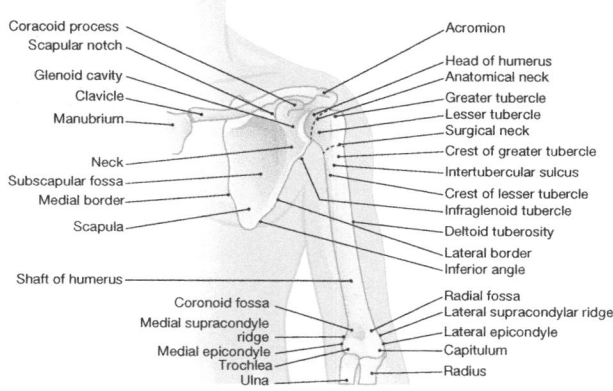

FIGURE 11.7 Bones of the shoulder.

- To test for full abduction ROM, have the patient externally rotate their arm to allow the humeral head to clear under the acromion.
- Passive ROM normal values are noted in **Figure 11.8**.
- Test all nine shoulder movements and compare bilaterally.

Special Tests of the Shoulder

- Shoulder tests should be completed in clusters, in contrast to completing a single test, to improve the reliability of results.
- **Hawkins–Kennedy test:** This test helps identify impingement of the supraspinatus. While holding the patient's elbow at 90° with one hand, and their wrist with the other hand, passively flex the shoulder to 90°, then internally rotate (**Figure 11.9**). The test is positive if it reproduces the pain.
- **Neer test:** Like the Hawkins–Kennedy, this test recreates impingement within the subacromial space in the shoulder joint. With a hand on the shoulder to eliminate extraneous movement, and with the patient's arm pronated (with the thumb pointing downward), the clinician passively flexes the arm forward to 180° (**Figure 11.10**). The Neer test is positive for impingement if it reproduces shoulder pain between 70° and 100° of flexion.
- **Empty can (or Jobe) test:** This test identifies supraspinatus weakness due to a tear, subacromial impingement, or a nerve injury.

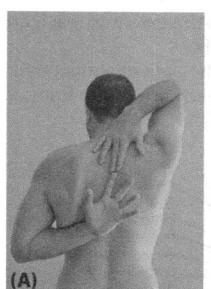
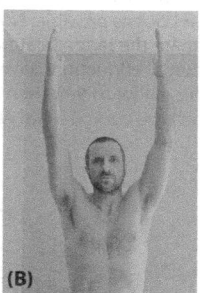
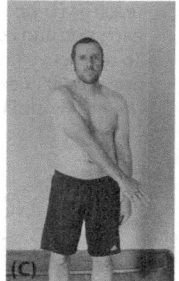
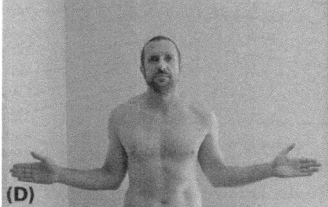

FIGURE 11.8 Shoulder range of motion. (**A**) Apley's scratch test. (**B**) Abduction: 180°. (**C**) Adduction: 45°. (**D**) External rotation: 90°.

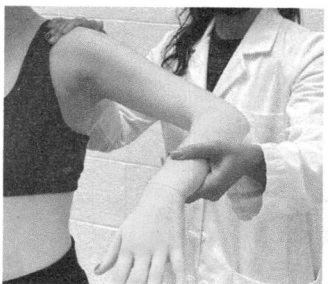

FIGURE 11.9 Hawkins–Kennedy test.

Have the patient abduct both of their arms to 90° at approximately 30° flexion. Next, have them internally rotate the shoulder so their thumbs are pointing to the ground (as if emptying a can of liquid in their hand; **Figure 11.11**). Then, have the patient try to actively resist adduction as the examiner applies downward pressure on the distal arms. The test is positive for supraspinatus weakness or impingement if the patient is unable to maintain their arm position or has pain.

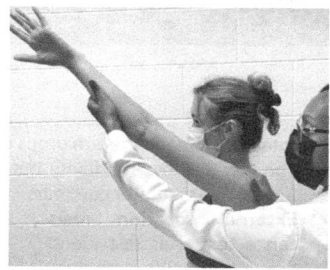

FIGURE 11.10 Neer test.

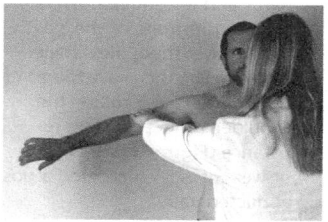

FIGURE 11.11 Empty can test.

- **Painful arc test:** Ask the patient to actively abduct their arms to 180° (**Figure 11.12**). The result is positive for subacromial impingement if the patient has pain within the range of 60° to 120° of abduction. Pain will often be worse with internal rotation and somewhat relieved with external rotation. A positive test indicates subacromial impingement.
- **Drop arm test:** This maneuver is another simple test for a supraspinatus rotator cuff tear. Passively abduct the patient's arm on the affected side to 90°. Release the arm and ask the patient to maintain the arm position against gravity. The test is positive for a

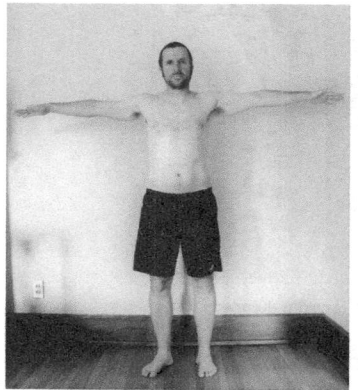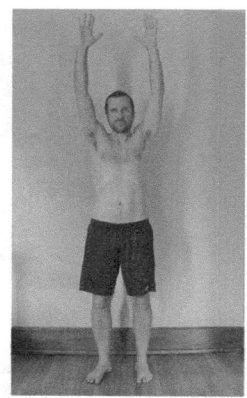

FIGURE 11.12 Painful arc test.

rotator cuff tear if the arm drops or the position is not maintained. The test has low sensitivity but high specificity for partial- and full-thickness rotator cuff tears.

- **External rotation resistance test:** This test identifies rotator cuff pathology, particularly of the infraspinatus and teres minor. While standing in front of the patient, have them flex their elbow to 90°, then have them try to externally rotate the shoulder while providing resistance (**Figure 11.13**). Pain or weakness is considered a positive result. Repeat with the arm abducted to 90°.

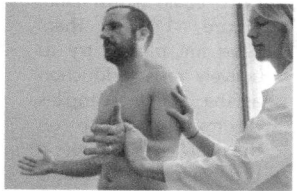

FIGURE 11.13 External rotation resistance test.

- **Apprehension test:** Have the patient lie supine with the arm flexed and the shoulder abducted to 90°. The clinician applies anterior force on the shoulder to displace the humerus anteriorly. The test is positive if the patient experiences apprehension or instability. This test assesses for glenohumeral instability.
- **Sulcus sign:** This test also assesses for glenohumeral instability. Have the patient stand comfortably as the clinician tugs downward on the affected arm. If there is shoulder instability, the humeral head will be displaced inferiorly, creating a sulcus, or dip, in the subacromial area.

Elbow

- Examine the elbow in both flexion and extension. Identify the carrying angle with the elbow in extension. A normal carrying angle is considered to be between 5° and 15° valgus. An increase in the angle is known as cubitus valgus. Cubitus varus is a decrease in that angle, also known as *gunstock deformity*; in children, this can be a sign of a fracture affecting the rotation of the distal end of the humerus. Also, look for edema at the tip of the elbow, over the olecranon fossa, as olecranon bursitis is a common complication of falling onto the tip of the elbow.
- Palpate the following bony landmarks: medial and lateral epicondyles, origins for the wrist flexors and extensor bundles, medial and lateral supracondylar lines of the humerus, olecranon, olecranon fossa, ulnar border, and radial head (which is palpated an inch distal to the lateral epicondyle during pronation and supination).
- Palpate the medial side of the elbow, feeling for the origin of the flexor bundle (pronator teres, flexor carpi radialis, palmaris longus, and flexor carpi ulnaris) and the ulnar nerve. Palpate for any tenderness over the ulnar collateral ligament. On the lateral side, palpate the extensor bundle (brachioradialis, extensor carpi radialis longus, and the extensor carpi radialis brevis) and feel for any tenderness over the radial collateral and the annular ligaments. The hand should be moved anteriorly to find the insertion of the biceps tendon and the brachial artery, which lies just medial to the biceps insertion point. The median nerve is found medial to the brachial artery.
- Passive ROM normal values are noted in **Figure 11.14**.

Special Tests of the Elbow

- **Cozen test:** This test identifies lateral epicondylitis (tennis elbow). Have the patient pronate the forearm, make a fist, and deviate the hand radially; while supporting the patient's elbow, provide resistance as the patient extends their wrist. The test is positive if the maneuver reproduces the pain.
- **Golfer elbow test:** This test identifies medial epicondylitis (golfer's elbow). With the patient's forearm supinated, the clinician extends the arm at the elbow and extends the wrist. Pain over the medial epicondyle is suggestive of epicondylitis. Epicondylitis can also cause weakened grip strength.
- **Varus and valgus stress tests:** These tests identify injury to the radial (lateral) collateral ligament of the elbow. These tests assess instability or excess laxity of the radial (lateral) collateral ligament (LCL) and the ulnar (medial) collateral ligament (MCL) of the elbow. Have the patient flex the elbow to about 30°. Stabilize the wrist and apply valgus stress to test the MCL. Apply varus stress to test the LCL. Pain or excess motion compared with the contralateral side is a positive test.

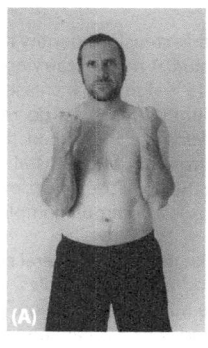
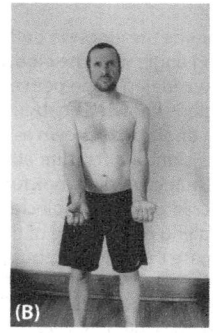
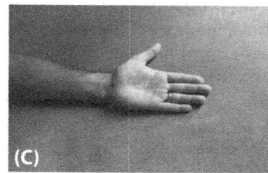
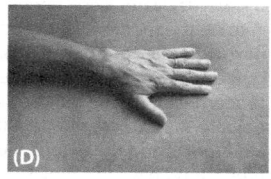

FIGURE 11.14 Elbow range of motion. (**A**) Flexion: 135°. (**B**) Extension: 0°–5° hyperextension. (**C**) Supination: 90°. (**D**) Pronation: 90°.

- **Tinel sign:** This test identifies compression of the ulnar nerve. With the elbow relaxed and the wrist supported, tap the ulnar nerve in the groove between the olecranon and the medial epicondyle (**Figure 11.15**). This version of the Tinel sign is a test for compression of the ulnar nerve. Tingling or pain along the ulnar distribution is considered a positive test.

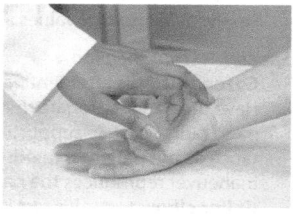

FIGURE 11.15 Tinel sign.

Wrist/Hand

- Inspect the wrist and hand (**Figure 11.16**). Ensure all five fingers are present; missing digits or parts of digits are not always noticeable at first glance. Observe the creases on the hands. Note the thenar eminence, thick muscle belly at the base of the thumb, and hypothenar eminence, at the base of the little finger.
- Inspection of the fingers and nails is essential for a thorough exam. With the fingers extended, look for rotation or crossing

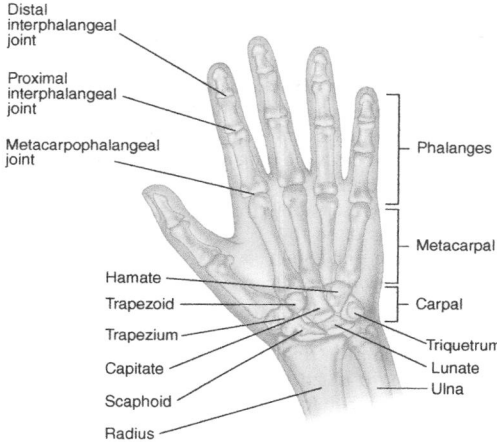

Distal interphalangeal joint

Proximal interphalangeal joint

Metacarpophalangeal joint

Phalanges

Metacarpal

Hamate

Trapezoid

Trapezium

Capitate

Scaphoid

Radius

Carpal

Triquetrum

Lunate

Ulna

FIGURE 11.16 Bones of the hand and wrist.

over of the fingers. This could be a sign of a phalange or metacarpal fracture. With a closed fist, the fingers should lay next to each other and not cross one another.

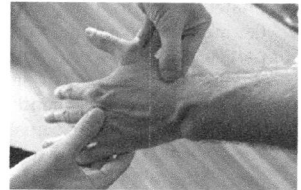

FIGURE 11.17 Area of snuff box tenderness.

- Palpate the styloid processes of both the radius and the ulna. Move to the anatomic snuffbox, the depression on the radial side of the wrist bordered by the abductor pollicis longus and the extensor pollicis brevis tendons (**Figure 11.17**). Tenderness is a sign of a possible scaphoid fracture. Feel for fullness and good muscle tone in the thenar and hypothenar eminences.

- Palpate the entire length of each metacarpal, feeling for any tenderness or deformity. Finish the bony palpation at the fingers with each phalange and interphalangeal (IP) joint.

- The following are the passive ROM normal values: wrist extension, 70°; wrist flexion, 80°; radial deviation, 20°; ulnar deviation, 30°; metacarpophalangeal (MCP) flexion, 80° to 90°; MCL extension, 30° to 45°; proximal interphalangeal (PIP) flexion, 100°; PIP extension, 0°; distal interphalangeal (DIP) flexion, 90°; DIP extension, 20°; finger abduction, 20°; finger adduction, 0°; thumb MCP flexion, 50°; thumb MCP extension, 20°; thumb abduction, 70°; thumb adduction, 0°.

Special Tests for the Wrist and Hand

- **Finkelstein test:** This test identifies tenosynovitis of the abductor pollicis longus and extensor pollicis brevis tendons, also known as *De Quervain syndrome*. With the patient's forearm supported on a flat surface and the wrist resting at the edge, ask the patient to slowly deviate the hand in the ulnar direction while the examiner flexes the thumb across the patient's hand. Pain over the tendons is considered a positive test.

- **Eichhoff test:** This is an additional test that is often misidentified as the Finkelstein test but is somewhat easier to conduct. For the Eichhoff test, the patient actively closes the thumb in their fist, then performs ulnar deviation of the hand (**Figure 11.18**). The test result is positive if it elicits pain. When conducting these tests, be sure to ask the patient to slowly deviate the hand, as a positive test result can be exquisitely painful.

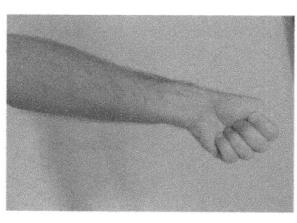

FIGURE 11.18 Eichhoff test.

- **Phalen test:** This test identifies median nerve pathology, particularly carpal tunnel syndrome. Have the patient sit with the dorsum of the hands pressed together in maximal wrist flexion for a full 60 seconds (**Figure 11.19**). Numbness or tingling in the median nerve distribution indicates a positive test result. One variation of the test is the reverse Phalen test where the hands are pressed together in front of the body in a prayer position. Another variation is having the patient stretch their arms forward and actively flex their wrists; the clinician can apply force to ensure flexion is maintained.

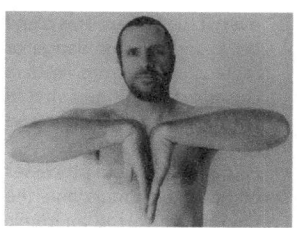

FIGURE 11.19 Phalen test.

- **Varus/valgus test:** As with the elbow, the collateral ligaments in the fingers can be tested with a varus or valgus force applied while the joint is relaxed and supported. Pain or excess motion compared with the contralateral side is considered a positive test. This test is particularly useful at the MCP joint of the thumb to identify skier's thumb, or a tear of the ulnar collateral ligament at the base of the thumb with increased motion or pain with a valgus force.

Lower Extremities
Hip

- Assess gait patterns. Look for altered gait patterns as these can be a clue to a variety of lower extremity conditions. A Trendelenburg gait could be a sign of weak abductors. Shuffling of the feet or a wide base gait can be signs of Parkinson or cerebellar disease. Watch several gait cycles (focusing on a different joint for each cycle) to determine which part of the lower extremity is causing the gait disturbance. If needed and after patient permission, the patient's gait could be recorded and reviewed repeatedly or at a slower speed to enhance evaluation.
- Inspect the bony landmarks including the levels of the iliac crests, PSIS, ASIS, gluteal folds, and medial malleoli to determine the symmetry of the lower limbs, leg length, or possible pelvic obliquity (**Figure 11.20**). Note the bony landmarks while the patient is standing and supine.
- A measurement from the ASIS to the medial malleolus is considered a true leg length measurement and should be done bilaterally for comparison. A measurement from the umbilicus to the medial malleolus is considered an apparent leg length measurement and can be compared with the true leg length measurement to help identify possible soft tissue adaptations that can result in apparent leg length differences even when true ones do not exist.

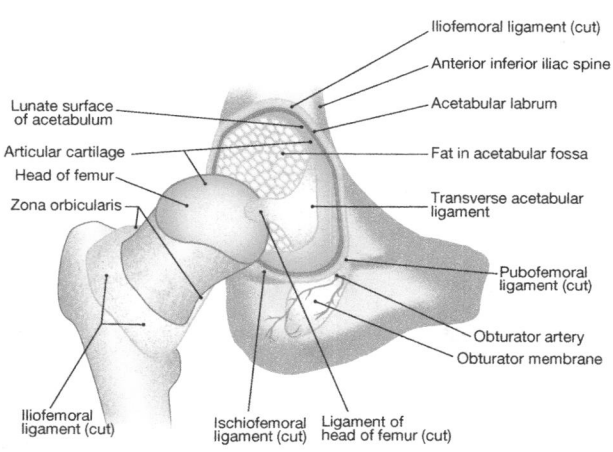

FIGURE 11.20 Hip anatomy.

- Palpate the hip. True hip joint pathology typically presents as pain and tenderness in the groin. Pain on the lateral hip, over the greater trochanter, is more commonly a trochanteric bursitis or abductor tendinitis, possibly related to a tight iliotibial (IT) band. Palpate the muscles to evaluate for tenderness or atrophy.
- Palpate the ischial tuberosities deep in the gluteal folds as this is the origin of the hamstrings and a common area of injury.
- Passive ROM normal values are noted in **Figure 11.21**.

Special Tests for the Hip

- **Thomas test:** This test identifies hip flexor contracture and tightness. With the patient supine, have them bring one knee to their chest. Control for lumbopelvic movement (i.e., pelvic tilt) by stabilizing the pelvis. Passive flexion in the contralateral leg is considered positive for hip flexor tightness/contracture of the contralateral side. The **FABER test** identifies hip flexor, sacroiliac, or hip intra-articular pathology. FABER stands for **F**lexion, **AB**duction, and **E**xternal **R**otation—the simultaneous movements performed during the test. With the patient supine, have them flex, abduct, and externally rotate the hip until the ankle rests upon the contralateral knee. Apply downward pressure, moving the knee closer to the table (**Figure 11.22**). Pain or decreased ROM is considered a positive test.
- **Log roll:** This test identifies intra-articular pathology, particularly symptomatic arthritis. With the patient supine, hold the ankle or knee and passively internally and externally rotate the leg. Pain in the groin is considered a positive test.
- **Stinchfield test:** This test identifies intra-articular hip pathology. With the patient supine, have them flex the hip to 30° or 45°.

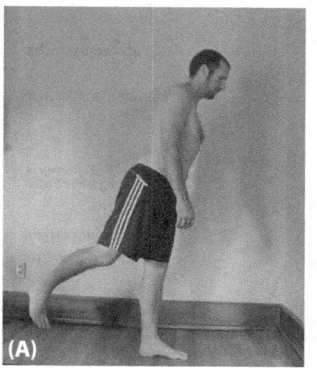 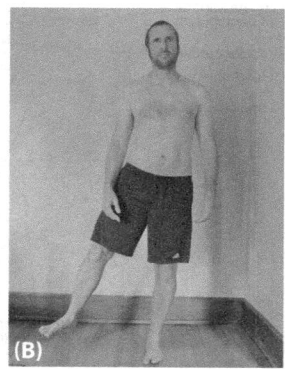

FIGURE 11.21 Hip range of motion. (**A**) Extension: 20°–30°. (**B**) Abduction: 40°.

Apply a downward pressure on the ankle with the patient resisting. Pain in the groin is considered a positive test.

* **Trendelenburg test:** This test identifies weakness of the hip abductor muscles. Have the patient stand on one leg for 10 seconds, then switch legs (**Figure 11.23**). Weakness of the gluteus medius on the standing side will lead to a drop of the pelvis on the unsupported side—a positive test.

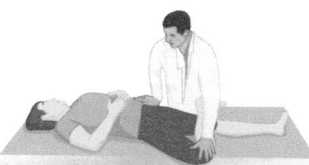

FIGURE 11.22 Flexion, abduction, and external rotation test.

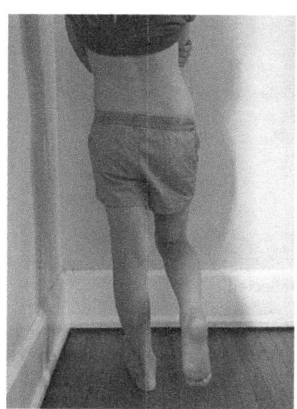

FIGURE 11.23 Negative Trendelenburg test. No drop of the pelvis noted on the unsupported side.

Knee

* Inspect the knee. Inspection of the knee is usually performed in the sitting position. However, evaluation for genu valgus (knock knee) and genu varus (bow-legged) should be done while the patient stands. Look for any deformity, effusion, asymmetry, and/or edema. A prominent tibial tuberosity can be a sign of Osgood–Schlatter disease, which is common in adolescence.
* Palpate the knee (**Figure 11.24**). On the lateral side of the knee, palpate the fibular head, lateral joint line, lateral femoral condyle, IT band, and Gerdy's tubercle, biceps femoris insertion, and LCL. On the medial side, palpate the medial joint line, MCL origin and insertion, pes anserine bursa, and bellies of the semitendinosus and semimembranosus muscles. Feel anteriorly for the patella and its borders, the tibial tuberosity, and the patellar and quadriceps tendons. On the posterior side, feel in the popliteal fossa for a possible fluid collection (a Baker's cyst), a sign of a meniscus tear, or osteoarthritis in the knee as can pain in the popliteal fossa.
* The following are the passive ROM normal values: flexion, 130° to 140°; extension, 0° to 5° hyperextension.
* Perform strength testing with the patient in a seated position.

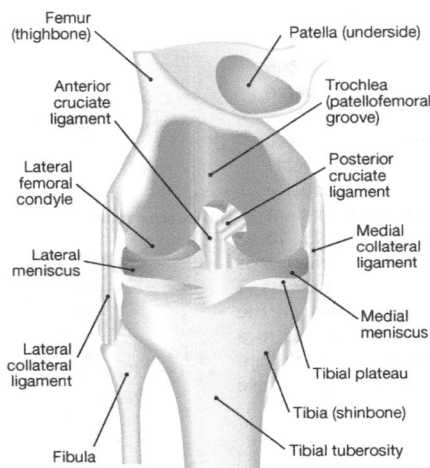

FIGURE 11.24 Knee anatomy. Frontal view of the right knee (with the patella reflected).

Special Tests for the Knee

- **Valgus stress test (Figure 11.25):** This test identifies injury to the MCL. With the patient supine and relaxed, hold the ankle and apply valgus stress to the lateral knee. Test in full extension and 20° to 30° of knee flexion. Pain/excessive laxity is considered a positive test.

- **Varus stress test (Figure 11.26):** This test identifies injury to the LCL. With the patient supine and relaxed, hold the ankle and apply varus stress to the medial knee. Test in full extension and 20° to 30° of knee flexion. Pain/excessive laxity is considered a positive test.

- **Anterior drawer test (Figure 11.27A):** This test

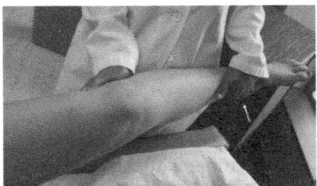

FIGURE 11.25 Valgus stress test.

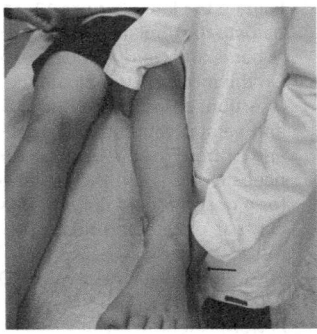

FIGURE 11.26 Varus stress test.

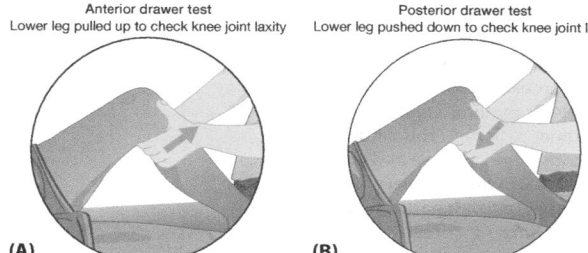

Anterior drawer test
Lower leg pulled up to check knee joint laxity

Posterior drawer test
Lower leg pushed down to check knee joint laxity

(A)   **(B)**

FIGURE 11.27 Drawer tests. (**A**) Anterior. (**B**) Posterior.

identifies injury to the anterior cruciate ligament (ACL). With the patient supine, have them flex their hip to 45° and flex knee to 90°, resting their foot on the table. The clinician should sit on the patient's foot to stabilize the leg and place their hands behind the proximal tibia, resting their thumbs on the tibial tuberosity. Use the index fingers to ensure relaxation of the hamstring muscles. Apply an anterior force. Increased anterior translation is indicative of an ACL tear.

- **Posterior drawer test (Figure 11.27B):** This test identifies injury to the posterior cruciate ligament (PCL). With the patient supine, have them flex their hip to 45° and flex the knee to 90°, resting their foot on the table. Sit on the patient's foot to stabilize the leg. The hands should be placed behind the proximal tibia, resting the thumbs on the tibial tuberosity. Use the index fingers to ensure relaxation of the hamstring muscles. Apply a posterior force. Increased posterior translation is indicative of a PCL tear.

- **Lachman test (Figure 11.28):** This test identifies a tear to the ACL. With the patient supine and relaxed, place the outside or prox- imal hand over the distal thigh and the inside hand (distal hand) over the prox- imal tibia. Allowing the hip

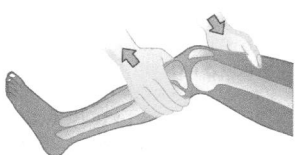

FIGURE 11.28 Lachman test.

to externally rotate can help ensure the patient is relaxed. Apply anterior translation force on the tibia with the distal hand while stabilizing the thigh with the proximal hand. Excessive anterior tibial translation is indicative of an ACL tear. This test can be chal- lenging if the patient is guarding.

- **Pivot shift:** This test also identifies ACL tears. The pivot shift test is completed while the patient is supine. The clinician starts with the knee in full extension and simultaneously applies a valgus and internal rotation force as the knee is slowly flexed. The clinician should note whether there is anterior subluxation of the lateral femoral condyle as the knee is flexed. This finding is considered positive and is most accurate with complete tears as compared with partial tears.

- **McMurray's test (Figure 11.29):** This test identifies meniscus pathology. With the patient supine, use one hand to grasp the patient's ankle and the other hand to stabilize the patient's knee. With the knee flexed, externally rotate the tibia and apply a valgus force while extending the knee. Move the knee from flexion while internally rotating the tibia and applying varus force. Pain or clicking over the medial or lateral joint lines is considered a positive test.

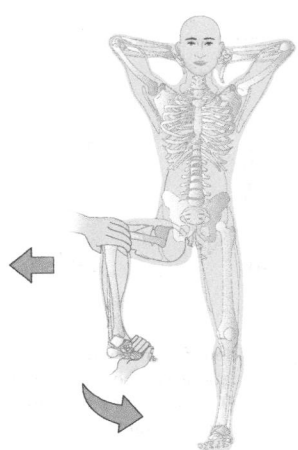

FIGURE 11.29 McMurray's test.

- **Thessaly test:** This test identifies meniscal injuries. Ask the patient to stand. The clinician should hold the patient's hands or the patient can grasp a table for balance. The patient is asked to then balance on the unaffected leg with the knee flexed to 5°. Then the patient should be instructed to twist with the leg in a manner that causes the femur to rotate back and forth (medially and laterally) three times. Then the patient is asked to perform this same movement using the affected leg. Pain in the knee of the standing leg is a positive test.

- **Apprehension test (Figure 11.30):** This test identifies patellar laxity or subluxations/

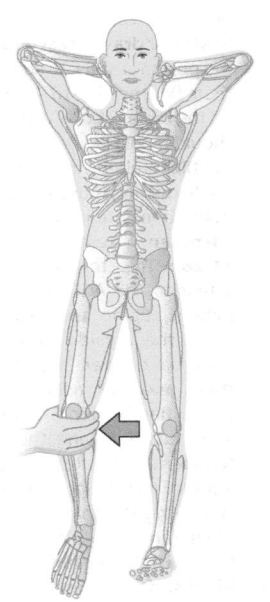

FIGURE 11.30 Apprehension test.

dislocations. With the patient supine and relaxed, place the knee in full extension. Apply a lateral force to the medial border of the patella. Pain or guarding is considered a positive test.

- **Ballottement test:** This test identifies joint effusion in the knee, which is most commonly caused by trauma to the knee. The test can help diagnose knee injuries and distinguish effusion from swelling due to injury involving extra-articular structures in the knee area. The patient should lie in the supine position with their legs extended. The clinician should place one hand superior to the patella and use the other hand to apply downward pressure in an anterior to posterior "milking" motion. If there is fluid, the clinician will feel it against their lower hand. Gently push down on the patella. If it can be depressed, it means that it was "floating" in fluid and signifies a positive test.

- **Bulge sign:** This is commonly used to test for knee effusion. Gently press slightly medial to the patella, then move the hand in an ascending motion and apply pressure firmly on the lateral aspect of the knee. A positive test is a "bulge" seen on the medial aspect of the knee after lateral pressure was applied, which indicates that a moderate amount of fluid is present. A medial aspect that does not bulge but tensely reflects lateral pressure is consistent with a large amount of fluid.

Ankle/Foot

- Inspect the patient's footwear. Shoes can provide information on wear patterns and show where a person is putting pressure on their feet throughout their gait cycle, which provides information about possible foot deformities or gait patterns.

- Observe the foot and ankle of the patient both in standing and sitting positions. Look for deformities and asymmetries as with any other joint, as well as any areas of calluses or corn formations. Calluses can indicate abnormal weightbearing or improperly fitting shoes. The skin should be the thickest around the heel, at the lateral border, and over the metatarsal heads.

- Look at the arches in the patient's feet. The arches should be more pronounced when the patient is not bearing weight. Observe the metatarsals (**Figure 11.31**). Note deformities, including claw toes, hammertoes, and mallet toes, on inspection.

- Palpate the medial side of the ankle and foot. Palpate over the medial malleolus, then down the foot to the navicular bone (the most prominent bone on the medial side). Palpate the medial head of the talus, which is just proximal to the navicular bone. Move down the foot to the first metatarsal, then distally to the first phalange and the IP joint. On the lateral side, start palpation at the lateral malleolus, then move inferiorly to palpate the peroneus longus and brevis. Just distal to the lateral malleolus

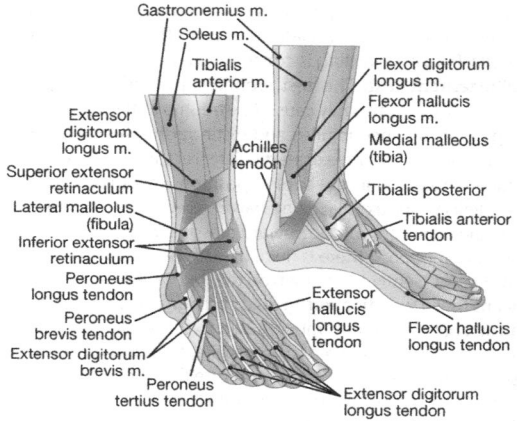

FIGURE 11.31 Foot and ankle anatomy.

is the area of the anterior talofibular ligament. Palpate down the foot and feel for the styloid process at the base of the fifth metatarsal. This is a common area of avulsion or stress fractures. Lastly, palpate the shaft of the metatarsals and phalanges, feeling for the metatarsophalangeal (MTP) and IP joints.

- On the posterior foot, palpate the Achilles tendon and its insertion site, feeling for any crepitus or nodularity. Then move to the plantar surface and the calcaneus. Continue moving distally and palpate the metatarsal shafts and heads, feeling for any tenderness.
- Palpate for pedal pulses. The posterior tibial artery can be palpated just posterior to the medial malleolus, and the dorsalis pedis artery can be palpated between the extensor hallucis longus and the extensor digitorum longus tendons. Absent or diminished pedal pulses can indicate peripheral vascular disease (PVD), compartment syndrome, or other pathology.
- The following are the passive ROM normal values: dorsiflexion, 20°; plantar flexion, 50°; inversion, 30°; eversion, 20°; abduction, 10°; adduction: 20°; first MTP flexion, 45°; first MTP extension: 70°.

Special Tests for the Ankle/Foot

- **Squeeze test (Figure 11.32):** This test identifies syndesmotic (or high) ankle injuries or fractures. With the patient relaxed, squeeze the midshaft of the tibia and fibula together. Pain over the ankle syndesmosis is considered a positive test; however, results should be interpreted with caution due to limited research to support its accuracy.
- **Talar tilt:** This test identifies ankle ligamentous injury. With the patient relaxed and foot in a neutral position, passively

move the foot into an adducted position; pain or increased motion is considered positive and a sign of damage to the LCL of the ankle. Next, passively move the foot into an abducted position. Pain or increased motion is considered a positive test and indicates pathology of the MCLs of the ankle.

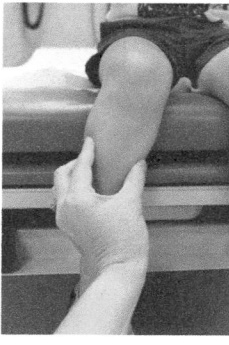

FIGURE 11.32 Squeeze test.

- **Thompson test:** This test evaluates the integrity of the Achilles tendon complex. With the patient prone or seated with the foot unsupported, squeeze the belly of the gastrocnemius. With an intact complex, the foot should passively plantar-flex when the calf is squeezed. No plantar flexion of the foot is considered a positive test.

ADDITIONAL PEDIATRIC EXAMS

Barlow–Ortolani Maneuvers

- These maneuvers are designed to test for hip dislocations and subluxations in 0- to 1-year-olds. With the infant supine, flex the hips and knees to 90°. The clinician's thumbs should rest on the medial side of the knees, with the fingers resting on the greater trochanters. Adduct the thighs and put gentle pressure through the femurs, trying to shift them out of the acetabula. A "clunk" is considered positive. Slowly abduct the thighs and use the fingers to put pressure on the trochanters to guide the femoral head back into position. Again, a clunking sensation is considered a positive test and could be a sign of hip subluxation or dislocation. If dysplasia is suspected within the first 6 months of life, an ultrasound evaluation is preferred to x-ray. If any tests are abnormal, refer to a pediatric orthopedic clinician for intervention(s) and/or treatment options (**Figure 11.33**).

Scoliosis

- Have the patient stand and observe them from the front. Note the symmetry of the patient's shoulders; the shoulders should be even. Uneven shoulder height can be a clue to scoliosis. Ask the patient to turn around and bend at the waist. The clinician should observe the patient from the rear. The spine should be straight without curvature and centered over the sacrum. Angles fewer than 10° can often be followed with periodic radiographs. Angles of up to 30° typically show no lasting effects into adulthood. Angles over 50° will lead to complications later in life. In more severe cases, a unilateral rib hump may be present. Routine screening for scoliosis is not recommended. See **Figure 11.34**.

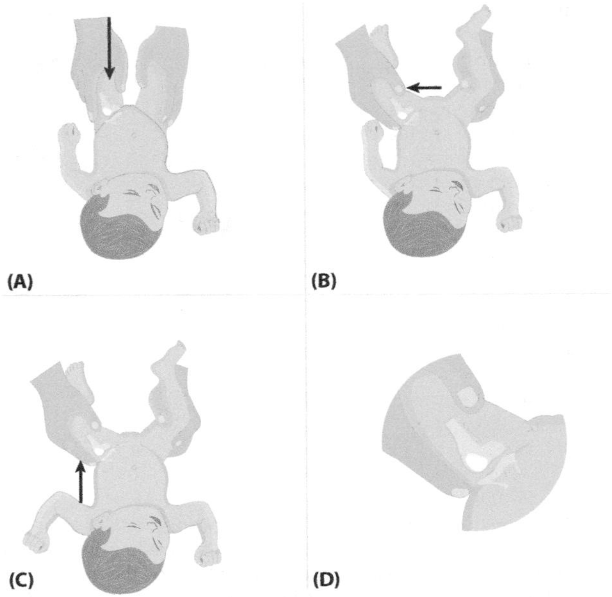

(A)

(B)

(C)

(D)

FIGURE 11.33 Barlow–Ortolani maneuvers. (**A**) Barlow testing: From an abducted (thighs outward) position, flex the infant's knees to 90° and apply posterior pressure or force. Ortolani testing: From the knee-bent position, abduct each of the infant's legs by moving the thigh outward (**B**) and apply anterior, upward pressure or force (**C**). (**D**) Testing is positive when maneuvers result in a felt or heard "clunk" or when limited motion in either hip or thigh is noted. Positive testing indicates that the femoral head is partially or completely dislocated from the acetabulum.

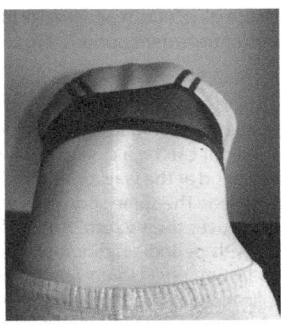

FIGURE 11.34 Scoliosis.

ABNORMAL FINDINGS

CARPAL TUNNEL SYNDROME

An inflammation and compression of the median nerve as it moves through the carpal tunnel of the wrist (**Figure 11.35**)

History
- Numbness and tingling over the median nerve distribution into the hand (thumb and index, middle or ring fingers); numbness and pain worse at night
- History of repetitive activity such as writing or typing
- Reports pain with gripping objects
- Symptoms induced or exacerbated by pregnancy in some cases

Physical Examination
- Decreased grip strength
- Atrophy of thenar eminence (later stages)
- Positive Phalen and Tinel tests
- Weakness of thumb strength and opposition

COMPARTMENT SYNDROME

Compartment syndrome occurs when pressure increases in the muscle compartment due to edema or bleeding. The fascia does not stretch, which causes compression of the surrounding capillaries, nerves, and muscles. This compression impedes blood flow to and from the affected tissues.

History
- History of fracture, burns, severe injury, surgery, casting, or during critical illness

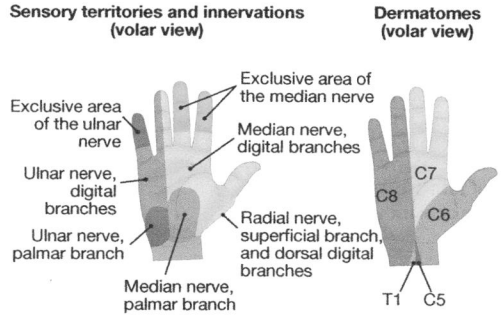

FIGURE 11.35 Median and ulnar nerve distribution (volar view).

- Prolonged compression of a limb during a period of unconsciousness
- Blood clot in an arm or leg
- Extreme, vigorous exercise (seen with chronic compartment syndrome)
- Taking anabolic steroids
- Five Ps (pain, pallor, paresthesia, pulselessness, paralysis)
- Feeling of muscle tightness
- Reports pain and paresthesia to the area (included in the five Ps of compartment syndrome)
- Burning sensation in the affected area

Physical Findings
- Legs, arms, and abdomen the most common sites, with the lower leg being most often affected
- Pallor and paralysis of the affected limb (included in the five Ps)
- Inability to find a pulse in the affected limb
- Swelling to the muscle

DE QUERVAIN SYNDROME
A tenosynovitis of the abductor pollicis longus and extensor pollicis brevis tendons

History
- History of repetitive thumb movements
- Reports a "sticking" sensation in the thumb when moving it

Physical Examination
- Pain and edema over the radial styloid
- Exacerbated with active wrist ulnar deviation
- Difficulty moving the thumb and wrist when performing activities that involve grasping or pinching
- Positive Finkelstein test

DUPUYTREN CONTRACTURE
A progressive nodularity and flexion contracture of the palmar fascia and digital flexors in the hand

History
- Occurs slowly over years; usually seen in people over the age of 50
- Use of tobacco and alcohol
- History of diabetes

Physical Examination
- Commonly affects the fourth and fifth digits
- Inability to completely straighten the affected finger(s)
- Nodules present on flexor tendons on the palmar side of the hand

- Without intervention, can progress to skin puckering and flexion contracture of the MCP and PIP joints

GOUT

An inflammatory arthritis associated with high levels of serum uric acid that then crystalizes and deposits into the synovial fluid

History
- Commonly seen in middle-aged men
- History of alcohol use and diets high in purines
- Acute onset with no known injury

Physical Examination
- Red, inflamed, exquisitely tender joint; most often the thumb, great toe, or knee
- Joint discomfort that lasts several weeks
- Limited ROM in the affected joint
- Joint aspiration analysis positive for monosodium urate crystals
- Possible elevation in serum erythrocyte sedimentation rate (ESR) and C-reactive protein (CRP) during acute attack
- Elevation of serum uric acid

LATERAL EPICONDYLITIS (TENNIS ELBOW)

An inflammation and eventual chronic degeneration of the common extensor bundle on the lateral elbow

History
- History of repetitive wrist extension
- Reports pain that may radiate from the lateral side of the elbow into the forearm and wrist

Physical Examination
- Pain over the lateral epicondyle of the humerus with activation of wrist extensors; pain worse when shaking hands, squeezing objects, holding the wrist stiff, or moving the wrist with force
- Decreased grip strength
- Positive Cozen test

LEGG–CALVE–PERTHES DISEASES

This occurs when the blood supply to the femoral head is temporarily severed, then eventually restored. Over time, this causes bone weakening and breakdown, causing the round, ball-like femoral head to lose its shape.

History
- Typically affects boys aged 4 to 10
- Pain in the groin, hip, thigh, or anterior knee
- Reports stiffness in the hip joint
- Family history of Legg–Calve–Perthes

Physical Examination
- Limited ROM in the hip joint
- Patient limping

Considerations
- The cause of Legg–Calve–Perthes is unknown. On imaging, the femoral head will appear mottled and sclerosed.
- Treatment can vary depending on the patient's age and the progression of the disease. Treatments can range from bracing and observation to femoral osteotomy.

MUSCULAR DYSTROPHY
A rare group of diseases that cause muscle weakening

History
- Family history of muscular dystrophy
- Males
- Usually starts in early childhood (before age 5)
- Learning to walk late (older than 18 months)
- Progressive muscle weakness and degeneration

Physical Examination
- Decreased muscle strength
- Difficulty walking; waddling gait, or walking on the toes or balls of the feet
- Difficulty running or jumping due to weakness in leg muscles
- Frequent falls, stumbling, and difficulty climbing stairs
- Difficulty standing from a lying or sitting position
- Reduced endurance
- Enlarged calf muscles
- Gower's sign (**Figure 11.36**)
- May gradually lose the ability to walk and do other everyday activities

Considerations
- Conditions are sex-linked (X-linked) disorders that typically pass from the mother (who has no symptoms) to their son. Girls are rarely affected.
- The average life expectancy is in the early 30s.

OSGOOD–SCHLATTER DISEASE
A condition common in adolescents that can develop when the growth plates are still open and excess force is generated through the patellar tendon to the tibial tuberosity in the area of the growth plate, causing an apophysitis injury

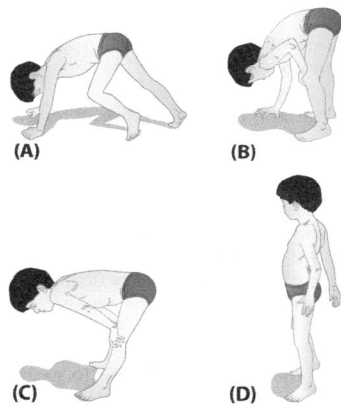

FIGURE 11.36 Gower's sign. In a positive test, the child will move from the hands and knees (**A**), to the hands and feet (**B**), then move the hands to their knees (**C**) to help push themselves to a standing position (**D**).

History
- Common in children and adolescents during puberty
- Reports anterior knee pain, centered over the tibial tubercle or distal patellar tendon
- History of sports participation that involves running, jumping, and swift changes of direction
- Can last from weeks to months
- Pain often worsened during activity and resolves with rest
- Typically unilateral

Physical Examination
- Painful, bony bump on the tibia just below the knee
- Pain and edema just below the knee over the tibial tuberosity on palpation

Consideration
- Similar injuries can be seen at the inferior pole of the patella (Sinding-Larsen–Johansson disease) and at the calcaneus (Sever disease).

OSTEOARTHRITIS
Wear of the articular cartilage at the end of the long bones or between spinal processes leads to joint space narrowing, osteophyte formation, and sclerosis of the bones.

History
- Often found in older adults
- History of previous trauma or injury
- Pain isolated to single joint
- Pain worse in the morning and improves throughout the day; will often improve with mild to moderate activity
- Worsens with prolonged activity

Physical Examination
- Pain typically with active and passive ROM
- Decreased ROM in the affected joint(s)
- Tenderness to palpation over joint line (if applicable)
- Positive x-ray showing joint cartilage degeneration

OSTEOPOROSIS/OSTEOPENIA
This is a condition that causes the bones to weaken and become porous and brittle, increasing fracture risk. Early stages of bone loss are considered osteopenia. As disease progresses, osteoporosis can develop.

History
- Typically asymptomatic in the beginning
- Diet low in calcium and/or vitamin D
- Females affected more than males
- Menopausal women
- Lack of weightbearing exercise
- Smoking history
- History of fractures
- Taking certain medications such as glucocorticoids, proton pump inhibitors, antiepileptic drugs, medroxyprogesterone acetate, aromatase inhibitors, and androgen-deprivation therapies

Physical Examination
- Loss of height over time
- Bone fracture, often with no associated trauma
- tA t-score <−2.5 (indicates osteoporosis) or between −1.0 and −2.5 (indicates osteopenia) on dual-energy x-ray absorptiometry (DEXA) scan

RADIAL HEAD SUBLUXATION (NURSEMAID'S ELBOW)
Partial dislocation of the head of the radius at the level of the radiohumeral joint

History
- Seen in young children, aged 1 to 4
- History of arm jerking injury motion
- History of a fall while holding onto an object, such as monkey bars

Physical Examination
- Pain is palpated at the elbow or wrist.
- Child will not want to move the arm.
- Child is holding their arm in a flexed and pronated position.

Consideration
- Hyperpronation or a supination-flexion technique may be used to reduce a radial head subluxation. It is easier to reduce the subluxation soon after the injury occurs and can be more difficult to reduce after more time has passed.

RHEUMATOID ARTHRITIS
A chronic autoimmune inflammatory disease affecting the joints; can lead to debilitating pain and deformity, most commonly of the MCP and PIP joints of the hands

History
- More common in women
- Onset typically in middle age
- History of smoking
- Positive family history of rheumatoid arthritis
- Morning stiffness typically lasting more than 1 to 2 hours
- Symptoms ongoing (present for at least 6 weeks)
- Anorexia, fatigue
- Reports pain in three or more joints (smaller joints typically affected first)

Physical Examination
- Tender, warm, edematous joints
- Commonly affects the PIP and MCP joints first
- Firm lumps (rheumatoid nodules) under the skin that form close to joints
- Ulnar deviation of the fingers (later sign)
- Positive rheumatoid factor (RF) and anticyclic citrullinated peptide (anti-CCP) serum levels
- Possible short-term elevation of CRP, possible long-term elevation of ESR

ROTATOR CUFF TEAR
Tear in the rotator cuff muscles, the supraspinatus, infraspinatus, subscapularis, and teres minor

History
- Increased risk with age
- History of traumatic injury or repetitive movements
- Reports pain and weakness with overhead activities
- Described pain as a dull ache
- Often causes significant deficits in completing ADLs

Physical Examination
- Pain affecting the dominant arm
- Pain characterized as a dull ache
- Decreased ROM, including forward flexion and internal and/or external rotation, in the affected arm
- Decreased shoulder strength in the affected arm
- Positive empty can test, external rotation resistance test, and/or lag test

Consideration
- Degenerative tears can be exacerbated insidiously.

SLIPPED CAPITAL FEMORAL EPIPHYSIS

The femoral head of the femur slips backward at the growth plate, causing a shift in the normal alignment of the femoral head of the femur and the neck section of the femur.

History
- Affects boys more often than girls
- Typically occurs in adolescents
- Reports pain in the hip, thigh, or knee
- Usually develops gradually
- Pain worsens with activity

Physical Examination
- Being overweight or obese
- Hip, thigh, or knee pain
- Leg length discrepancy
- Limp
- External rotation of affected leg

Consideration
- The x-ray will have the appearance of ice cream falling off a cone. Treatment is surgical unless the disease has significantly progressed and growth plates are closed. Referral to orthopedics is necessary.

PHYSICAL EXAMINATION DOCUMENTATION

Documentation should include results of inspection, palpation, ROM, strength, reflexes (and/or applicable neuro exam components), and any special tests completed.

EXAMPLE OF NORMAL FINDINGS (BACK EXAM)

No visible deformity of spine, or upper or lower extremities. Scapulae, iliac crests, and gluteal crease symmetric. No visible dermal cysts or hairy patches. No limp or alteration of gait or leg length abnormality. Muscle circumference equal throughout the lower extremities bilaterally. No paraspinal musculature or spinal processes tenderness; no tenderness to percussion of spinous processes. Muscle strength: 5/5 with hip flexion, knee flexion, knee extension, plantar flexion, and dorsiflexion. Toe and heel walking intact. Sensation intact and equal bilaterally in lower extremities throughout to light touch, as well as sharp and dull stimuli. No saddle anesthesia. Spine: flexion: 60°, extension: 30°, lateral bending: 20° bilateral, lateral rotation: 10° bilateral, straight leg test negative bilateral, patellar and Achilles reflexes 2+ symmetric bilaterally.

REFERENCES
References for this chapter draw from Chapter 18, Evidence-Based Assessment of the Musculoskeletal System, of the textbook *Evidence-Based Physical Examination: Best Practices for Health and Well-Being Assessment (Second Edition)*. The references may be accessed in the digital version of the handbook at https://connect .springerpub.com/content/.

12

Evidence-Based Assessment of the Abdomen and Gastrointestinal and Urological Systems

- Assessment of the abdomen requires an understanding of the bony and muscular architecture of the abdomen and the organs, muscles, and structures contained within it.
- Abdominal pain is one of the most common subjective chief concerns. Most individuals with abdominal pain have a benign or self-limiting condition. The initial goal of assessment is to identify individuals with a serious etiology.
- Abdominal pain can be challenging to diagnose due to the non-specific neuroreceptors found in the visceral cavity.
- Abdominal pain can be referred pain from outside the gastrointestinal/genitourinary (GI/GU) system, so other systems should always be considered and ruled out.
- Any painful areas of the abdomen should be examined last to prevent muscle guarding and decrease patient anxiety due to fear of pain during palpation.
- It is important for the clinician to know and understand red flags for the history and physical examination so appropriate referrals including emergency evaluation can be initiated (**Box 12.1**).

SUBJECTIVE HISTORY

COMMON REASONS FOR SEEKING CARE
- Abdominal pain
- Nausea and vomiting
- Diarrhea or constipation
- Urinary problems (dysuria, incontinence)

> ## BOX 12.1 Red Flags in History and Physical Exam
>
> - Arthritis
> - Bilious emesis
> - Deceleration of linear growth
> - Delayed onset of puberty
> - Dysphagia
> - Family history of inflammatory bowel disease, Lynch syndrome, celiac disease, peptic ulcer disease, Barrett's esophagus, or hepatobiliary disease
> - Hematuria
> - Hematemesis
> - Hepatosplenomegaly
> - Nighttime pain or diarrhea
> - Oral ulcers
> - Perianal skin tags/fissures
> - Persistent right upper quadrant or right lower quadrant pain
> - Persistent vomiting or diarrhea
> - Recurrent unexplained fever
> - Rectal bleeding or melena
> - Severe flank pain or groin pain
> - Unexplained anemia
> - Unintentional weight loss

HISTORY OF PRESENT ILLNESS

- **Onset:** When did the symptoms start? What was the individual doing when they became symptomatic? Did this occur suddenly, or has it been developing gradually?
- **Location:** Does the symptom have associated pain or discomfort? If so, where is the discomfort located? Does the pain radiate anywhere?
- **Duration:** How long do the symptoms last? Over what period of time has the abdominal/GI/GU symptom developed? Have these symptoms occurred in the past?
- **Characteristics:** How would you describe the pain? Is it aching, burning, sharp, cramping, squeezing, dull, shooting, stabbing? Does the vomitus have undigested food, partially digested food, bile, or blood? What is the frequency, volume, and consistency (hard/watery/soft/unformed) of the stool? Would you describe the stool as greasy, bulky, foul-smelling, or bloody?
- **Associated symptoms:** Is there any associated fever, nausea/vomiting, diarrhea/constipation, arthritis/arthralgias, rashes, headaches, anorexia, passage of flatus, jaundice, dysuria, urgency

and/or frequency of urination, hematuria, straining, bloating, sense of incomplete evacuation, urinary infection, urinary incontinence, heartburn, early satiety, or weight loss/gain?

- **Aggravating factors:** What actions, activities, types of food, or body positions make the symptoms worse?
- **Relieving factors:** What actions, activities, or body positions decrease the symptoms? If relieved, how long does the relief last?
- **Treatment:** What medications has the individual taken to help with the symptoms, including acid suppressives, laxatives, or over-the-counter (OTC) pain relief? Clarify the dosage and frequency of any medications.
- **Severity:** How severe are the symptoms on a scale of 0 to 10? Do the symptoms interfere with sleep or daily function? Are the symptoms worsening? How often are the symptoms causing you to miss work/school?

HEALTH HISTORY

Past Medical History

- History of GI/GU illnesses throughout the life span
  - History of abdominal or urological surgeries
  - History of *Helicobacter pylori*
  - Last colonoscopy (results, interventions)
  - History of urinary tract infection (UTI) and/or pyelonephritis (any untreated UTIs)
  - Incontinence (current, acute, chronic)
  - Recent, previous, or traumatic vaginal childbirth
  - Pelvic or rectal prolapse
  - Benign prostatic hypertrophy
  - Hematuria
- Comorbidities or risk factors related to GI or urological diseases
  - Chronic diseases (cancers, congenital disorders, autoimmune disorders)
  - Cardiovascular (CV) disease (history of myocardial infarction)
  - Mental health conditions, including substance abuse
  - Diabetes and/or hypertension (HTN)
  - Disability related to mobility
  - Neurologic disease or disorders, including neurogenic bladder
  - Dementia and/or confusion
  - Overweight/obesity
  - Recent illness, trauma, or travel

Medications

- Prescribed and OTC medications or supplements, including dose and frequency
- Recent antibiotic use

Allergies
- Allergies to medications, or seasonal, environmental, and/or food allergies? If yes to being allergic to any substance or environmental trigger, clarify reaction:
  - ○ Nausea, intestinal upset? Vomiting?
  - ○ Skin rashes, itching? Hives?
  - ○ Swelling of tongue, lips, face?

Immunizations
- **Risks for vaccine-preventable illnesses:** Vaccine status (rotavirus, hepatitis A, hepatitis B)

Pediatric Considerations
- **Neonate:** Birth history, meconium passage, intolerance to eating (e.g., vomiting, diarrhea, little interest in eating)
- **Infants:** Breast-/bottle-fed, type of formula (frequency and amount per feeding), introduction of solid food (what kind, when given), other fluid intake
- **Toddlers/young children:** Diapers or toilet-trained, difficulty with toilet training (e.g., methods used, challenges), overflow soiling, retentive posturing during stooling, known food sensitivities, current diet, liquid intake, change in eating patterns
- **All ages:** Where does the child fall for growth and development based on pediatric growth charts? Has the trend been stable or has there been a recent change in the trajectory?

FAMILY HISTORY
- Family history of GI disease (celiac disease, inflammatory bowel disease [IBD], gastroesophageal reflux disease [GERD], eosinophilic esophagitis, liver disease, irritable bowel syndrome [IBS], peptic ulcer disease [PUD], Barrett's esophagus, or hepatobiliary disease)
- Cancer (esophageal, gallbladder, liver, pancreatic, gastric, small intestine, colon, rectal)
- Autoimmune disorders (thyroid disease, diabetes mellitus type 1, IBD)
- Polyposis syndromes (including Lynch syndrome)
- Cystic fibrosis
- Migraines
- Mental health disorders (mild, moderate, or severe anxiety, depression, or mental illness)

SOCIAL HISTORY
- Current dietary patterns, including fiber intake
- Recent change in diet
- Access to healthy food, clean water

- Family dynamics/environment
- Life event stress
- Emotional/behavioral symptoms
- Recent travel out of the country
- Exposure to lakes/streams
- Contact with animals
- Caffeine intake (type, amount, frequency)
- Sexual activity and practices
- Water/fluid intake
- Smoking history/history of tobacco use
- Substance use, including alcohol

REVIEW OF SYSTEMS

- **General:** Fever, fatigue, malaise, anorexia, weight loss, weight gain
- **Cardiovascular:** Chest pain, ankle edema, dyspnea
- **Respiratory:** Shortness of breath, pain with inhalation, cough, history of pneumonia
- **Gastrointestinal:** Abdominal pain, nausea, vomiting, constipation, diarrhea, heartburn, increased abdominal girth, irritable bowel symptoms, and/or dysphagia
- **Genitourinary:** Dysuria, urinary frequency and/or urgency, suprapubic pain, lower back pain (flank pain), hematuria, turbid or cloudy urine, foul-smelling urine, concentrated or dilute urine, nocturia
- **Reproductive:** Vaginal or urethral discharge, dyspareunia, recent or current pregnancy, menstrual history
- **Neurologic:** Memory loss, confusion, disorientation, mental/physical disability, decreased sensation of lower extremities or perineum, decreased reflexes in lower extremities
- **Musculoskeletal:** Back pain, muscle aches, arthritic joints, arthritis pain, history of exercise or back strain
- **Mental health:** Mild, moderate, or severe anxiety, depression, or mental illness

PHYSICAL EXAMINATION

In the abdominal exam, the sequence is inspection, auscultation, percussion, and palpation. Palpation should occur last since there is the possibility that pain can be elicited during this aspect of the exam and can alter the clinical findings that occur following the occurrence of pain.

PREPARATION FOR THE EXAM

- Ensure adequate lighting. Ensure the patient has been adequately draped with the abdomen exposed while maintaining privacy of the genitalia and breasts.

- Ask the patient to empty their bladder prior to the exam, which can help relax the abdominal musculature, maintain comfort, and assist in all elements of the abdominal exam, especially palpation.
- Place the patient in a supine position with their arms at the side and their knees bent. Positioning the patient with the arms above the head can cause tension in the abdominal muscles, making the exam difficult.
- Use of a warm room and stethoscope can also help to relax tense abdominal muscles.

GENERAL SURVEY
- Vital signs, including temperature, pulse rate, respiratory rate, and blood pressure
- Posture and position
- Presence of abdominal guarding and/or evidence of pain (facial expressions, body movements, vital signs)
- Toxic versus nontoxic appearance

INSPECTION
- Use tangential lighting while seated next to the patient to highlight skin characteristics/color, as well as the contour of the abdomen and any underlying organs or masses.
- Inspect the abdomen from the side as well as while looking down at the abdomen for symmetry and contour. Note any jaundice.
- Inspect the contour and the skin for bruises, discoloration, spider angiomas, scars, or lesions. Look for any visible pulsations, dilated abdominal veins, edema, or ascites (**Figure 12.1**).
- Ask the patient to take a deep breath and hold it; this helps to lower the diaphragm and move abdominal organs downward to better assess bulges or masses that may

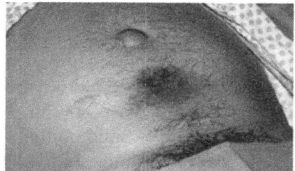

FIGURE 12.1 Cullen's sign.
Source: Image courtesy of Herbert L. Fred, MD and Hendrik A. van Dijk.

not have been previously noted. Ask the patient to raise their head off the exam table, which allows the abdominal muscles to contract and the clinician to assess for previously undetected masses, bulges, or nodules.

AUSCULTATION
- The majority of available evidence does not recommend auscultating bowel sounds.
- Auscultate the abdomen for bruits over the aorta, renal, and femoral arteries (**Figures 12.2** and **12.3**). Normally, no bruits

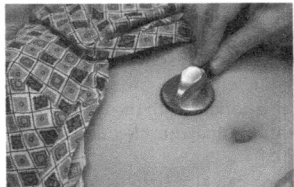

FIGURE 12.2 Auscultation of the abdominal aorta.

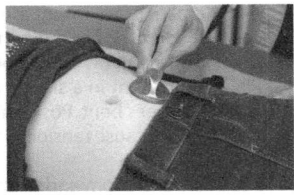

FIGURE 12.3 Auscultation of the renal arteries.

are auscultated. Abdominal bruits (during systole) heard in the epigastric region of the abdomen are likely a normal finding in a healthy person; however, continuous bruits (across systole and diastole) or bruits heard away from the midline are more concerning and deserve a more focused assessment.

PERCUSSION

- Percussion helps assess the size, density, and location of abdominal organs and structures. In addition, percussion can help detect fluid or air in the abdomen. To percuss, place the distal joint and tip of the middle finger of the nondominant hand firmly on the abdomen, avoiding the ribs. Do not place any other

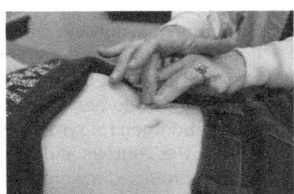

FIGURE 12.4 Abdominal percussion technique.

portion of the hand on the abdomen as this will dampen percussion notes. Use the middle finger of the dominant hand to strike the distal interphalangeal (IP) joint of the stationary finger on the abdomen (**Figure 12.4**). Use short, quick motions while listening for the percussion tone produced from vibration of the underlying organs and structures.
- Percuss lightly in all four quadrants of the abdomen. Generalized tympany is found over the majority of the abdomen due to gas. Dullness occurs over fluid, organs, masses, or distended bladder.

Percussion of the Liver

- Percussion can be used to estimate liver size; however, this technique is a general estimation of the size of the liver, or the liver span. It is often inaccurate due to difficulty of the technique, especially for individuals with breast tissue. Enlargement of the liver associated with hepatitis or ascites may be easier to detect than normal liver size. Current evidence indicates that liver percussion is as accurate as scratch testing. The scratch test, discussed later in this chapter, for identifying the lower liver edge is at least as accurate as percussion and is significantly more effective for young patients. While percussion of the liver may be useful in determining the location of the lower border of the liver, percussion findings should be interpreted with caution.

- Dullness is typically heard over the liver when percussed. To estimate the size or span of the liver, percussion should be used to determine both the lower and upper borders. Start percussion at the right midclavicular line over an area of lung resonance. Percuss at the interspaces between the ribs and move down the right midclavicular line, listening for a change in percussion tones from resonance to dullness. Mark this change in tone associated with the upper border of the liver, typically at the fifth intercostal space (ICS), with a tape or an appropriate writing device. Start percussion at an area of tympany in the abdomen at the right midclavicular line. Percuss upward along the midclavicular line, noting the change from tympany to dullness, and mark this spot associated with the lower border of the liver. Measure the distance between the two marks; the normal liver span at the right midclavicular line is 6 to 12 cm (2–5 inches) at the right midclavicular line.

Percussion of the Spleen

- The spleen is difficult to percuss due to the stomach and intestine, which lie in the abdominal cavity. Listen for dullness of the spleen while percussing just posterior to the left midaxillary line. Splenic dullness may be heard from the sixth to the tenth rib. Dullness at Traube's space (**Figure 12.5**) has been shown to have moderate sensitivity and specificity in association with splenomegaly; however, this finding is less accurate when patients are overweight or obese. There is limited evidence for the use of spleen percussion techniques to rule out splenomegaly (specificity 32.6%–87%, sensitivity 22%–85.7%).

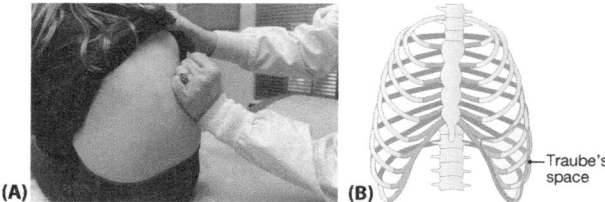

(A) **(B)**

FIGURE 12.5 (**A**) Percussion of the costovertebral angle to assess for tenderness. (**B**) Traube's space. Surface markings: left sixth rib, left midaxillary line, left costal margin.

- The spleen can also be assessed by percussing the lowest ICS in the left anterior axillary line before and after the patient takes a deep breath. Using this method, the area should remain tympanic with the patient's breathing. If the spleen is enlarged, tympany changes to dullness as the spleen moves forward and down with inspiration.

Percussion of the Kidneys
- Percuss the right and left costovertebral angle (CVA) to assess for tenderness or pain, indicating kidney inflammation or musculoskeletal problems. Direct fist percussion, when the clinician directly strikes the CVA using the ulnar surface of the fist, can be used (see **Figure 12.5**). Conversely, indirect fist percussion may be used by placing the palm of the right hand on the back and striking this hand with the ulnar surface of the fist of the left hand.

PALPATION
- Similar to percussion, palpation can be used to assess for masses, tenderness, and fluid in the abdomen. In addition, abdominal organs can be evaluated for size, shape, mobility, and consistency using palpation techniques (**Figure 12.6**).
- Remember to review techniques that allow the patient to relax, especially during the palpation portion of the exam. Pressing too firmly, having cold hands, and/or having used a cold stethoscope may cause the abdominal muscles to tense or cause voluntary guarding to occur, which may interfere with deep palpation. Palpate the painful areas last as examining these areas will cause pain and muscle tension that skew palpation findings.

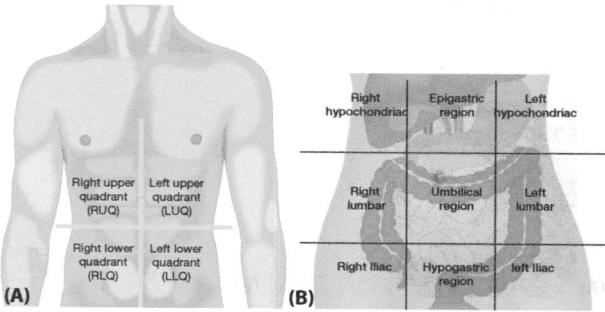

FIGURE 12.6 Quadrants of the abdomen to describe the location and symptoms of pain. (**A**) Four quadrants. (**B**) Nine quadrants.

Light Palpation

- Start with light palpation of the abdomen, moving in a systematic way through all four quadrants (see **Figure 12.6**). The clinician should place the palmar surface of their hand lightly on the abdomen with the fingers outstretched and close together (**Figure 12.7**). Press down on the abdominal wall no more than 1 cm with light palpation. Keep the hands low and parallel to the abdomen; keeping the hands high and pointing downward increases the likelihood of the patient tensing the abdomen. Use a light and circular motion, avoiding disjointed, jabbing, or hurried motions. Pick up the hand when moving to the next area of the abdomen; do not drag the fingers. The abdomen should normally feel soft and smooth.

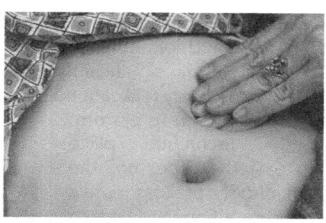

FIGURE 12.7 Abdominal palpation.

Deep Palpation

- Deep palpation requires the clinician to depress the abdomen 5 to 8 cm. Similar to light palpation, move in a systematic way through all four quadrants of the abdomen. Deep palpation can help determine abdominal organs and masses that may not be large enough to detect with light palpation. It also may reveal tenderness not evident with light palpation. When performing deep palpation, note any masses, tenderness, and pulsations.
- Exam findings of guarding, rigidity, rebound tenderness, percussion tenderness, and pain with coughing nearly double the likelihood of peritonitis. Review the Special Tests for the Abdomen section for information on how to elicit rebound tenderness. Rigidity alone makes the diagnosis of peritonitis almost four times as likely.

Liver Palpation

- Because the rib cage covers most of the liver, it is difficult to palpate. Normally, the liver is not palpable, although it may be palpated in thin patients without any underlying disease and in children. Place the left hand under the patient at the 11th and 12th ribs while pressing up in order to elevate the liver toward the abdominal wall. The right hand should be placed on the abdomen, fingers parallel to the midline. Using the right hand, push deeply under the right costal margin. Ask the patient to take a deep breath while trying to feel the edge of the liver as the diaphragm brings it down to the fingertips of the clinician's right hand. If the liver edge is palpated, it should feel smooth, non-tender, and without nodules. A palpable liver edge below the costal margin significantly increases the likelihood of detecting hepatomegaly (+likelihood ratio = 233.7).

- **Scratch test:** To perform this technique, place a stethoscope on the xiphoid process while using a finger to scratch the abdominal surface (**Figure 12.8**). Note differences in sound transmission over solid and hollow organs. When the liver is reached, the

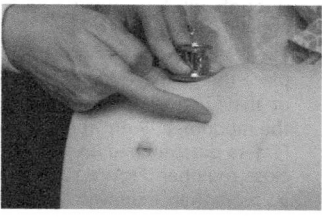

FIGURE 12.8 Scratch test.

sound of the finger scratching the abdominal surface becomes louder. This test has shown high reproducibility and moderate agreement between scratch test findings and ultrasound; obesity can jeopardize results.

Palpation of the Spleen

- There is moderate evidence for the use of palpation tests to confirm an enlarged spleen (specificity 82%–93%, sensitivity 31%–85.6%). Normally, the spleen is not palpable, although approximately 3% of the population have a palpable spleen tip. The

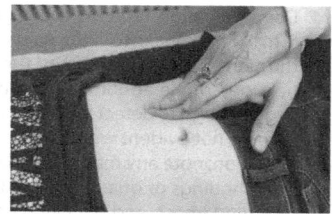

FIGURE 12.9 Palpation of the spleen.

clinician places their left hand across and behind the patient's left side at the CVA, lifting up the spleen (**Figure 12.9**). The right hand is placed on the patient's abdomen below the left costal margin, pressing the fingers toward the spleen. Ask the patient to take a deep breath while attempting to feel the spleen as it comes toward the clinician's fingers. If the spleen is palpable, it is considered an abnormal exam if it is greater than 2 cm below the costal margin. A palpable spleen increases the likelihood of detecting splenomegaly (+LR = 8.5). The spleen must be enlarged three times before it is palpable. See **Table 12.1** for the Hackett's grading system for a palpable spleen.

Palpation of the Kidneys

- To palpate the right kidney, stand at the right side of the patient and place one hand on the patient's right flank and the other

TABLE 12.1 Hackett's Grading System for Palpable Splenomegaly

Grade 0	Spleen is normal and impalpable.
Grade 1	Spleen is palpable only on deep inspiration.
Grade 2	Spleen is palpable on the midclavicular line, halfway between the umbilicus and the costal margin.
Grade 3	Spleen expands toward the umbilicus.
Grade 4	Spleen goes past the umbilicus.
Grade 5	Spleen expands toward the pubis symphysis.

Note: Modest correlation ($r \leq 0.62$, $p < .001$).

hand at the right costal margin. Press the two hands together and ask the patient to take a deep breath (**Figure 12.10A**). The kidney edge may be felt between the fingers or not palpated at all; both findings are normal. To palpate the left kidney, reach across the patient and behind the left flank with the left hand. Press the right hand into the abdomen while asking the patient to inhale (**Figure 12.10B**). Press firmly between the two hands; there should be no change with inhalation.

Palpation of the Aorta

• Palpate the aorta with the opposing thumb and fingers slightly left of the midline in the upper abdomen. As an alternative, assess the width of the aorta by pressing on either side of the aorta in the upper abdomen with one hand on each side of the aorta. The ability to palpate the aorta is related to the size of the aneurysm, but the inability to palpate the aorta is not efficient at ruling out an aneurysm in patients with obesity or in those who cannot relax their abdomen to facilitate the examination. The normal aorta is 2.5 to 4.0 cm wide in the adult.

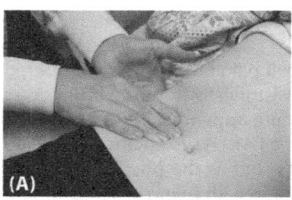 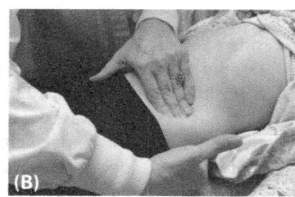

FIGURE 12.10 Palpation of the (**A**) right kidney and (**B**) left kidney.

Palpation of the Gallbladder

- If the gallbladder is palpable during an abdominal exam, this is an abnormal finding. A palpable and tender gallbladder suggests acute cholecystitis and has a positive likelihood of detecting obstruction of the bile ducts (+LR = 26.0). If enlarged, the gallbladder can be felt behind the smooth liver border in the right upper quadrant (RUQ) of the abdomen. Compared with the smooth liver, an enlarged gallbladder feels like a firm mass. If palpable, an inflamed gallbladder is exquisitely tender, making palpation difficult due to abdominal muscle guarding.

SPECIAL TESTS FOR THE ABDOMEN

The following tests are typically considered positive when pain is associated with the maneuver. Therefore, these specialized tests need to be completed last since the pain response may cause peritoneal irritation and could jeopardize any future exam findings. Similar to other clinical exam tests, combinations of findings from the clinical examination are **more powerful** than any single finding.

McBurney's Point

- Pain with palpation of the right lower quadrant (RLQ) of the abdomen indicates a positive McBurney's point (sometimes called McBurney's sign).
- A positive test can be associated with a diagnosis of appendicitis.

Rebound Tenderness or Blumberg's Sign

- Palpate the abdomen by applying slow and steady pressure to the suspected area, followed by abrupt removal of the pressure.
- The test is considered positive if pain is worsened upon release of the hands (vs. application of the pressure) when the underlying structures shift back into place. A positive sign indicates peritoneal irritation. The odds of appendicitis triple in children who exhibit rebound tenderness (LR, 3.0; 95% confidence interval [CI], 2.3–3.9) and reduce the likelihood of its occurrence if rebound tenderness is absent (summary LR, 0.28; 95% CI, 0.14–0.55). The results do not appear as favorable for adults (LR+, 1.59; 95% CI, 1.22–2.06; LR– 0.65; 95% CI, 0.54–0.61) and the test was not found to reliably identify pathology that required intervention.

Rovsing's Sign

- Deeply palpate the left iliac fossa. If pain is felt, this is considered a positive sign (**Figure 12.11**). Historically, a positive Rovsing's sign has been associated with acute appendicitis; it has a sensitivity of 30.1% and a specificity of 84.4%. A systematic review and meta-analysis identified Rovsing's sign as the physical examination finding most strongly associated with ruling in acute appendicitis (LR+ = 3.52, 95% CI, 2.65–4.68).

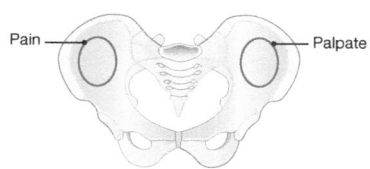

FIGURE 12.11 Rovsing's sign. Location of the iliac fossa and eliciting the Rovsing's sign.

Psoas Test
- With the patient in the supine position, place one hand just above the patient's right knee. Ask the patient to raise their leg while applying downward pressure on the leg (**Figure 12.12**).
- Pain indicates irritation of the psoas muscle due to inflammation of the appendix. Some sources advise that a positive test can indicate a retrocecal (behind the cecum) appendicitis presentation due to retroperitoneal inflammation (LR+ 2.38, 95% CI, 1.21–4.57; LR– 0.90, 95% CI, 0.83–0.86).

Heel Drop Test (Also Called the Markle Test or Heel Jar Test)
- Have the patient stand on their toes and then abruptly release back onto their heels, creating a jarring sensation to the body. Pain in the RLQ is a positive test and contributes information toward a possible diagnosis of appendicitis (LR+ 1.95, 95% CI, 1.51–2.52; LR– 0.48, 95% CI, 0.38–0.61).

Digital Rectal Examination
- Digital rectal examinations (DREs) are sometimes warranted when the patient has a GI or urinary concern. See Chapter 13, Evidence-Based Assessment of the Male Genitalia, Prostate, Rectum, and Anus.

Murphy's Sign
- Place one hand at the costal margin in the RUQ and ask the patient to breathe in deeply (**Figure 12.13**). If the gallbladder is inflamed,

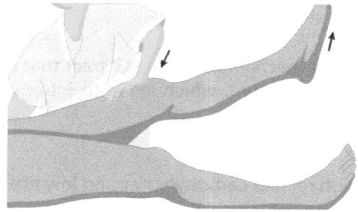

FIGURE 12.12 Psoas test.

the patient will experience RUQ pain upon palpation and will have abrupt cessation of breath (i.e., catch their breath) due to pain as gallbladder descends and contacts the palpating hand.

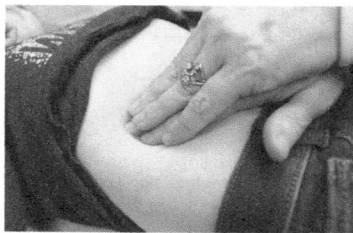

FIGURE 12.13 Murphy's sign.

- Murphy's sign (LR+ 2.8, 95% CI, 0.8–8.6) is considered positive when the patient experiences RUQ pain with palpation. Sensitivity is 80% for a diagnosis of cholecystitis.

PEDIATRIC CONSIDERATIONS

- In the infant, the contour of the abdomen is protuberant due to undeveloped abdominal musculature and may reveal respiratory movement and peristalsis. The liver predominates in the RUQ, and the liver edge may be palpated at the right costal margin or slightly below. The spleen, kidneys, and bladder may be palpated in the infant.
- In children 4 years and older, the liver is still palpable as is the spleen. The liver span is 3.5 cm at age 2 years, 5 cm at age 5 years, and 6 to 7 cm during adolescence. The right and left kidney may also be palpated. Modifications in how the abdominal exam is performed may be necessary in young children.

CONSIDERATIONS FOR THE OLDER ADULT

- Palpation of the abdominal organs may be easier due to thinning of the abdominal wall and weakness of the abdominal musculature.
- The liver is easier to palpate and may be found 1 to 2 cm below the costal margin with inhalation.
- Decreased motility occurs with aging, which in turn means symptoms of gas and distention, as well as tympany upon percussion.

ABNORMAL FINDINGS

CONSTIPATION

Abnormal transport mechanisms of the GI tract that cause slow motility in the intestinal lumen, which leads to infrequent, hard, and difficult-to-pass stools

History
- Diets with high refined carbohydrates and low fiber intake
- History of prolonged laxative use
- Drug usage (e.g., opiates)
- Decreased physical activity

- At least a 3-month duration of symptoms
- Straining with bowel movements
- Hard stool
- Incomplete evacuation
- Fewer than three bowel movements a week

Physical Examination
- Dried, hard, small stools palpated in the rectal cavity
- Mass palpated in the left lower quadrant (LLQ)

Considerations
- Most often, the decreased motility is noted in the large intestines.

DIARRHEA

Abnormal and rapid transport of chyme in the GI tract, causing increased intestinal motility and changes in the osmotic mechanism that results in abnormal absorption, leading to loose, watery stools

History
- Reports loose, watery stools
- Frequent bowel movements
- Cramping due to inflammation
- Increased intestinal motility of the GI tract
- Gas formation
- Can cause dehydration
- Other symptoms may be present based on underlying etiology and can include vomiting, fever, lethargy/malaise, and diffuse abdominal pain

Physical Examination
- Abdominal tenderness may be present or absent.

Considerations
- The rapid transport can be triggered by numerous causes that include bacterial, viral, organic, or functional. Viral gastroenteritis is the most common cause of diarrhea.
- Most often, the episodes are self-limited and resolve within a few days without intervention.
- When the diarrhea is accompanied by high fever and intractable vomiting, dehydration can occur. This complication occurs particularly frequently in children and older adults and can require hospitalization.

ABNORMAL FINDINGS BASED ON LOCATION OF ABDOMINAL PAIN

The location of abdominal pain and tenderness often provides the clinician with valuable insight into possible GI and urological differential diagnoses (**Figure 12.14**).

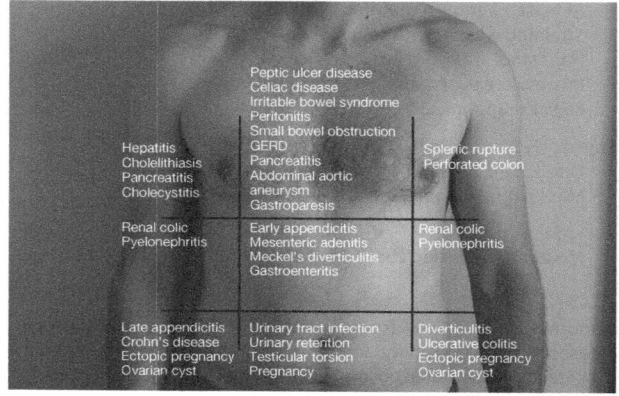

FIGURE 12.14 Differential diagnoses according to localization of pain. GERD, gastroesophageal reflux disease.

RIGHT UPPER QUADRANT PAIN: DUODENUM/ LIVER/GALLBLADDER/PANCREAS

The RUQ of the abdomen has several underlying organs, the dysfunction of which can cause pain and pathology. RUQ pain encompasses a variety of diagnostic possibilities. The most common etiologies are diseases of the liver, gallbladder, or pancreas. A careful history and physical exam can help the clinician differentiate the etiology of the pain, but all underlying structures need to be considered.

Acute Pancreatitis
Inflammation of the pancreas; can be acute or chronic, with symptoms ranging from mild to severe

History
- RUQ or epigastric abdominal pain that is described as piercing/ penetrating
- Pain radiating to the back
- Reported nausea and vomiting

Physical Examination
- Fever
- Tachycardia
- Shallow respirations
- Postural HTN
- Diaphoresis
- Tenderness with palpation of the RUQ

Consideration
- It can be the result of a variety of disorders including gallstones, biliary disease, alcohol abuse, cystic fibrosis, autoimmune diseases, certain heredity diseases, or as a side effect of medication administration.

Cholecystitis/Cholelithiasis
This is an occlusion of the bile duct due to either infection or stones. The term *cystitis* implies infection as a result of bacteria, whereas *lithiasis* refers to any obstruction as a result of stones.

History
- Affects female patients more than male patients; often occurs in the 40s
- Overweight/obese
- Acute, colicky RUQ pain with radiation to the back or right shoulder or epigastric pain
- Anorexia
- Nausea and vomiting
- Sudden and rapidly intensifying pain

Physical Examination
- RUQ abdominal pain and/or epigastric pain on palpation
- Positive Murphy's sign
- Low-grade fever
- Occurrence of jaundice if obstruction is present

Hepatitis
Hepatitis is an inflammatory condition of the liver that often occurs from a viral infection or, in some cases, occurs as a secondary result of medications, drugs, toxins, and alcohol. There are five types of viral hepatitis (A, B, C, D, and E). A different virus is responsible for each type of virally transmitted hepatitis. The history and physical exam findings are different based on the type of hepatitis that is contracted. The signs and symptoms in the list that follows are general for most types of hepatitis but can vary.

History
- Fatigue, flu-like symptoms
- Nausea/vomiting
- Anorexia
- Clay-colored bowel movements
- RUQ abdominal pain
- Dark urine

Physical Examination
- Jaundice
- Low-grade fever
- RUQ pain with palpation

- Palpable liver border on abdominal exam; abnormal liver function tests (LFTs) including alanine aminotransferase (ALT), aspartate aminotransferase (AST), alkaline phosphatase (ALP), bilirubin, albumin, total protein, prothrombin, and gamma-glutamyl transpeptidase (GGT)
- Abnormal hepatitis panel
- Thrombocytopenia
- Jaundice
- Hepatomegaly on ultrasound

RIGHT LOWER QUADRANT PAIN: APPENDIX/ASCENDING COLON

Important to consider in the evaluation of RLQ pain is the potential for radiated or referred pain from a different site or to another part of the body. Pain referred to the back is commonly associated with RLQ pain. Always consider a female GU etiology when a female patient presents with LLQ pain. See Chapter 14, Evidence-Based Assessment of the Breasts, Female Genitalia, and Reproductive System.

Appendicitis

An inflammation of the appendix that can result from a variety of elements that can obstruct the appendix lumen and cause subsequent bacterial growth

History

- Most common between the ages of 10 to 30 years
- Pain initially vague and around the umbilicus, but migrates within hours to RLQ (LR+ 4.81, 95% CI, 3.59–6.44)
- Feeling of constipation
- Nausea/vomiting

Physical Examination

- Low-grade fever (LR+ 3.4, 95% CI, 2.4–4.8; applicable to children only)
- Positive McBurney's point tenderness (RLQ pain)
- Pain with coughing/hopping (LR+ 7.64, 95% CI, 5.94–9.83)
- Rovsing's sign tenderness (LR+ 3.52, 95% CI, 2.65–4.68)
- Rectal tenderness
- Elevated white blood cell (WBC) count
- Positive psoas sign
- A graded compression ultrasound, CT scan, or MRI showing acute appendicitis
- History of SARS-CoV-2 (applicable to children only)

Consideration

- Appendicitis is a surgical emergency and can cause significant morbidity and mortality if not identified early. Perforation, gangrene, and peritonitis can result within the first 36 hours.

Regional Ileitis/Crohn's Disease

An autoimmune, IBD of the terminal ileum, characterized by a sub-acute or chronic necrotizing inflammation and intermittent exacerbations of mucosal inflammation and ulceration

History
- Intermittent, cramping abdominal pain
- Severe diarrhea usually with blood, pus, and mucus
- Fatigue and malaise, arthralgias

Physical Examination
- Fever
- Weight loss
- Decreased hemoglobin and hematocrit; high WBC count
- Elevated erythrocyte sedimental rate (ESR) and C-reactive protein (CRP) levels usually high during exacerbation
- Can affect other body systems
- Low levels of sodium, potassium, chloride and carbon dioxide can be found with chronic diarrhea
- Low albumin and prealbumin levels, but otherwise normal LFTs unless there is concomitant liver damage or poor liver functioning
- Positive hemoccult stool test
- Positive fecal biomarkers, including calprotectin and lactoferrin
- Imaging that indicates thickened bowel wall, areas of inflamed bowel, and potential complications including fistulas, abscesses, and obstructions
- Skip lesions and discrete ulcers on colonoscopy

LEFT UPPER QUADRANT PAIN: SPLEEN/ STOMACH/CARDIAC

Left upper quadrant (LUQ) pain can be associated with splenic, gastric, or cardiac diseases. Always rule out a cardiac etiology when a patient presents with LUQ pain. See Chapter 3, Evidence-Based Assessment of the Heart and Vascular System.

Perforated Colon

An opening that occurs anywhere in the intestinal tract that results in stool contents leaking into the viscera or peritoneal cavity

History
- History of trauma, an abdominal surgery, or swallowing a foreign object (should always be a consideration in young children)
- Possible complication from various disease states such as diverticulitis, IBD, PUD, strangulated hernia, or toxic megacolon
- Reports gradual-onset, but worsening, abdominal pain

- Nausea/vomiting
- Chills

Physical Examination
- Abdominal pain on palpation (location can vary based on affected area)
- Board-like abdomen distention
- Fever

Consideration
- A perforated colon is a surgical emergency.

Splenomegaly/Ruptured Spleen
This refers to enlargement of the spleen due to infections, inflammatory diseases, or neoplasms. Motor vehicle accidents, sports injuries, and fighting are common causes of splenic rupture. Splenic rupture is a medical emergency that causes life-threatening internal bleeding.

History and Physical Findings
Splenomegaly
- Asymptomatic in some
- Pain and/or fullness in the LUQ that can radiate to the left shoulder
- Fatigue
- Frequent infections
- Anemia
- Ultrasound or scintigraphy showing splenomegaly (both imaging tests should be used if the diagnosis is an important clinical concern)

Splenic Rupture
- Often occurs due to blunt trauma or injury
- Reports lightheadedness and dizziness
- Sudden-onset abdominal pain
- Splenomegaly and/or tenderness in the LUQ on abdominal exam
- Hemodynamic instability
- Confusion

LEFT LOWER QUADRANT PAIN: DESCENDING COLON
LLQ pain is usually associated with diseases originating in the descending colon or sigmoid colon region.

Sigmoid Diverticulosis/Diverticulitis
Diverticulosis is the herniation or outpouching of the walls of the colon. This herniation creates small pouches. When these pouches fill with food particles or feces, it causes inflammation and/or the bacteria count to increase, causing infection.

History
- LLQ pain, occasionally abdominal pain can be in RLQ
- History of chronic constipation or, less commonly, diarrhea
- Nausea/vomiting

Physical Examination
- Fever
- Tenderness to the LLQ abdominal quadrant with palpation
- Leukocytosis

Ulcerative Colitis
An autoimmune disorder that can affect any area of the large colon and is characterized by intermittent inflammation and ulceration of the colon mucosal lining

History
- Periods of exacerbations and remissions
- Urgency when having bowel movement
- Abdominal pain, often in the LLQ
- Diarrhea with blood or pus
- Can affect other systems (symptoms include arthralgias, eye irritation, rashes)

Physical Examination
- Weight loss
- LLQ abdominal pain with palpation
- Rectal pain and bleeding
- Anemia
- Stool cultures with WBCs
- Cobblestoning on colonoscopy
- In severe cases, signs of systemic toxicity including fever, tachycardia, anemia, elevated ESR, and rapid weight loss

PERIUMBILICAL/EPIGASTRIC PAIN: STOMACH/ TRANSVERSE COLON/AORTA
Epigastric or periumbilical pain is a very common concern of discomfort stemming from digestive structures, but cardiac differentials should always be considered.

Abdominal Aortic Aneurysm
Abdominal aortic aneurysm (AAA) should be considered and ruled out when abdominal pain is in the epigastric area as it can be a life-threatening condition. See Chapter 3, Evidence-Based Assessment of the Heart and Vascular System.

Celiac Disease

This is an autoimmune disorder with strong genetic predisposition where the ingestion of gluten leads to damage of the small intestinal wall, eventually leading to malabsorption of all nutrients.

History
- Constipation, diarrhea, bloating, flatulence
- Depression
- Fatigue
- More than half the adults with celiac disease with signs and symptoms unrelated to the digestive system, including arthralgias; loss of bone density (osteoporosis) or softening of the bone (osteomalacia); itchy, blistery skin rash (dermatitis herpetiformis); mouth ulcers; headaches and fatigue; nervous system injury, including numbness and tingling in the feet and hands; possible problems with balance; and cognitive impairment

Physical Examination
- Weight loss
- Iron deficiency anemia
- Pain with palpation of the abdomen (diffuse or in the epigastric region)
- May have abnormal celiac disease antibody tests, including tissue transglutaminase antibody, deaminated gliadin peptide antibodies, antiendomysial antibodies, antireticulin antibodies, and quantitative immunoglobulin A
- Shortened or flattened intestinal villi seen on endoscopy, which is the gold standard test for diagnosis

Consideration
- Children with celiac disease are more likely than adults to have digestive problems.

Gastroparesis

Gastroparesis occurs when peristalsis of the intestinal tract is delayed or has stopped working completely. The cause of gastroparesis is typically unknown but can be due to an underlying condition (e.g., diabetes, past surgeries) or a causative agent (e.g., medications).

History and Physical Findings
- Severe abdominal pain primarily in the upper or central midline abdomen, described as cramping or sickening
- Persistent nausea and vomiting
- Anorexia
- Abdominal bloating
- Fullness after eating just a few bites
- GERD

- Weight loss and malnutrition
- Variability in blood sugar levels

Gastroesophageal Reflux Disease/Dyspepsia
A condition in which stomach acid flows back into the esophagus due to the inadequate closure of the lower esophageal sphincter; often called *heartburn, ingestion, or reflux*

History
- A burning sensation in the chest (heartburn), usually after eating; symptoms worse at night in supine position; worse after meals and with certain foods and medications
- Chest pain
- Difficulty swallowing, globus sensation
- Abdominal bloating, regurgitation of food or sour liquid
- Certain medications including theophylline, dopamine, diazepam, calcium channel blockers, anticholinergics, and opioids
- Triggers including caffeine, alcohol, chocolate, or fatty foods
- Relieved with antacids
- Tobacco use
- Pregnancy
- Hiatal hernia

Physical Examination
- Pain with palpation of the epigastric area
- Negative *H. pylori* test
- Cough, hoarseness

Irritable Bowel Syndrome
A functional bowel (motility) disorder characterized by intermittent, mild to severe abdominal pain with a change in bowel habits

History
- Recurrent abdominal pain, at least 1 day/week in the last 3 months, with an altered bowel pattern
- Diarrhea, constipation, alternating diarrhea and constipation
- Bowel movements that generally occur during waking hours, most often in the morning or after meals
- Abdominal bloating, increased gas production (belching and/or flatulence)
- Exacerbated with emotional stress and/or eating
- Abdominal pain relieved with defecation
- Periods of exacerbations and remissions
- Mucus in the stool
- History of food intolerances or sensitivities

Physical Examination
- Diffuse abdominal pain with palpation

Considerations
* The cause is unknown but can be associated with other conditions, such as celiac disease, parasitic infection, or IBDs.
* The Rome IV criteria are the most widely used diagnostic criteria.

Peptic Ulcer Disease
An inflammation and ultimate ulceration of the stomach or duodenal lining

History
* History of chronic use of nonsteroidal anti-inflammatory drugs (NSAIDs)
* Asymptomatic in some
* Abdominal pain, often in the epigastric region, but can be in the LUQ or RUQ of the abdomen
* Pain described as gnawing or burning, can radiate to the back, and worsens with immediate food intake (gastric) or 2 to 5 hours after food intake (duodenal)
* Heartburn, belching, bloating, and nausea

Physical Examination
* Pain with palpation of the epigastric area of the abdomen
* Positive guaiac test and *H. pylori* testing
* Gastroduodenal lesions found on endoscopy

Considerations
* Some patients may initially present only with complications like GI bleeding, gastric outlet obstruction, fistulas, and perforation.
* In rare cases, PUD can be due to Zollinger–Ellison syndrome.

Peritonitis
An inflammation of the peritoneal lining of the abdomen as a result of bacterial infection from a perforation in the bowel or as a result of surgical contamination

History
* History of advanced cirrhosis
* Diffuse abdominal pain

Physical Examination
* Fever
* Guarding, rebound tenderness
* Rigidity and distention of abdomen
* Altered mental state
* Leukocytosis

Consideration
* Spontaneous bacterial peritonitis primarily occurs in patients with advanced cirrhosis. It usually manifests with severe abdominal pain and is considered a medical emergency, requiring

immediate intervention. If it is not found early in the course of infection, shock ensues, rapidly followed by multisystem organ failure.

Small Bowel Obstruction

A condition that occurs when the normal flow of intraluminal contents is interrupted, causing partial or complete blockage of the GI contents

History

- History of previous abdominal surgery, postoperative adhesions, and hernias
- Stools that have decreased in diameter and frequency
- Abrupt onset of periumbilical abdominal pain; paroxysmal, cramping abdominal pain
- Nausea/vomiting
- Abdominal distention
- Obstipation

Physical Examination

- Dehydration, causing tachycardia, orthostatic hypotension, and reduced urine output
- Abdominal/inguinal hernias on exam

ABNORMAL FINDINGS OF THE URINARY SYSTEM

LOWER URINARY TRACT INFECTION

Infection of the lower urinary tract including the bladder and urethras

History

- Female patients more often affected, older adults can be more susceptible
- Sexually active
- Having a urinary catheter
- Incomplete bladder emptying due to an enlarged prostate, prolapsed bladder or uterus, kidney stones, or pregnancy
- Dysuria (pain often worse at the end of urination), nocturia
- Urinary frequency or urgency
- Suprapubic or lower back pain

Physical Examination

- Gross hematuria
- Appearance of turbid urine
- Low-grade fever
- Urethral discharge (primarily in men)
- Mild abdominal tenderness over the bladder with palpation
- No CVA tenderness

- Positive nitrites, pyuria, and hematuria on urinalysis (sensitivity of 74.02%)
- Positive urine culture result

Consideration
- Gram-negative organisms are most commonly the causative agent in UTIs, with strains of *Escherichia coli* accounting for the majority of cases.

PYELONEPHRITIS
An inflammation and infection of the upper urinary tract involving the renal pelvis and kidney

History
- History of untreated lower UTI
- Sudden onset of systemic symptoms (fever, chills, malaise)
- Urinary frequency or urgency, dysuria
- Unilateral flank pain, abdominal pain
- Nausea/vomiting

Physical Examination
- Gross hematuria
- Unilateral CVA tenderness
- Enlarged kidney (palpable on exam)
- Urinalysis showing pyuria, bacteriuria, and nitrites
- WBC casts on microscopy
- Urine culture (>10,000 CFU/mL of a uropathogen)

Considerations
- An infection of the upper urinary tract is more severe and can have more serious implications than an infection of the lower urinary tract.
- Acute pyelonephritis will classically present as a triad of fever, unilateral flank pain, and nausea or vomiting, but not all symptoms have to be present.

RENAL COLIC (UROLITHIASIS, URETEROLITHIASIS)
An obstructing calculus (renal/kidney stone) within the urinary system that causes severe pain

History
- Sudden-onset, unilateral, severe pain in the flank
- Intermittent, colicky pain (comes in waves and fluctuates in intensity)
- Pain radiating to the lower abdomen, groin, or genitals
- Nausea/vomiting
- Urinary frequency or urgency, dysuria
- Low voided volumes (distal ureteric stones)

Physical Examination
- Positive CVA tenderness
- Pink, red, or brown urine
- Tachycardia
- Patient often pacing and constantly moving due to pain
- Microscopic hematuria

Considerations
- The pain from renal colic is caused by dilation, stretching, and spasm of the ureters.
- Most kidney stones are formed from calcium oxalate. Kidney stones are treated in different ways depending on the location and size of the stones.

URINARY INCONTINENCE

Urinary incontinence is the involuntary leakage of urine. The four main types of incontinence are stress incontinence, urge incontinence, overflow incontinence, and functional incontinence. There can be overlap of two or more of these conditions, called mixed incontinence. See **Table 12.2** for the Historical Symptom Assessment tool.

History
- **Stress incontinence:** History of vaginal childbirth; being overweight or obese; history of pelvic prolapse; pregnancy; loss of urine when sneezing, laughing, coughing, jumping, exercising, or increasing abdominal pressure
- **Urge incontinence:** History of neurologic disease or injury, history of diabetes, urinary frequency, intense urinary urgency immediately followed by the involuntary loss of urine

TABLE 12.2 Urinary Incontinence: Historical Symptom Assessment

| Symptom | Types of Incontinence | | | |
	Stress	Urge	Mixed	Overflow
Leak with cough, sneeze, exercise	+	−	+	−
Leak with urgency	−	+	+	−
Frequent urination	−	+	+	−
Continuous leakage	−	−	−	+

- **Overflow incontinence:** History of benign prostatic hypertrophy, neurogenic bladder, diabetes, or any other condition that can damage the nerves or bladder; constant or frequent dribbling of urine
- **Functional incontinence:** Dementia, disabilities related to mobility, history of arthritis, diuretic medications, any physical or mental impairment that causes difficulty in effectively getting to the bathroom

Physical Examination
- Exam findings can be highly variable based on the individual, their medical/surgical history, and the type of incontinence they are experiencing.

PHYSICAL EXAMINATION DOCUMENTATION

Documentation should include results of inspection, auscultation, percussion, palpation, and special tests (if applicable).

EXAMPLE OF NORMAL FINDINGS
Abdomen flat. No visible pulsations, masses, or distention. Skin without rashes, lesions, ecchymoses, or scars. No bruits over the aorta, renal, or femoral arteries. Tympany noted on percussion and abdomen nontender to light and deep palpation of all four quadrants. No splenomegaly or hepatomegaly. No inguinal lymphadenopathy. Right and left kidneys nonpalpable. No CVA tenderness bilateral.

EXAMPLE OF ABNORMAL FINDINGS
Abdomen appears slightly distended. No visible pulsations or masses. Skin without rashes, lesions, ecchymoses, or scars. No bruits over the aorta, renal, or femoral arteries. Tympany noted on percussion over gastric bubble. Patient exhibiting abdominal guarding upon start of palpation. Abdomen tender to light palpation, which triggers tenderness at the RLQ between the iliac crest and umbilicus (McBurney's point). Unable to tolerate deep palpation. Muscle rigidity noted, positive rebound tenderness, and positive Rovsing's sign. Positive psoas test, positive heel drop test. No splenomegaly or hepatomegaly. No inguinal lymphadenopathy. Kidneys nonpalpable, nontender with direct percussion.

REFERENCES

References for this chapter draw from Chapter 19, Evidence-Based Assessment of the Abdominal, Gastrointestinal, and Urological Systems, of the textbook *Evidence-Based Physical Examination: Best Practices for Health and Well-Being Assessment (Second Edition)*. The references may be accessed in the digital version of the handbook at https://connect.springerpub.com/.

13

Evidence-Based Assessment of the Male Genitalia, Prostate, Rectum, and Anus

CLINICAL CONSIDERATIONS

- Care should be taken to provide sensitive, affirming, evidence-based assessment and counseling for individuals with respect for gender identity and sexual orientation. It is crucial to recognize that there are populations who are vulnerable to disparities in care related to implicit or unconscious bias and/or reluctance to share information for fear of bias.
- Gender identity can be determined only by the individual; it is imperative that individuals be given the opportunity to provide their preferred name and gender pronouns, and provided access to care that optimizes their overall physical health and emotional well-being.
- Sexual orientation is assessed to determine what preventive care should be recommended; however, the categorization of sexual orientation, for example, heterosexual, gay, lesbian, bisexual, or asexual, does not always predict types of sexual behaviors. Targeted questions regarding behavior, asked without judgment, will help the clinician elicit important information.
- Gender and ethnic disparities significantly influence men's health and wellness. As part of a well visit, assess for normal functioning of the genitourinary (GU) and reproductive systems and health promotion needs.
- Clinical examination of the adult male genitalia is not typically done as part of routine wellness examinations. However, a thorough exam is done for any individual presenting with GU concerns. In addition, genital exams should be performed during all infant and child wellness evisits, with a caregiver present.
- Male GU and anogenital conditions may be inflammatory, infectious, neoplastic, or traumatic in nature, or can be associated with developmental changes. For example, sexual function and testosterone levels wane during older adulthood; the prostate enlarges throughout a man's lifetime.

SUBJECTIVE HISTORY

COMMON REASONS FOR SEEKING CARE

- Reproductive health and/or sexual health concerns, including exposure to sexually transmitted infections (STIs), penile discharge, or lesions, as well as pubic area rash/itching
- Scrotal pain, swelling, or lesions
- Inguinal or groin swelling

HISTORY OF PRESENT ILLNESS

- **Onset:** When did the symptoms start? Are the symptoms recent? How did the symptoms begin?
- **Location:** Specific location of the symptoms?
- **Duration:** Are the symptoms persistent or transitory? Increasing or unchanged?
- **Characteristics:** How would you describe the symptoms? Is there itching, burning, discharge, pain, swelling, bruising, or redness?
- **Aggravating factors:** Worse with exercise, movement, activity, or straining? Are the symptoms associated with sexual activity?
- **Relieving factors:** What actions or activities decrease the symptoms?
- **Treatment:** What medications has the individual taken to help with the symptoms? Clarify the dosage and frequency of over-the-counter (OTC) and prescribed medications.
- **Severity:** How severe are the symptoms on a scale of 0 to 10?

HEALTH HISTORY

- Clinicians who establish trust, remain open-minded, and are careful about using unassuming language find that patients willingly share the information needed to provide evidence-based, sensitive, high-quality care that supports their health and well-being.

Script for Health History Assessment

Key health and well-being assessments pertinent to sexual orientation and gender identity, including past medical history, family, and social history, are included in the script that follows. This script can be adapted for age and gender identity and is intended to be inclusive of LGBTQIA+ populations. Note that the information being assessed includes all components of a health history.

Hello, my name is ____. How do you like to be addressed?

All individuals should have the opportunity to state their name and preferred pronouns.

Tell me about your health history. Have you ever been diagnosed with a chronic condition? Have you had surgery? Any hospitalizations? Do you take any prescribed medications? Over-the-counter medications?

Assessing past medical and surgical history should be conducted in a similar way for all patients, regardless of sexual orientation and/or gender identity.

Where do you live? Does anyone live in the home with you? Is your housing safe and stable?

Assessing social determinants of health is imperative, especially for individuals who identify with vulnerable minority groups.

To understand whether you have any inherited health risks, could you tell me about your biological parents' health? Any cancers, heart disease, diabetes ... ?

It may be important to ask specifically about genetic relationships, as many LGBTQIA+ people have chosen families that are not genetically related.

How is your relationship with your family of origin? Are they supportive of you? Who are your best supports?

Assessing family and social support systems is a key component of health assessment.

Do you now or have you ever smoked tobacco? Do you drink alcohol? Any past or present drug use?

Screening all patients for tobacco, alcohol, and drug use is an evidence-based priority.

Tell me about your gender identity.

It is important to allow the person the space to explain their identity to you, but you may need to ask specifically whether the person identifies as female, male, nonbinary, or some other description.

These follow-up questions are especially important for nonbinary, transgender, and gender fluid individuals:

Tell me about your gender journey. When did you first realize your identity differed from your sex assigned at birth? What steps have you taken to affirm your gender identity?

Allow the individual to share their history. Options include, but are not limited to, using a different name and/or gender pronoun, as well as changes in physical appearance, medical treatment, and/or surgical treatment; include dates of initiation of medical treatments such as puberty suppressors and hormones.

What organs were present at birth?

An organ inventory should be done to determine what organs the person has or had, including breast tissue, cervix, uterus, ovaries, penis, testes, prostate, and so forth. It should be performed for all patients, as cisgender people may also have had surgeries that alter their reproductive organs.

What organs are present currently?

Assess for surgical removal of the cervix, uterus, ovaries, breast tissue, penis, and testes.

Are organs enhanced with hormones?

Examples include clitoral tissue and breast tissue.

Are organs enhanced with surgery?

Examples include breast augmentation, vaginoplasty, facial feminization, metoidioplasty, phalloplasty, and testicular implants.

Have you shared your identity with friends? Family? Partners? School? Work?

Responses to these questions provide information related to social, family, community, and professional support and/or concerns.

Do you have safe access to bathroom facilities?

Urinary stasis from holding the bladder for extended periods of time is a risk factor for urinary tract infections (UTIs). This question also assesses for environmental safety.

Do you tuck?

Tucking is the process of moving the penis and testes between the legs to conceal the organs; this may be accomplished by wearing tight clothing or using some type of binder or strap. Sometimes, the testes are pressed up into the inguinal canal, risking incarceration/strangulation. *Escherichia coli* UTIs are more common in individuals who tuck.

Do you bind?

Binding is the process of flattening breast tissue so that the chest appears more masculine. This is typically achieved with medical-grade binders and can cause fungal infections and skin breakdown.

Do you need help changing legal documents to align with your identity?

Know where to refer patients, such as www.lambdalegal.org.

Are you sexually active? Do you have a regular partner?

Sexual health screening is a key assessment for all individuals.

How do you identify sexually? What is your sexual orientation?

If the person does not understand, provide options, such as "Do you identify as straight, gay, lesbian, bisexual, or something else?"

In order to know which screenings would benefit you, can you tell me with whom you have sex? What parts of your body do you use when having sex? How do your partners identify their gender and sexual orientation?

If the person does not understand, provide options, such as "Do you have sex with women, men, both? Are your partners cisgendered? Do you participate in oral sex (receptive/insertive), oral–vaginal contact, oral–anal contact, anal sex (receptive/insertive), vaginal sex (receptive/insertive)? Do you use shared sex toys or have any type of genital-to-genital contact?" Note: For individuals who identify as transgender, it may be important to first ask about "triggering" labels for body parts; for example, an individual who identifies as transgender male may prefer to use the term *frontal canal* instead of *vagina*, and may find that the term *vagina* triggers feelings of gender dysphoria. Reflecting preferred labels or terms within sexual health history questions is most appropriate.

Are you in a relationship?

Not all people who are sexually active, even with regular partners, are in a relationship, and a relationship is not always exclusively between two people.

Is your relationship open or closed?

Some relationships have consensual agreements that partners have other sexual partners outside of the relationship. Some relationships are between multiple people, rather than two.

Are you satisfied with your sexual function?

This is a key assessment for all individuals.

How do you protect yourself from STIs?

If using barrier protection such as condoms, ask "Do you wear protection 100% of the time? Are barriers used for oral–genital contact?"

When was the last time you had STI screening?

This is a key assessment related to sexual health for all individuals.

Do you use drugs or alcohol when having sex? Do you exchange sex for money, drugs, or a place to stay?

These questions are intended to identify behaviors and situations that increase risks to health and well-being.

Do you desire to have biological children? Do you desire pregnancy?

For transgender patients, also ask whether they desire to have preserved fertility, such as cryopreservation of sperm and eggs, prior to starting hormonal or surgical transition. This issue is especially complicated in individuals on puberty blockers as they are never exposed to natal hormones necessary for gamete development.

Have you felt isolated, trapped, or like you are walking on eggshells in an intimate relationship? Has someone pressured or forced you to do something sexual that you didn't want to do? Has someone hit, kicked, punched, or otherwise hurt you?

Screen for intimate partner violence, as well as past and/or current history of physical, sexual, emotional, economic, or verbal abuse.

REVIEW OF SYSTEMS

- **General/dermatologic:** Recent illness, weight loss, lesions or rashes, fever, chills
- **Head, eyes, ears, nose, throat:** Oral lesions, eye drainage or redness, pharyngitis
- **Lymphatic:** Lymphadenopathy, tender lymph nodes in the groin area
- **Cardiovascular/respiratory:** Chest pain, edema, dyspnea, cough
- **Gastrointestinal:** Localized pain, change in bowel habits, blood in the stool, pain with defecation, dyschezia

> **BOX 13.1** Red Flags in Subjective History That Indicate Possible Testicular Torsion
>
> - Sudden onset of testicular pain and swelling
> - Transverse testicular lie
> - Nausea, vomiting
> - Acute abdominal pain (which may be the presenting symptom in children and adolescents)

- **Genitourinary:** Urinary frequency, dysuria, weak urinary stream, "dribbling," urinary frequency, nocturia, hematuria, rectal bleeding, rectal pain, anal itching
- **Musculoskeletal:** Back pain, myalgias
- **Neurologic/mental health:** Worry; sadness, helplessness, hopelessness; fatigue or insomnia; change in mood, stress, coping; healthy lifestyle behaviors

RED FLAGS IN SUBJECTIVE HISTORY

- Testicular torsion occurs when a testicle rotates, twisting the spermatic cord and causing ischemia. Emergency surgery is required to preserve the viability of the testicle. **Box 13.1** includes a summary list of symptoms.

PHYSICAL EXAMINATION

- Maintain patient modesty by exposing the patient's groin and anogenital region only as required.
- Genital examination can be performed with the patient supine or sitting; the ideal approach is the patient standing with the clinician in a sitting position to best assess for hernia or testicular abnormalities.
- Anorectal examination can be performed with the male in a side-lying position with their hips and knees flexed.

INSPECTION

- Inspect the skin of the groin, pubis, penis, scrotum, and perineum for rashes, lesions, discoloration, or swelling. Note whether the penis is circumcised or uncircumcised. When adults present with GU concerns, retract the prepuce (foreskin) of the uncircumcised penis to inspect the glans and urethral meatus. Phimosis, inability to retract the foreskin, is normal during infancy and childhood and should not be forcefully retracted (**Figure 13.1**).
- Gently compress the glans penis between the thumb and the first finger to inspect for patency, inflammation, or urethral discharge.
- Following the genital examination, inspect the anus for skin tags, fissures, hemorrhoids, or other skin lesions.

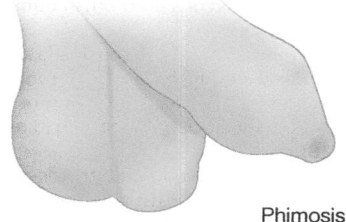

Phimosis

FIGURE 13.1 Phimosis.

PALPATION

- Palpate the shaft of the penis for nodules, plaques, or other soft tissue masses. The index or middle finger of the clinician's hand should be placed posteriorly while the thumb of the same hand is placed anteriorly.
- The testis should be gently palpated for nodules, hard masses, and abnormal shape. A normal testis should feel smooth, ovoid, and nontender. Palpate the epididymis along the posterior aspect of the testis and up along the spermatic cord. Note any swelling or soft tissue masses within the scrotal sac, epididymis, or spermatic cord.
- Palpate the inguinal nodes for enlargement and/or tenderness, especially when evaluating for concern of infection or malignancy of the genitalia.

ADDITIONAL ASSESSMENTS FOR SPECIFIC CONDITIONS

Cremasteric Reflex

- Attempt to elicit the cremasteric reflex when evaluating for certain testicular concerns that cause scrotal pain. The reflex is triggered by stroking the inner thigh with the index and middle finger. An intact reflex will cause the ipsilateral cremaster muscle to contract, thereby raising the testis. In some conditions, like testicular torsion, the cremasteric reflex will be negative because the cremaster muscles surrounding the spermatic cord are twisted and unable to contract.
- The absence of the cremasteric reflex for patients presenting with scrotal pain is a useful sign, indicating the need for emergent evaluation.

Transillumination

- Transillumination evaluates the scrotal sac for concerns such as scrotal swelling. Perform the procedure by dimming the lights of the exam room and shining a bright light (e.g., penlight, otoscope) through the wall of the scrotum. Fluid will illuminate; soft tissue masses will not.

Assessment for Hernia

- An hernia is a protrusion of a body organ through the wall of the cavity that contains it.
- An inguinal hernia occurs when there is a fascial defect in the inguinal canal that allows the bowel to protrude through the deep inguinal ring (indirect inguinal hernia; **Figure 13.2A**) and sometimes through the superficial inguinal ring (direct inguinal hernia; **Figure 13.2B**).
- When the bowel protrudes through the deep inguinal ring and becomes entrapped, it is considered an incarcerated inguinal hernia. If the bowel cannot be reduced (pushed back into the abdominal cavity), emergent surgery is required to preserve viability of the bowel. A femoral hernia, or direct inguinal hernia, enters the inguinal canal via a defect inferior to the deep inguinal ring.
- The examination for inguinal hernia should be performed with the patient in standing position and the clinician in a seated position facing the patient. With a gloved index or middle finger, gather loose skin from the scrotum and invaginate the scrotal sac with the finger upward along the inguinal canal until the external ring is reached (**Figure 13.3**).
- Ask the patient to cough or bear down as when making a bowel movement. If an hernia is present, a bulging sensation can be palpated/felt at the tip of the finger. While the patient bears down, also observe the inguinal area for bulging over the femoral canal that can indicate a femoral hernia.

Digital Rectal Examination

- Digital rectal examination (DRE) can be performed to evaluate the lower rectum and prostate. DRE is indicated for men presenting with concerns of abdominal, anal, or perianal pain; rectal bleeding or unexplained blood in the stool; unexplained weight loss; abnormal mass in the anus or rectum; significant change in bowel or bladder habits (incontinence or constipation); change in urinary

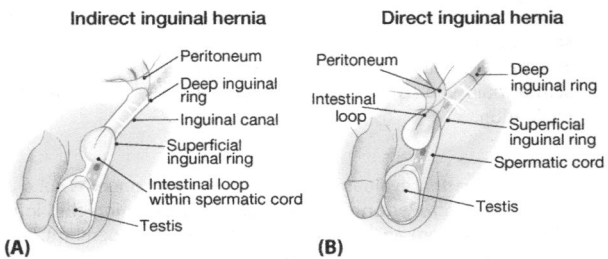

FIGURE 13.2 Inguinal hernias. (**A**) Indirect. (**B**) Direct.

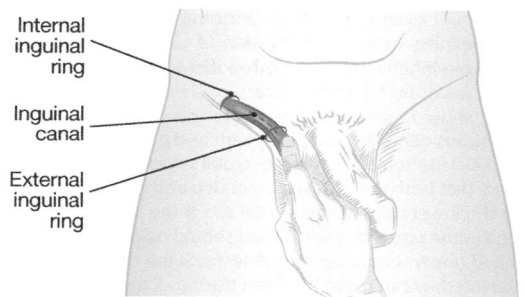

Internal
inguinal
ring

Inguinal
canal

External
inguinal
ring

FIGURE 13.3 Technique for assessing inguinal hernias.

stream; and/or urethral discharge or bleeding. Otherwise, DRE is not performed as a routine element of male wellness examinations.

- The patient should be unclothed from the waist down and in a gown and/or covered with a drape. The ideal positioning for the examination is either with the male standing with a forward bend at the waist or side-lying with their knees to the chest. Separate the buttocks and inspect for fissures, hemorrhoids, bleeding, skin tags, and rashes.
- Lubricate the index or middle finger of a gloved hand. Inform the patient that a finger will be inserted into the rectum. Ask the patient to take a deep breath and relax and breathe out while gently inserting the examining finger into the anal canal.
- Palpate the prostate anteriorly, noting the size, symmetry, and texture. A normal prostate is walnut-sized, symmetrical, and smooth with a cartilaginous texture (similar to the tip of the nose). The prostate has a midline groove (sulcus) that should be palpable.
- Rotate the finger 360° to palpate the span of the rectal wall for masses or irregularities. Stool may be palpated in the rectal vault; note consistency (hard or soft). Assess anal tone by asking the patient to tighten their anal sphincter on the finger. Once the patient relaxes, withdraw the finger and inspect for blood, stool, or mucus. Redrape the patient, provide tissues or cleansing cloths, and allow privacy so they can clean up and get dressed.

PEDIATRIC CONSIDERATIONS

- The anogenital examination of the infant or child should be performed with a caregiver present. If the caregiver is unable to be present, another healthcare clinician (chaperone) should be present. Some states have mandatory chaperone laws; it is important for clinicians to know their respective state laws. For adolescents, a chaperone can be a caregiver or another healthcare clinician, but this should be the adolescent's choice.

- Routine GU exams should be performed during all infant and child wellness exams. The foreskin of uncircumcised newborns and young infants may be tightly adhered to the glans penis and should never be forcefully retracted. The newborn exam, in particular, should include inspection for congenital malformations, ambiguous genitalia, and placement and patency of the anus.
- The clinician should palpate the scrotal sac for soft tissue masses to ensure that both testes have descended and can be brought down into the lower third of the scrotal sac. If the testis cannot be palpated in the scrotum, the clinician should palpate the inguinal canal and upper scrotal sac for the testis. Some testes are "retractile," meaning they can move between the inguinal canal and scrotum. A retractile testis can be located and brought down into the lower third of the scrotum. Retractile testes should resolve by puberty.
- For adolescents, the genital examination can produce anxiety. Adolescents can be unsure whether their developing bodies are "normal," and they have a greater need for modesty and privacy. Assessment of adolescent genitalia is similar to that for adults, except the clinician should assess for sexual maturity (Tanner staging). See Chapter 17, Evidence-Based Considerations for Assessment Across the Life Span to review assessment of sexual maturity and pubertal development.

CONSIDERATIONS FOR OLDER ADULTS

- Assess for physiologic changes in older adults, as sexual function wanes during older adulthood and erectile dysfunction becomes increasingly common. Pubic hair thins, the scrotum becomes more pendulous, and orgasms may develop more slowly. Testosterone levels decline. The prostate enlarges slowly throughout a man's lifetime, potentially leading to restriction or blockage of urine flow through the urethra. The risk of benign prostatic hypertrophy and prostate cancer increases with age.
- DRE has low sensitivity and specificity for detecting prostate cancer. The decision to screen for prostate cancer with prostate-specific antigen (PSA) testing must be individualized and evidence-based, as new recommendations about life expectancy and risks become available.

RED FLAGS IN OBJECTIVE EXAM

- Patients who present with urinary symptoms, including dysuria, frequency, straining, hesitancy, or urgency of urination, urinary incontinence, and/or erectile dysfunction should have an exam to evaluate for GU disorders, including bladder cancer, testicular cancer, prostatitis, and prostate cancer. Red flags indicating serious urological disorders are listed in **Box 13.2**.

> **BOX 13.2** Red Flags in Objective Exam That Are Indications of Serious Urological Disorders
>
> - Hematuria
> - Palpable bladder
> - Fever and flank pain or tenderness
> - Penile discharge and/or lesions
> - Painless testicular lump
> - Exquisite tenderness of a testicle
> - Exquisite tenderness of the prostate
> - Nodularity of the prostate
> - Loss of anal reflex
> - Loss of cremasteric reflex
> - Loss of bowel or bladder control

ABNORMAL FINDINGS

CONGENITAL OR DEVELOPMENTAL ABNORMALITIES

Anorectal Agenesis/Imperforate Anus

This is a congenital anorectal malformation in which there is an absence of or abnormal location of the anal opening. Not always readily evident on exam, the key finding is failure of the newborn to pass meconium within the first 24 to 48 hours following birth. Imperforate anus can be part of a cluster of findings of a more complex congenital syndrome. Surgical correction is required.

Epispadias and Hypospadias

Hypospadias is a congenital malformation of the male GU tract in which the urethral opening is abnormally located on the ventral aspect of the penis. Similarly, but less commonly, epispadias is an abnormal dorsal placement of the urethral meatus.

History
- Abnormal spraying during urination

Physical Examination
- Urethral meatus located on the glans, penile shaft, scrotum, or perineum

Consideration
- Varies in severity

Hydrocele

Hydrocele is a collection of peritoneal fluid in the scrotal sac resulting from a fascial defect in the inguinal canal. All males have this defect at some point during gestation, but when it persists it allows peritoneal fluid to travel back and forth. This can be normal up to 1 to 2 years of age.

History
- Painless scrotal swelling (unilateral or bilateral) that may fluctuate in size

Physical Examination
- Transillumination of the scrotum can be helpful in the diagnosis. Peritoneal fluid will illuminate in the scrotal sac, while bowel tissue will not.

Considerations
- Hydroceles that persist beyond 1 to 2 years of age require surgical correction.
- In older children and adults, a hydrocele can be idiopathic or develop secondary to infection, inflammation, trauma, or malignancy.

Phimosis/Paraphimosis

Phimosis is a condition in which the foreskin of an uncircumcised penis cannot be retracted over the glans. This condition (**Figure 13.1**) can be physiologic or pathologic. Physiologic phimosis occurs in almost all newborn males due to naturally occurring adhesions between the foreskin and the glans penis. The adhesions spontaneously resolve over time with intermittent erections and foreskin retraction. Physiologic phimosis is expected to resolve prior to puberty, but usually by age 3. Key findings of physiologic phimosis can vary from an inability to retract the foreskin far enough to view the urethral meatus to an inability to retract the foreskin fully past the corona of the glans penis. Pathologic phimosis is acquired as a result of distal scarring of the prepuce due to infection or inflammation. The key finding is a contracted fibrous ring around the opening of the distal prepuce with an inability to retract the foreskin. Pathologic phimosis requires medical treatment.

Paraphimosis is a condition that results from forcefully retracting tight foreskin back over the glans penis. The foreskin becomes entrapped behind the corona of the glans. Key signs and symptoms include painful swelling of the distal glans penis with a constricted band of tissue proximal to the corona. Paraphimosis is a medical emergency because it will eventually result in tissue ischemia and necrosis.

Testicular Torsion

Testicular torsion occurs when a testicle rotates, twisting the spermatic cord and causing ischemia.

History

- Review the "red flags" listed in **Box 13.1.**
- Symptoms include sudden onset of testicular pain and swelling.

Physical Examination

- Absent cremasteric reflex
- Transverse lie

Consideration

- A medical emergency; can result in testicular ischemia within 6 to 12 hours

Undescended Testes

History

- The testis fails to descend into the lower third of the scrotum by 4 months of age.

Physical Examination

- The testis may be located in the intra-abdominal space (cryptorchidism), the inguinal canal, or the upper third of the scrotum.

Consideration

- Surgical correction is required to preserve fertility and decrease the risk of testicular cancer.

Varicocele

Varicocele is a collection of dilated twisted veins surrounding the spermatic cord that typically occurs in the left hemiscrotum.

History

- Scrotal sac has a "bag of worms" texture and appearance (**Figure 13.4**).
- Most are asymptomatic, but some will present with a dull ache.

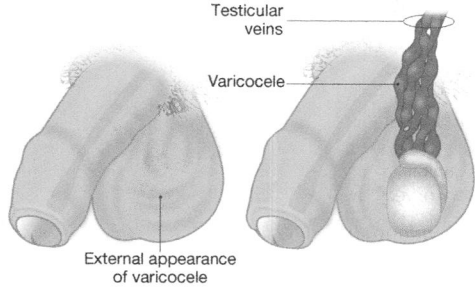

FIGURE 13.4 Varicocele.

Physical Examination
- Palpable testicular veins worsen with increased venous pressure (e.g., standing or performing Valsalva).

Consideration
- It does not require intervention unless there is atrophy of the testicle, which can lead to infertility.

INFECTION OR INFLAMMATORY DISORDERS

Balanitis and Balanoposthitis

Balanitis describes an inflammation of the glans penis, while balanoposthitis describes an inflammation of the glans penis and foreskin in uncircumcised males. Key signs and symptoms can include genital itching, pain, dysuria, exudate, erythema, swelling of the glans or the foreskin, foul odor, and phimosis. Causes include poor hygiene and infectious agents like STIs and other bacterial, fungal, and viral organisms.

Epididymitis, Orchitis, and Scrotal Cellulitis

Acute epididymitis is a clinical syndrome involving pain, swelling, and inflammation of the epididymis that can last up to 6 weeks. When the testis is also affected, it is referred to as *epididymo-orchitis* or *orchitis*. Scrotal cellulitis of the scrotum is an infection of the dermis of the scrotal tissue, which occurs from bacterial entry via a break in the integrity of the epidermal barrier. Scrotal cellulitis presents with scrotal pain, swelling, and inflammation (**Figure 13.5**). Urgent medical treatment is required to prevent an abscess or gangrene.

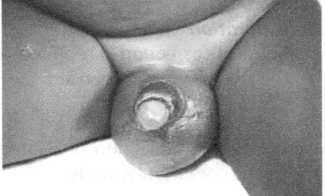

FIGURE 13.5 Scrotal cellulitis.
Source: Centers for Disease Control and Prevention/Robert S. Craig.

Male Genital Candidiasis

History
- Itchy genital rash caused by fungal or yeast infection

Physical Examination
- Potentially fissured, erythematous rash (**Figure 13.6**)

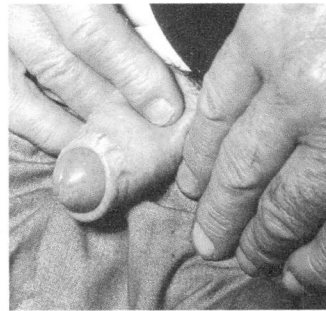

FIGURE 13.6 Male genital candidiasis.
Source: Centers for Disease Control and Prevention/Brian Hill.

- White, curd-like exudate possible, especially in uncircumcised males
- Can affect the glans, foreskin, scrotum, thighs, gluteal folds, and buttocks

Consideration
- More common among men with diabetes, uncircumcised males, and males with female sex partners with recurrent vaginal yeast infections

Nonspecific Urethritis
Urethritis describes an inflammation of the urethra. It can be caused by chemical irritants but is often a common indicator of STIs in males.

History
- Dysuria, itching, burning, and/or discharge
- Associated with unprotected sex; sexual activity with new partner

Physical Examination
- Erythema and/or discharge at the urethral meatus, which can be clear or purulent (**Figure 13.7**)

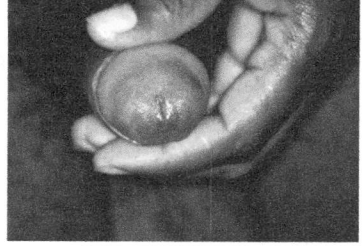

FIGURE 13.7 Nonspecific urethritis.

Considerations
- Purulent penile discharge is often associated with chlamydia and/or gonorrhea.
- Although secondary causes may exist, infectious organisms are the most common cause.

Sexually Transmitted Infections
History
- Discharge, burning with urination, itching
- May be asymptomatic
- Unprotected sex, increased risk with less than 100% condom use

Physical Examination
- Urethritis, urethral discharge
- May have associated inguinal lymphadenopathy, tenderness
- May have skin changes, including inflamed, erosive papules (scabies), vesicles/ulcers (herpes), chancre (syphilis), or genital warts (human papillomavirus [HPV])

Considerations

* Gonorrhea and chlamydia are the most common bacterial causes of STIs.
* HPV is the most common STI. There are numerous types of HPV; many types are associated with cancers, some are associated with genital warts or condyloma (**Figure 13.8**).

OTHER ABNORMALITIES OF MALE GENITALIA

Manifestations of Systemic Conditions

Systemic conditions can cause dermatologic symptoms in the male genitalia. In particular, reactive arthritis can manifest in part as vesicles and crusted plaques on the penis. Chronic, generalized pruritus and dermatologic changes can signify an underlying systemic disease; disorders such as connective tissue disease, lichen planus, seborrheic dermatitis, lichen sclerosus, atopic dermatitis, and psoriasis cause cutaneous findings.

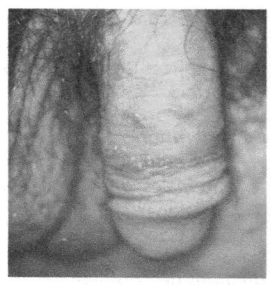

FIGURE 13.8 Condyloma. Note the presence of soft, wart-like growths about the penile shaft, known as *condylomata acuminate* or *anogenital warts*. *Source:* Centers for Disease Control and Prevention/MF Rein, MD.

Peyronie Disease

A condition in which dorsal fibrous plaques alter penile anatomy and impair function; etiology unknown but likely multifactorial and related to a postinflammatory healing process

History

* Penile curvature or deformity
* Erectile penile shortening
* Penile pain and sexual dysfunction
* Risk factors including genital injuries, urethral instrumentation, and prostatectomy

Physical Examination

* Penile curvature, nodules

Considerations

* Noncancerous, fibrous tissue causing curvature is likely scar tissue.
* Pain during erections usually improves within 1 to 2 years.

Skin Cancer

History

* The first sign of penile cancer is often skin change in the foreskin, glans penis, or penile shaft.

- Key symptoms may include thickening of skin, changes in skin color, and ulcers.

Physical Examination
- Well-defined, velvety red plaques
- Lesions or skin changes with or without lymphadenopathy

Consideration
- Initial assessment and evaluation should be guided on the likelihood of whether an infection or malignancy is more likely. While penile cancer is rare, 95% are squamous cell carcinomas.

Testicular Tumor/Malignancy
History
- Solid, firm lump within the testicle; often painless
- Males with history of cryptorchidism (undescended testicle) at increased risk

Physical Examination
- Solid, firm mass within the testes
- Testicular mass on scrotal ultrasound

Considerations
- The average age at time of diagnosis is 33 years old.
- Testicular cancer is not uncommon.

PROSTATE, RECTAL, OR ANAL ABNORMALITIES
Anal Fissures
An anal fissure is a small tear in the mucosal lining of the anus.

History
- Key symptoms can include bleeding or pain with bowel movements.

Physical Examination
- Visible cracks are seen in the skin around the anus.

Considerations
- Risk increases with history of constipation or straining during bowel movements.
- Risk increases with anal penetration during sexual intercourse.

External and Internal Hemorrhoids
Enlarged, bulging veins of the distal rectum and anus

History
- Painless, bright-red bleeding with bowel movements, anal itching, acute onset of perianal pain, and/or fecal soiling
- Risk factors including family history of hemorrhoids, obesity, pregnancy, chronic constipation, and straining with bowel movements

Physical Examination

- Erythema and tenderness of anal tissue and/or rectal mucosa; hemorrhoids may prolapse outside the anal sphincter.
- Internal hemorrhoids are located in the distal rectum.
- External hemorrhoids are located within the anus.

Consideration

- Acute onset of perianal pain may be indicative of a thrombosed hemorrhoid.

Prostate Cancer

Cancer of the prostate gland is typically detected at an asymptomatic stage. Key signs of prostate cancer include abnormal finding of the prostate on DRE, that is, nodules or asymmetry, and/or elevated PSA levels. PSA is not specific for prostate cancer, however, and can be elevated in other conditions. Abnormal DRE or urinary/rectal symptoms warrant further investigation.

Prostatic Enlargement

An enlargement of the prostate gland, which becomes more common as men age (**Figure 13.9**)

History

- Urinary frequency, impaired flow, weak urine stream, nocturia, urinary dribbling post urination

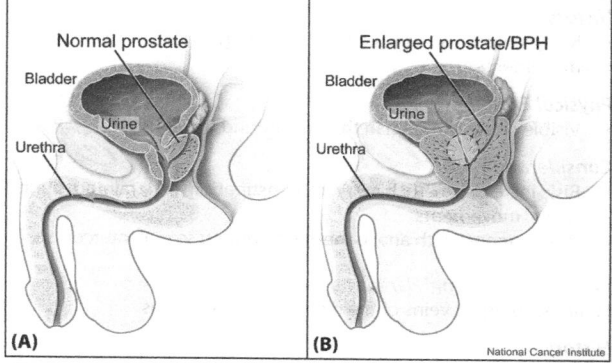

FIGURE 13.9 Benign prostatic hyperplasia. (**A**) Flow of urine with a normal prostate and (**B**) with an enlarged prostate/benign prostatic hyperplasia (BPH).
Source: Image courtesy of National Cancer Institute.

Physical Examination
- Normal anal sphincter tone
- Nontender prostate, no palpable distinct nodules

Considerations
- Medications may contribute to symptoms (e.g., antihistamines, decongestants, diuretics).
- Comorbidities also contribute to symptoms (diabetes, heart failure, prostate or bladder cancer).

Rectal Polyps and Rectal Cancer
Rectal polyps refer to a protrusion of the rectal mucosa into the lumen of the rectum. Hyperplastic polyps can be precancerous. Nearly all colon and rectal cancers begin as polyps.

History
- Usually asymptomatic
- May have persistent bowel pattern changes (diarrhea, constipation, or narrow stools)

Physical Examination
- Palpable rectal mass
- Occult or frank blood in the stool

Consideration
- Polyps are usually asymptomatic but may ulcerate and bleed if they become enlarged and obstruct the colon. Polyps can be benign, inflammatory lesions or neoplastic lesions. Inflammatory polyps are an endoscopic physical finding of inflammatory bowel disease like Crohn's disease or ulcerative colitis. Neoplastic polyps are an endoscopic physical finding of rectal cancer.

PHYSICAL EXAMINATION DOCUMENTATION

Documentation should include results of inspection, palpation, and special tests.

EXAMPLE OF NORMAL FINDINGS
No palpable inguinal hernias or lymphadenopathy. Scrotal sacs pendulous without swelling, tenderness, palpable masses, discoloration, or lesions. Penis without erythema, lesions, tenderness, or urethral discharge. Anus no hemorrhoids, fissures, or lesions. Rectal wall intact, no masses or tenderness. Prostate smooth, without palpable nodules or enlargement.

EXAMPLE OF ABNORMAL FINDINGS: ADOLESCENT MALE
Mild tenderness and lymphadenopathy of two inguinal nodes, right groin. No skin changes or lesions noted. Scrotum without tenderness

or palpable masses. Mucopurulent penile discharge; lab specimen of urethral discharge obtained and sent for sexually transmitted infection (STI) testing. No penile lesions or tenderness. Rectal exam deferred. Tanner stage 4.

REFERENCES

References for this chapter draw from Chapter 20, Evidence-Based Assessment of Sexual Orientation and Gender Identity, and Chapter 22, Evidence-Based Assessment of the Male Genitalia, Prostate, Rectum, and Anus, of the textbook *Evidence-Based Physical Examination: Best Practices for Health and Well-Being Assessment (Second Edition)*. The references may be accessed in the digital version of the handbook at https://connect.springerpub.com/.

14

Evidence-Based Assessment of the Breasts, Female Genitalia, and Reproductive System

CLINICAL CONSIDERATIONS

- The personal nature of discussions about sexual and reproductive health requires recognition that populations are vulnerable to disparities in care related to implicit or unconscious bias. Care should be taken to provide sensitive assessment using respectful terminology and counseling for individuals with respect for gender identity and sexual orientation.

- Consider conducting the health history while the patient's clothes are on. Sitting naked on an exam table under a flimsy gown increases the likelihood of the patient feeling vulnerable.

- Always carefully and fully listen when patients share concerns about breast/chest lumps or masses, even when the clinical level of suspicion is low. Regardless of age, gender, or positive/negative family history of cancer, the presence of a breast mass should never be dismissed.

- Ideally, patients should have an opportunity to speak with a clinician privately, without anyone else in the room. Sometimes practices have a policy to meet with a patient alone. Discussion can include review of whether clinical breast exam (CBE), vaginal/cervical inspection, or pelvic exam is warranted.

- A wellness exam or a well-woman examination includes a comprehensive, thorough, evidence-based history and physical examination. Testing to consider includes Pap and human papillomavirus (HPV) testing; sexually transmitted infection (STI) screening; wet prep; and breast, ovarian, endometrial, cervical, and colon cancer screening.

- For the individual who presents with reproductive or sexual health concerns, a sensitive, patient-centered, detailed history will inform what physical exam needs to be done.

- Understanding the anatomy and physiology of the female genitourinary (GU) and reproductive systems, menstrual cycle, and reproductive life span is key to providing sexual and reproductive health guidance.

SUBJECTIVE HISTORY

COMMON REASONS FOR SEEKING CARE

- Well-woman exam
- Vaginal discharge, itching
- Menstrual cycle irregularities, including amenorrhea, heavy menstrual bleeding
- Pelvic pain, dysmenorrhea
- Breast lump, breast pain

HISTORY OF PRESENT ILLNESS

- **Onset:** When did the symptoms start? Are the symptoms recent? How did the symptoms begin?
- **Location:** Specific location of the symptoms: vaginal, suprapubic, lower abdomen, adnexal, umbilical; highly localized (the patient can point to one place) versus a more generalized discomfort or pain that moves around? Specific area of a breast or axilla, or bilateral breast symptoms?
- **Duration:** Are the symptoms persistent or transitory? Increasing or unchanged?
- **Characteristics:** Describe the symptoms. Is there itching, burning, discharge, odor, changes in urination, changes in menstrual cycle, cramping, pain, and/or tenderness? If pain or tenderness, is the pain burning, stinging, sharp, dull, throbbing, or causing a feeling of heaviness or bloating? Any associated changes in skin or lymph nodes?
- **Aggravating factors:** Are symptoms associated with sexual activity? Menstrual cycle? Traumatic event? Urination?
- **Relieving factors:** What actions or activities decrease the symptoms?
- **Treatment:** What medications has the individual taken to help with the symptoms? Clarify the dosage and frequency of over-the-counter (OTC) and prescribed medications.
- **Severity:** How severe are the symptoms on a scale of 0 to 10? Do the symptoms limit participation in activities at work, school, or home?

HEALTH HISTORY

- Clinicians who establish trust, remain open-minded, and are careful about using unassuming language find that patients willingly share the information needed to provide evidence-based, sensitive, high-quality care that supports their health and well-being.
- Review the script provided in Chapter 13, Evidence-Based Assessment of the Male Genitalia, Prostate, Rectum, and Anus, as an example of how to ask assessment questions related to gender identity and reproductive and sexual health. The script can be adapted for all populations, including LGBTQIA+ individuals.
- For a comprehensive wellness exam or well-woman exam, include assessment of menstrual, gynecologic, obstetric, and sexual health, as well as past medical, family, and social history.

Menstrual History
- **Date of last menstrual period:** If cycles are irregular, date of last normal menstrual period
- **Regularity of menstrual cycle:** Description of any irregularities (e.g., spotting between cycles, missed periods); cycle length (from the first day of one to the first day of the next)
- **Duration of flow:** Irregularities related to bleeding (e.g., heavy bleeding, spotting)
- **Symptoms that accompany menstruation:** Breast tenderness or pain, dysmenorrhea or cramping, headaches, nausea
- Age of menarche (first episode of menstruation), and last menstrual cycle if postmenopausal

Gynecologic History
- Breast history
  - Current or previous malignant or nonmalignant conditions
  - Breastfeeding history (chestfeeding history)
  - Presence of breast implants, including length of time, type, and complications
  - Self-exam concerns, practices
  - Last mammogram
- Gynecologic history
  - Last pelvic examination
  - Last Pap test
    - History of abnormal Pap testing
    - Treatment related to abnormal Pap testing (i.e., loop electrosurgical excision procedure [LEEP] or cone biopsy)
    - Last HPV testing and result
- History of STI, noting when and how it was treated
- Gynecologic surgery, including year and rationale
- Fertility or infertility treatment
- Exposure to diethylstilbestrol

Obstetric History
- The obstetric history tells the story of every pregnancy that an individual has had. The clinician should document the year and duration of each pregnancy (in weeks), the method of delivery, and any complications during or after the pregnancy for the mother and the infant. It is important to obtain details about each child born (e.g., gender, weight, current condition of each child today). The GTPAL system is used to summarize these assessment findings.
  - **Gravida:** Number of pregnancies
  - **Term:** Number of full-term births (≥37 weeks' gestation)
  - **Preterm:** Number of preterm births (≥20 weeks' gestation, <37 weeks' gestation)

- ○ **Abortions:** Number of abortions (spontaneous, elective, ectopic) <20 weeks' gestation
- ○ **Living:** Number of living children

SEXUAL HISTORY

Sexual history is an opportunity for the clinician to acknowledge the importance of sexuality, relationships, and sexual behavior to one's overall health. This part of the exam should not be limited to a disease-oriented perspective, but should provide an opportunity to further the patient–clinician relationship and support behaviors that encourage sexual health across the life span. Assess the six Ps as listed:

1. **Partners:** Currently sexually active, ever sexually active; number of recent partners, number of partners in the last year, lifetime partners; gender of partners
2. **Practices:** Genital (vaginal, penile), oral, anal
3. **Protection from STIs:** Use of condoms or other protection against STIs, typical use, comfort level in discussing protection with partner
4. **Past history of STIs:** Diagnosis, treatment, recurrent symptoms; ever tested for STIs including HIV; status of partner(s)
5. **Pregnancy prevention:** Assessment of reproductive life plan (e.g., desire for pregnancy, use of family planning methods, currently attempting to be pregnant or avoid pregnancy, partner support, and need for contraception or fertility counseling)
6. **Plus additional questions:** Allowing time for questions about sexual health, which may include necessary screenings, intimacy, or sexual expression

Past Health History
- Hospitalizations, surgeries, ED visits
- Hypertension, cardiovascular disease, stroke, clotting disorders
- Cancer; treatment with chemotherapeutics, radiation
- Diabetes, insulin resistance, polycystic ovarian syndrome (PCOS)
- Endocrine or autoimmune disorders, including thyroid disorders
- Anxiety, depression, trauma, or mental health disorders

Medications
- Prescribed and OTC medications or supplements, including dose and frequency

Allergies
- Allergies to medications, or seasonal, environmental, and/or food allergies? If yes, clarify reactions.

Preventive Health Behaviors
- Physical activity and exercise
- Typical diet; nutritional concerns

- Sleep and rest; concerns or disorders
- Stress and coping
- Vaccine history

FAMILY HISTORY
- Breast, ovarian, cervical, colon cancers
- Genetic disorders or congenital malformations; recurrent pregnancy losses
- Diabetes, hypertension, heart disease
- Preeclampsia

SOCIAL HISTORY
- Review social determinants of health (SDOH)
- Home situation
  - Married/single/divorced/widowed/partnered?
  - Who lives in the home? Is partner supportive?
  - Is housing/home/neighborhood safe? Risk or current victim of violence?
- Substance use
  - Tobacco use? If yes, assess smoking history, readiness to quit.
  - Alcohol use? If yes, screen for binge drinking, problematic use.
  - Other substances (e.g., medications not prescribed, illicit drugs)?
- Occupation or school safety
  - Exposure to hazards (e.g., fumes, radiation, chemicals, viruses)
  - Stress, anxiety, burnout related to workplace culture, school, or work expectations

REVIEW OF SYSTEMS
- **General/endocrine:** Recent illness, weight loss or gain, fever, chills, hair loss, acne, facial hair, night sweats, hot flashes
- **Head, eyes, ears, nose, throat:** Headaches, changes in vision, congestion, pharyngitis, oral lesions
- **Lymphatic:** Lymphadenopathy, tender lymph nodes in the axillae or groin area
- **Cardiovascular/respiratory:** Chest pain, edema, dyspnea, cough
- **Breasts/dermatologic**: Nipple discharge, skin lesions or rashes, pruritus, palpable lumps, pain or tenderness, breast fullness
- **Gastrointestinal:** Nausea, vomiting, localized or generalized abdominal or pelvic pain, change in bowel habits, blood in the stool
- **Genitourinary:** Urinary frequency, dysuria, hematuria, dyspareunia, vaginal or anal itching, painful genital lesions
- **Musculoskeletal**: Back pain, myalgias
- **Neurologic/mental health:** Worry; sadness, helplessness, hopelessness; fatigue or insomnia; change in mood, stress, coping; syncope; history of trauma

RED FLAGS IN SUBJECTIVE HISTORY

- Gynecologic cancers (ovarian, uterine, and cervical cancer) often present with vague and nonspecific symptoms, especially in early stages. Recognize red flag symptoms for prompt referral and treatment (**Box 14.1**).

PHYSICAL EXAMINATION

- For a well-woman examination, a thorough head-to-toe examination is recommended. While this chapter reviews the breast and female genitalia exams only, components of the well-woman exam include assessing the lymphatic, cardiac, respiratory, and integumentary systems, in addition to physical exam of the mouth, throat, thyroid, breasts, abdomen, pelvis, and genitalia.
- The presence of a chaperone during physical examination should be offered to all women, especially when performing breast and/ or pelvic exams, which can be a source of anxiety for women. The clinician's approach should be respectful and caring.

CLINICAL BREAST EXAM

CBE includes visual inspection and palpation of the breasts and axillae. Despite the controversy regarding the population health benefit of CBE for screening breast cancer, considerations for performing the exam include that it may:

- Identify a small proportion of breast malignancies not detected with mammography
- Be requested by an individual who has concerns

BOX 14.1   Red Flags in Subjective History That Indicate Possible Gynecologic Cancers

- Abdominal distention or bloating
- Early satiety with loss of appetite
- Unexplained pelvic or abdominal pain
- Increased urinary urgency or frequency
- Postcoital bleeding
- Postmenopausal bleeding
- Unexplained weight loss or fatigue
- Unexplained change in bowel habits
- Over 50 years of age with new symptoms of irritable bowel syndrome

- Allow for documentation of the presence of palpable masses and cysts in young individuals who are not typical candidates for mammography

Inspection of the Breasts

With the patient sitting and disrobed to the waist, note breast size, shape, and contour. Inspect the breasts and nipples for symmetry. Note any changes to the skin of the breasts, including dimpling, peau d'orange appearance, erythema, or edema. Have the patient raise their arms overhead, place their hands at the hips, and sit with their hands pressed together; observe for a shift in nipple position, as well as significant asymmetry or any unusual dimpling or bulging of breast tissue.

Palpation of the Breasts and Axillae

- Palpate the axillary lymph nodes while the patient is still in a seated position; each arm should be supported while the nodes are palpated. Palpation should be completed with the pads of the fingers, using a fluid, circular motion. Care should be taken to ensure the entire surface area of the lymphatic region is palpated, both lightly and deeply.
- Palpate each breast with the patient in the supine position with one hand above their head. The entire breast is examined from the second to sixth ribs and from the left sternal border to the midaxillary line. Imagine the breast divided into four quadrants with vertical and horizontal lines intersecting at the nipple (**Figure 14.1**). The upper outer quadrant encompasses the axillary tail of breast

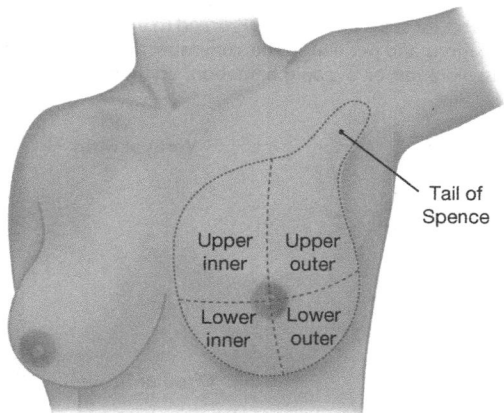

FIGURE 14.1 Breast quadrants. This figure shows the four quadrants of the breast. This anatomic system is commonly used to describe exam findings in breast conditions.

tissue that extends into the axilla. Palpate in all four quadrants of both breasts by compressing breast tissue between the pads of the three middle fingers and the chest wall.

- Proper breast palpation technique entails the use of the finger pads in a continuous rolling, gliding circular motion in the vertical strip, circular, or wedge pattern (**Figure 14.2**). Pressure of the fingers should be varied from light to medium to deep palpation. The areolas and nipples are included inherently in the palpation of the breast; however, nipple expression to assess for nipple discharge is not recommended unless the patient describes spontaneous discharge that requires evaluation.

PHYSICAL EXAMINATION OF THE FEMALE GENITALIA

- This is most commonly performed with the patient in the lithotomy position, a supine position with the legs separated, flexion at the hips and knees, and feet resting in foot rests. Use of optional positioning may be helpful in patients with mobility limitations.
- Regardless of the chosen positioning, attention should be paid to the appropriate draping of the patient during the examination. Care should be taken to preserve modesty and warmth. Ideally, the clinician should drape the patient to ensure eye contact with them throughout the examination.

Inspection and Palpation of the External Genitalia

- Begin with a thorough exam of the external genitalia. Starting with the mons pubis, evaluation should include the pattern and quality of hair distribution on both the mons and the labia majora. Inspect for signs of infection. Proceed to inspection of the skin of the mons and perineum. The skin inspection should evaluate for discoloration or hypopigmentation, erythema, and excoriation.

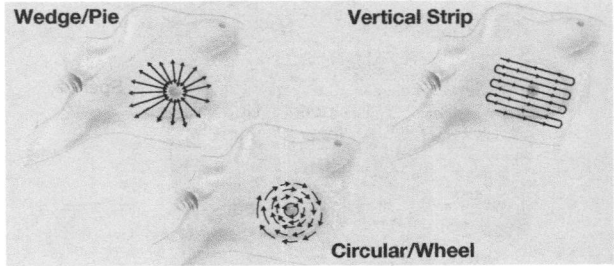

FIGURE 14.2 Breast palpation methods. Breast palpation should be completed in one of these three ways (*clockwise, left to right*): wedge/pie, vertical strip, or circular/wheel. These examination techniques provide a systematic way to ensure the clinician palpates the entire breast.

Note any visible ulcerations, pustules, vesicles, growths, lesions, nevi, varicosities, or scars.

- Evaluate the labia and clitoris for development or atrophy. Inspect the introitus, noting its shape—closed or gaping—in the lithotomy position. The Bartholin and Skene glands should be inspected for swelling and purulent exudates. The perineal body should then be assessed. This area begins with the posterior aspect of the labia and extends to the anus. The inspection of the perineal body should include the items previously described.
- The perianal area should be examined. Inspect for injury, lesions, warts, hemorrhoids, or other abnormalities. Evidence of trauma should prompt further investigation.

Internal Inspection: Speculum Examination

- Performing a speculum examination allows for direct visualization of the cervix and the surrounding vaginal walls. A speculum examination for the sole purpose of screening for STIs is not necessary as other methods for sample collection are available. An appropriately sized speculum should be chosen prior to starting the examination.
- By convention, the speculum examination is performed first, followed by the bimanual examination. The speculum should be warmed with warm water or a warming device. Current recommendations suggest that a small amount (dime-sized) be applied to the introitus and bills of the speculum for ease of insertion.
- Begin by separating the labia with the thumb and the first finger of the nondominant hand for visualization of the introitus. The traditional approach to insertion of the speculum recommends holding the speculum with the bills completely closed facing the lateral aspects of the vagina. With the speculum angled slightly downward, apply gentle pressure toward the coccyx and direct the speculum inward. Avoid a severe downward angle as this will cause the base of the speculum to compress the sensitive structures of the upper genitalia. Upon full insertion of the speculum, rotate the handle of the speculum downward so the bills are in the inferior/superior position and open the speculum for visualization of the cervix. Open the speculum only as wide as needed for visualization. It is not necessary to open it completely.
- An alternative method involves inserting the speculum directly into the vagina with the bills in the inferior/superior position. Application of a gentle downward pressure on the vaginal wall aids in the insertion of the speculum.
- If the clinician has difficulty finding the cervix or determining the appropriately sized speculum to use, consideration should be given to performing a bimanual examination first for assessment of anatomy and position of the cervix.

- Vaginal tissue should be inspected during both insertion and removal of the speculum. If using a plastic speculum, the bills are clear, which can aid in visualization. Use of a metal speculum will require tilting the position of the bills, so visualization of the entirety of the vaginal vault can be performed. The vagina should be inspected for color, tissue appearance, moisture, discharge, moles, or lesions, and any unusual odors should be noted.
- The speculum should be positioned to allow for visualization of the entire surface of the cervix (**Figure 14.3**). Inspection should include the size/shape of the os, color, bleeding or discharge; evaluation of the squamocolumnar junction; and assessment for any lesions or growths. Normal cervical variations are depicted in **Figure 14.4**.

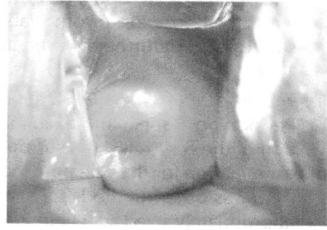

FIGURE 14.3 Cervix as viewed using a speculum.

- Carefully complete the collection of endocervical and cervical cells

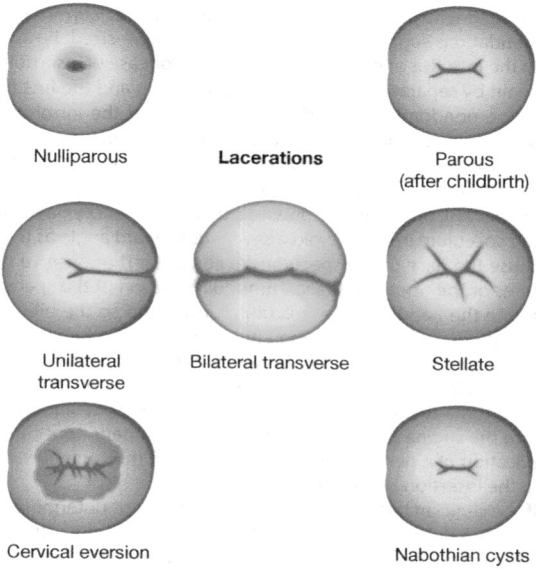

Nulliparous	**Lacerations**	Parous (after childbirth)
Unilateral transverse	Bilateral transverse	Stellate
Cervical eversion		Nabothian cysts

FIGURE 14.4 Normal variations of the cervical os.

(**Figure 14.5**) by meticulously following the technique recommended. This is required if an adequate specimen is to be evaluated for cellular changes. These techniques vary depending on the collection tools used.

- Upon completion of the inspection of the cervix and collection of necessary specimens, the speculum lock should be released and the speculum should be opened slightly while simultaneously drawing upward with the handle of the speculum, following the same plane used with insertion. This allows the bills of the speculum to release the cervix. A final inspection of the vaginal walls should be performed if needed. The bills of the speculum should be allowed to fall closed naturally, which avoids pinching the vaginal tissue and labia in the bills. Gently remove the speculum from the vagina.

Palpation: Bimanual Exam
- The bimanual examination is performed to assess the uterus and adnexa. The index and the middle finger of the dominant hand are lubricated with a water-soluble lubricant and inserted into the vagina until the cervix is palpable, moving the fingers to the posterior fornix, located below the cervix. Take care to tuck the thumb out of the way to avoid compressing the sensitive structures of the pubic symphysis, mons pubis, and clitoris.
- The clinician should place the same leg as the dominant hand on the step of the examination table, leaning forward slightly so weight is shifted forward a bit. The nondominant hand is placed on the lower abdomen, above the pubic symphysis. Using the flat surface of the fingers, a sweeping downward motion toward the internal fingers is used to isolate the uterus. The internal fingers

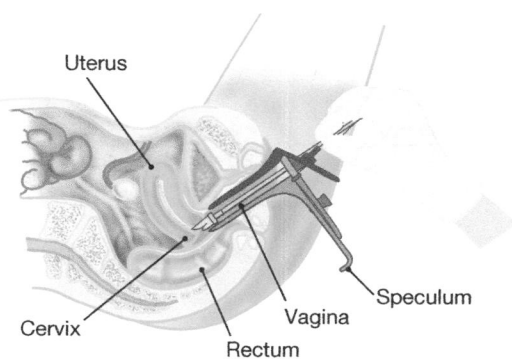

FIGURE 14.5 Collection of cervical specimen for Pap testing.

direct the uterus up to the fingers, gently compressing the uterus. This procedure allows for palpation of the uterine size and position in the pelvis.

- The size, shape, and symmetry of the uterus should be documented, as well as the position and consistency of the uterus. In normal circumstances, palpation of the uterus is not painful; any discomfort should be noted and may warrant further evaluation.
- See **Figure 14.6** for a cross-sectional view of a bimanual examination and **Figure 14.7** to review the normal variations in uterine position.
- Palpation of the adnexa serves to assess the ovaries and fallopian tubes. To assess the right adnexa, shift the internal fingers to the patient's right side, moving the fingers to the right vaginal fornix. The flat surface of the fingers of the nondominant hand is placed just medial to the right anterior superior iliac spine and directed downward to meet the internal fingers. The goal is to capture the adnexa between the internal and external fingers for palpation. The ovary is approximately 3 × 2 cm and is often compared with the size of a walnut. This maneuver is repeated on the left side for assessment of the left adnexa. Documentation should include a description of the size and mobility of the adnexa, as well as consistency.
- Palpation of the ovaries in postmenopausal women is not considered a normal finding; if this should be identified on examination, it requires further evaluation.

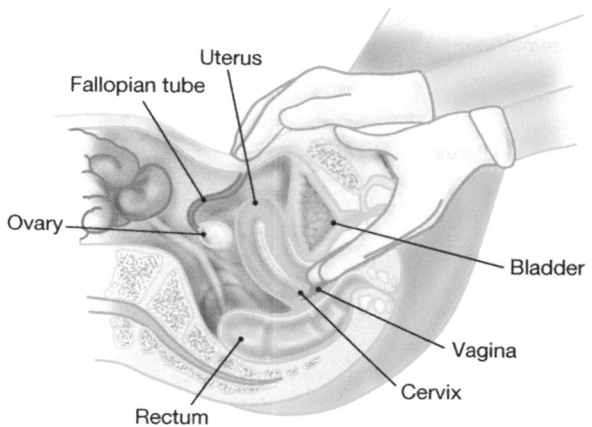

FIGURE 14.6 Bimanual examination.

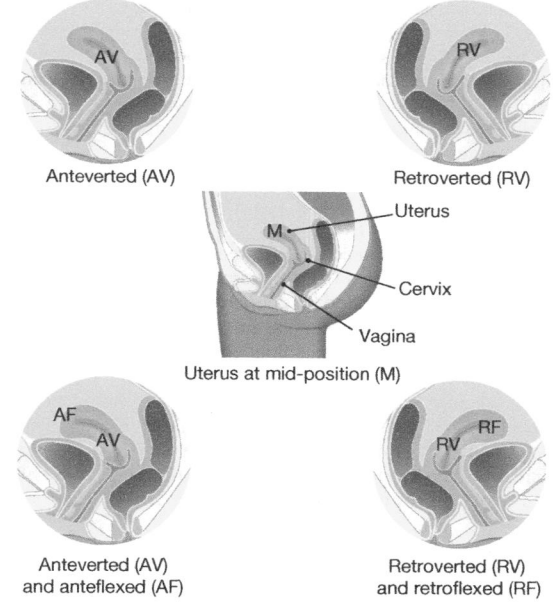

FIGURE 14.7 Normal variations in the position of the uterus.

- Cervical motion tenderness (CMT) is found in several pathologic conditions (e.g., pelvic inflammatory disease [PID], appendicitis, and ectopic pregnancy). It is performed by placing the index and middle fingers on either side of the cervix and gently pulling the cervix to one side, then the other. Pain with traction on the adnexa is a positive CMT. Interrater reliability for CMT is low, but there is still evidence that suggests its clinical significance in assisting with the diagnosis of PID.

Rectovaginal Examination
- Rectovaginal examination (RVE) can be used for additional evaluation, if needed, and is typically performed after bimanual examination is completed. It is used to further assess the uterus, uterosacral ligaments, and rectovaginal septum.
- Clean gloves should be donned prior to completing the RVE. The first finger of the dominant hand is placed into the vagina and the middle finger of the same hand is placed into the rectum.

Gentle upward pressure of the middle finger allows for the assessment of the rectovaginal septum. The uterosacral ligaments can be palpated by locating them along the posterior wall of the cervix, lateral to the sacrum. A retroverted uterus can be examined using this method. Examination should evaluate for any abnormalities, including tenderness, nodules, or apparent thickening or thinning.

LIFE-SPAN AND SPECIAL POPULATION CONSIDERATIONS
Pediatric and Adolescent Exams
- Routine GU exams should be performed during all infant and child wellness examinations. The newborn examination, in particular, should include inspection for congenital malformations, atypical or ambiguous genitalia, and placement and patency of the anus. The pediatric anogenital examination should be performed with a caregiver present.
- For adolescents, a chaperone can be a caregiver or another healthcare clinician, but this should be the adolescent's choice. See Chapter 17, Evidence-Based Considerations for Assessment Across the Life Span, for additional information about assessment of sexual maturity for female adolescents.

Trauma-Informed Care
- Approximately 45% of women in the United States have experienced sexual violence (e.g., rape, sexual coercion, and/or unwanted sexual contact). Before midadolescence, one out of every five girls have been sexually abused. Nearly one in three adult women experience at least one physical assault by a partner during adulthood. Given the significance of this problem, clinicians caring for women of all ages should be aware of the potential for a history of violence or other trauma.
- Trauma-informed care provides a framework for engaging with individuals who have had a history of trauma. There are four basic principles that direct trauma-informed care: an awareness of the prevalence of traumatic events, an ability to recognize the signs and symptoms of trauma, development of policies and practices that integrate knowledge regarding trauma, and avoiding retraumatizing the individual during the history and patient examination.
- The pelvic exam can be an anxiety-inducing experience and is often more problematic for women who have experienced sexual violence. It is important to have an open dialogue with the patient during all portions of the exam. Obtain permission to perform each part of the exam, explaining what the examination entails and the purpose for doing it. Give the patient permission to stop the exam at any time. Identification and a sensitive approach

to individual concerns and needs will strengthen the clinician–patient relationship and allow for appropriate referrals for further assessment, support, and treatment.

Postmenopausal Considerations

The decrease in estrogen levels during the menopause transition results in thinning of the vaginal tissue. This thinning causes decreased elasticity of the tissue, a paler appearance, and more fragile tissue, which can result in vaginal dryness and petechiae. These changes can range from asymptomatic to moderate to severe dyspareunia, vaginal discomfort, and irritation. As a result of these changes, speculum examination may be uncomfortable for the postmenopausal patient. Consider use of water-based lubrication and a speculum of smaller size.

RED FLAGS IN OBJECTIVE EXAM

- The red flags indicating possible breast malignancy are listed in **Box 14.2**. All breast masses require imaging for full evaluation. Regardless of age, gender, or family history of cancer, the presence of a breast mass should never be dismissed.
- The primary screening imaging modality for breast cancer is mammography. Other imaging should be considered on the basis of current evidence available, patient presentation, and breast specialist recommendation.

BOX 14.2   Red Flags in Objective Exam Indicating Possible Breast Malignancy

- Mastitis in nonpregnant, nonbreastfeeding female
- Axillary or supraclavicular lymphadenopathy
- Breast lump or mass palpated with indistinct, irregular borders
- Breast lump with hard, asymmetric texture
- Painless, immobile breast lump (fixed to adjacent structure)
- Skin dimpling associated with breast lump
- Palpable mass with localized thickening of surrounding tissue
- New onset of nipple retraction
- Unilateral nipple discharge in nonpregnant individual
- Unilateral, spontaneous, bloody nipple discharge, originating from one breast duct with or without a breast mass

ABNORMAL FINDINGS OF THE BREAST AND AXILLAE

ACCESSORY BREAST TISSUE

Accessory or additional mammary tissue remote from the primary breast tissue can occur along "milk lines" anywhere from the axilla to the groin.

History
- May present as a soft subcutaneous lump near or in the axillae
- May present as a supernumerary or "third" nipple; may be mistaken for a freckle or mole

Physical Examination
- Accessory tissue is present with/without an observable accessory nipple.
- Area of the accessory breast tissue can be tender and enlarged in response to the hormonal fluctuations of the normal menstrual cycle and can become full and active with pregnancy and lactation.

Consideration
- Accessory breast tissue is benign; this finding is common.

BENIGN BREAST MASS OR LUMP
- The self-detection of a breast mass or lump is the most common reason for women presenting for clinical breast evaluation in reproductive healthcare practices. The goal in evaluating any breast abnormality or patient concern is to exclude the presence of a malignancy and to find the most efficient path to an accurate diagnosis and management. Most breast lumps are benign. However, the presence of a breast mass should never be dismissed based solely on physical exam.
- Breast tissue can be rope-like or lumpy in texture as a result of glandular or fibrocystic breast tissue. More than half of women experience fibrocystic breast changes at some point in their lives. Benign breast disorders encompass a large group of nonmalignant conditions; most of these conditions are not pathologic and stem from exaggerated physiology of normal breast development and involution. The two most common benign conditions that are associated with distinct, palpable masses or lumps are fibroadenomas and breast cysts.

Breast Cyst
Breast cysts are fluid-filled, round-to-ovoid structures, and are nonproliferative lesions with a minimal breast cancer risk.

History
- Tender breast lump that is round and mobile
- Can be unilateral or bilateral

Physical Examination
- Palpable cysts vary greatly in size, and present as single or multiple entities.

Considerations
- Breast cyst formation can be related to hormonal changes induced by hormone fluctuations of the menstrual cycle, hormone replacement therapy, or medications.
- It is more common in women over the age of 40 years.

Fibroadenoma
Fibroadenomas are composed mainly of parenchymal/stromal tissue and are proliferative lesions that have the propensity to change over time.

History
- Palpable lump; may be tender to touch

Physical Examination
- Single well-defined mobile ovoid and discrete mass palpable on exam

Considerations
- Multiple fibroadenomas can be present.
- It is more common in women younger than 25 years old.

BREAST CANCER
Breast cancer is the most common female cancer and the second leading cause of cancer death in women in the United States. Invasive breast cancers constitute a heterogeneous group of lesions that differ with regard to their clinical, radiographic, and histologic features. The most common histologic types of invasive breast cancers are invasive (infiltrating) ductal carcinoma and invasive lobular carcinoma.

Inflammatory Breast Cancer
A rare, highly aggressive malignant breast condition

History
- Sensation of fullness/heaviness, burning, or tenderness
- Unilateral presentation of an erythematous or purplish, edematous, or inflamed appearing breast involving one-third or more of the breast area
- Rapid change in breast size (<3 months)

Physical Examination
- Has axillary or supraclavicular lymphadenopathy.
- Breast mass may or may not be palpable.
- Breast changes may include inverted nipple; unilateral, localized area of erythema and edema; and peau d'orange skin changes of the affected breast (**Figure 14.8**).

Considerations
- Risk factors include race/ethnicity, younger age at menarche, and obesity.
- Metastatic disease is present in one-third of patients at diagnosis.

Invasive Ductal Carcinomas
History
- Often presents as a discrete firm mass on palpation

Physical Examination
- There are no clinical characteristics that are specific to invasive ductal carcinomas.
- It is more likely to present as an abnormality, such as spiculated mass, on a mammogram.

Consideration
- Prognosis varies and depends on tumor size, histologic grade, hormonal receptor expression, lymph node status, and whether lymph-vascular invasion has occurred.

Invasive Lobular Carcinomas
History
- May present as a palpable mass or a mammographic abnormality similar to those of invasive ductal carcinoma, but findings often more subtle and underestimated

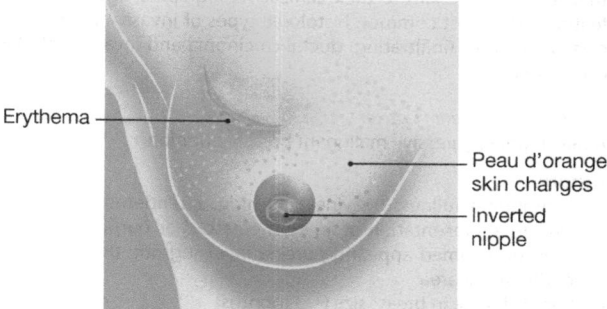

FIGURE 14.8 **Inflammatory breast cancer.**

Physical Examination
- On exam, there may be only an area of thickening or induration, without distinct margins.
- Mammogram may show no more than a poorly defined area of asymmetric density with architectural distortion, even in the presence of a palpable mass.

Consideration
- Prognosis is similar and reliant on the same factors as with ductal carcinoma.

Paget Disease of the Breast
This is a rare type of breast cancer affecting the skin, nipple, and areola; it can occur in men or women from adolescence through the eighth decade of life.

History
- Itching, tingling, or erythema of the nipple and/or areola

Physical Examination
- Thickening, flaking, or crusting of the skin on/around the nipple
- Flat nipple
- Yellowish or bloody nipple discharge
- Breast lump(s) in the same breast

Consideration
- Owing to the benign appearance of Paget disease in early stages, this cancer is often initially mistaken for dermatitis or eczema.

BREAST PAIN: MASTALGIA OR MASTODYNIA
Breast pain is extremely common; majority of all women experience this symptom during their reproductive years. Mastalgia is not correlated with malignancy; it is correlated with hormonal fluctuations. Breast pain, tenderness, and fullness are often early signs of pregnancy.

History
- Bilateral breast pain, often cyclic, that is, associated with menstrual cycle
- Often generalized and described as heaviness and tenderness
- If unilateral, more likely associated with musculoskeletal strain, injury, or overuse

Physical Examination
- There is tenderness of the breast and/or of chest wall.
- Nodularity may be palpable if pain is associated with normal fibrocystic breast changes.

Considerations
- If the breast pain is cyclic, it is more likely to be related to hormonal fluctuations.

- Noncyclic pain is more likely to be musculoskeletal in origin; the pain may originate from the breast or the chest wall since the pectoral muscle lies beneath the breast.

MASTITIS

Mastitis is an infection in the breast that occurs in up to 10% of women who are lactating. Note that mastitis is not common in women who are not breastfeeding and not pregnant; breast tissue that appears infected or inflamed in nonlactating women should be evaluated for conditions other than mastitis, including malignancy.

History
- Fever (over 100°F)
- Fatigue, chills, arthralgia, myalgias, malaise, and/or poor appetite
- Unilateral presentation most likely
- Abrupt onset of symptoms

Physical Examination
- Warm, tender, erythematous, firm area of the breast
- Possibly complicated with a palpable abscess

Considerations
- May result from trauma/chafing to the nipple associated with breastfeeding, piercings
- Prolonged breast engorgement a risk factor

NIPPLE DISCHARGE, GALACTORRHEA

- Nipple discharge in women of reproductive age is a relatively common occurrence and may represent either benign or pathologic conditions.
- Nipple discharge is more likely to be pathologic if it is unilateral, occurs spontaneously, persists, appears to be coming from one duct, or is clear/colorless, bloody, or serous.
- Milky nipple discharge (galactorrhea) in nonlactating individuals (male or female) warrants further evaluation. Tumors are the most common pathologic cause of galactorrhea; for a woman with amenorrhea and nipple discharge who is not pregnant, assessment of their prolactin level is imperative.

History
- Nipple discharge (unilateral or bilateral, milky or clear/serous/bloody)
- Pregnancy status (recent or current)
- Menstrual cycle regularity, or amenorrhea
- Medications, such as hormonal therapies, antipsychotics, antidepressants, or antihypertensives

- History of endocrine disorders or tumors, pituitary or hypothalamic disease
- Other substance use, such as herbal supplements, opiates, sedatives, cocaine, and cannabis

Physical Examination
- Presence or absence of breast mass
- Milky, serous, bloody, or clear discharge from one or both breasts
- Skin changes to either breast

ABNORMAL FINDINGS OF THE FEMALE GENITALIA

SEXUALLY TRANSMITTED INFECTIONS
Gonorrhea
Gonorrhea is an STI caused by the bacterium *Neisseria gonorrhoeae*, which most commonly infects the cervix, uterus, fallopian tubes, and urethra. It is transmitted by sexual contact via the mouth, penis, vagina, or anus of an infected partner and is the second most commonly reported STI.

History
- Asymptomatic in majority of women
- Midcycle vaginal bleeding
- Vaginal discharge
- Dysuria

Physical Examination
- Vaginal discharge
- Cervicitis

Consideration
- In severe or untreated cases, the patient may develop PID infertility, increased risk for ectopic pregnancy, and chronic pelvic pain.
- Untreated infections may lead to disseminated gonococcal infection, which can present as arthritis, tenosynovitis, and/or dermatitis, and can be fatal.

Chlamydia
Chlamydia is the most commonly reported bacterial STI. Caused by the bacterium *Chlamydia trachomatis* and transmitted through sexual contact similar to gonorrheal infections, chlamydia is a common cause of cervicitis in women.

History
- Asymptomatic in majority of women
- Vaginal discharge
- Dysuria, pyuria, urinary frequency

Physical Examination
- Vaginal discharge
- Friable cervix (i.e., easily induced endocervical bleeding)

Consideration
- Severe or untreated infections can result in PID, infertility, increased risk for ectopic pregnancy, and chronic pelvic pain.
- Perinatal transmission can occur and cause significant conjunctivitis or pneumonia in newborns.

Trichomoniasis
Trichomoniasis is caused by an infection with the protozoal parasite *Trichomonas vaginalis.*

History
- Asymptomatic in majority of women
- Vaginal discharge and itching
- Dysuria
- Irritation and itching of the vulva

Physical Examination
- Greenish-yellow, frothy, and malodorous vaginal discharge
- Erythematous vulvar tissue and vaginal mucosa
- "Strawberry cervix" a rare but pathognomonic finding that results from punctate hemorrhages on the cervix and vaginal tissue (**Figure 14.9**)

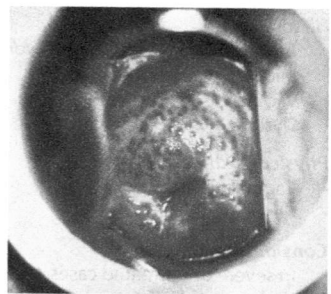

FIGURE 14.9 *Trichomonas vaginalis* infection and characteristic strawberry cervix.
Source: Centers for Disease Control and Prevention.

Consideration
- Trichomonads may be noted on microscopy.

Syphilis
Syphilis is an STI caused by the bacterium *Treponema pallidum* that can present in a variety of ways depending on the stage of infection. Syphilis is spread by direct contact with a painless sore, known as a *chancre.*

Primary Stage
- Chancre (raised lesion, with an indurated margin, approximately 1–2 cm in size)
- Painless chancre, which may be found on the genitals, mouth/throat, anus, or vagina
- Typically occurs 21 days after exposure

Secondary Stage
- Palmar rash on the hands and bottoms of the feet; typically appears rough and red and does not usually cause itching (**Figure 14.10**)
- Fatigue, fevers, lymphadenopathy
- Hair loss, weight loss, myalgias
- Resolution of symptoms eventually even without treatment.

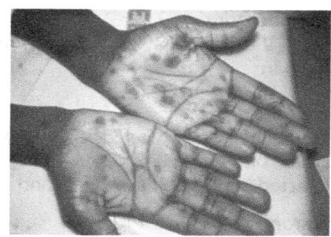

FIGURE 14.10 Palmar rash on palms of the hands due to secondary syphilis.
Source: Image courtesy of Centers for Disease Control and Prevention.

Latent Stage
- Time when no symptoms are present that can last for years
- Continues to be contagious

Tertiary Stage
- This typically occurs 10 to 30 years after initial infection and can be fatal.
- Symptoms of tertiary syphilis depend on the organ system affected; it can cause infection in the nervous system, eyes, vascular and cardiac systems, liver, bones, and joints.

Genital Warts (Condyloma Acuminata)
HPV types 6 and 11 are the most common cause of genital warts. As noted in this chapter, HPV is the most common STI. There are numerous types of HPV; many types are associated with cancers, whereas some are associated with genital warts or condyloma.

History
- Nonitchy, nontender lesions may appear as flesh tones, white, pink, or red.
- It can appear as a single lesion or grouped together, as depicted in **Figure 14.11**.

Physical Examination
- Flat, papular, or pedunculated growths on the genital mucosa and the surrounding skin of the perineal area, including the groin, suprapubic or perianal region, and vulva

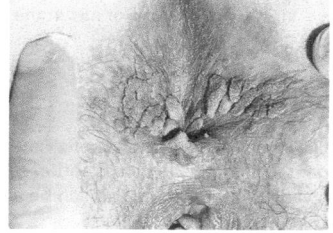

FIGURE 14.11 Genital warts found on the perineum.
Source: Image courtesy of SOA-AIDS Amsterdam.

Consideration
- HPV vaccines have significantly reduced the incidence of genital warts.

Genital Herpes
Genital herpes is a viral STI caused by the herpes simplex virus (HSV) type 1 or type 2. HSV infections can be transmitted via contact with infected herpes lesions, genital and oral secretions, or mucosa.

History
- Painful "blister" lesions are located around the mouth or genital area.
- Patient may have flu-like symptoms including body aches, fever/chills, headache, and lymphadenopathy during a primary infection.
- If symptoms recur, the outbreaks usually have shorter duration and less severe symptoms.

Physical Examination
- Vesicular lesions; one or more may be ulcerated

Considerations
- A primary herpes infection occurs when a patient without antibodies to HSV develops an infection.
- The virus can be shed from normal-appearing skin/tissues, and many people have no symptoms and are not aware they are infected.
- Although there is no cure for a viral herpes infection, there are treatment options available to help manage outbreaks.

Pubic Lice (Pediculosis Pubis)
These are translucent parasites that are usually spread through sexual contact; transmission through fomites (e.g., towels, clothing, or linens) is possible, but much less likely.

History
- Itching in the pubic area

Physical Examination
- Visible live lice and/or nits in the pubic hair

Consideration
- Condoms do not provide protection against pubic lice infestation.

Pelvic Inflammatory Disease
PID involves infection and inflammation of the upper genital tract organs, including the uterus and/or fallopian tubes. PID can arise from a variety of infections and can be a complication of gonorrheal and chlamydial infections.

History
- Lower abdominal/pelvic pain
- Vaginal discharge

- Pain with intercourse
- Frequent urination

Physical Examination
- Fever, abdominal tenderness, rebound tenderness
- Tenderness on bimanual examination, including CMT
- Positive culture for gonorrhea, chlamydia, trichomoniasis, and/or bacterial vaginosis

Consideration
- The symptoms of PID range from mild to severe; infertility can result from damage to the upper genital tract organs.

VAGINITIS/VAGINOSIS
Bacterial Vaginosis
Bacterial vaginosis is a vaginal infection caused by an imbalance in the vaginal flora; it is the most common vaginal infection in women aged 15 to 44 years.

History
- Often asymptomatic
- Vaginal itching or irritation
- Strong fishy odor that is particularly noticeable after intercourse

Physical Examination
- White or gray vaginal discharge with pH >4.5
- Positive whiff test
- Clue cells on microscopy

Consideration
- Known risk factors for bacterial vaginosis include having a new sexual partner or multiple sexual partners and douching.

Candidiasis
Vulvovaginal candidiasis (VVC) is an inflammation of the vulvar and vaginal tissues owing to an infection with *Candida* yeast. Approximately half of all women will experience a yeast infection at least once during their lifetime. There are several different species of *Candida* that cause VVC; however, *Candida albicans* is by far the most common.

History
- Vulvar itching/irritation
- Thick, white discharge
- Dysuria
- Dyspareunia

Physical Examination
- Curd-like discharge adherent to the vaginal walls
- Erythematous vagina and vulvar tissue
- Blastospores and pseudohyphae on microscopy

Consideration
- Risk factors include sexual debut, pregnancy, immunosuppression, and uncontrolled or undiagnosed diabetes.

Genitourinary Syndrome of Menopause
A constellation of symptoms that affect the vulvovaginal and urethra areas during menopause or postmenopause as a result of decreased levels of estrogen

History
- **Genital symptoms:** Vaginal dryness, burning, and irritation
- **Sexual symptoms:** Dyspareunia, lack of lubrication, postcoital bleeding
- **Urinary symptoms:** Dysuria, urgency, frequent or recurrent urinary tract infections

Physical Examination
- Thinning of the epithelial tissue of the vagina, pallor, loss of rugae
- Labia minora resorption, introital retraction
- Decrease in elasticity and vascularity of vagina, tissue fragility

Consideration
- Care should be taken to use water-soluble lubrication when performing a speculum exam as insertion of the speculum can be painful.

VULVAR/VAGINAL/URETHRAL LESIONS

Lichen Planus
A chronic, inflammatory autoimmune condition of unknown etiology that affects the skin and mucous membranes, including the vulva and vagina

History
- Dysuria
- Irritation of vulvar area, itching
- Dyspareunia, postcoital bleeding
- Itchy rash likely to affect other areas of the body

Physical Examination
- White papules, plaques, and erosions
- Vagina can be friable; speculum exam painful

Consideration
- The most common type, erosive lichen planus, causes painful ulcers and scarring.

Lichen Sclerosus
Lichen sclerosus is one of the most common vulvar dermatoses. Similar to lichen planus, it is an autoimmune-mediated, chronic, and inflammatory disease; however, lichen sclerosus is progressive,

most often occurs postmenopause, and vaginal involvement almost never occurs.

History
- Vulvar itching, typically worse at night
- Dysuria
- Urine/stool retention

Physical Examination
- Initial appearance of the skin may be white, thickened, excoriated, and edematous.
- As disease progresses, the skin loses pigmentation and becomes very thin with wrinkled appearance, and the anatomic features of the external genitalia become distorted.
- Patient may have anal fissures, ulcerations, lichenification, and scarring.

Consideration
- Women with lichen sclerosis are at increased risk of squamous cell carcinoma of the vulva.

Intertrigo
An inflammatory condition of the skin in warm moist areas; occurs in places where two skin surfaces rub together; common skin rash that occurs throughout the life span

History
- Between skin folds or in genital areas, skin surfaces are irritated, red, and macerated.
- It typically occurs in larger skin fold areas such as the axilla, groin folds, inner thighs, and breast and abdominal folds.

Physical Examination
- Cracked or crusty skin, erythema, edema

Considerations
- Intertrigo is susceptible to secondary infections.
- Factors increasing risk of development include hot and humid conditions, obesity, diabetes, incontinence, malnutrition, and poor hygiene.

Vulvar Cancers and Vulvar Intraepithelial Neoplasia
Vulvar cancers are relatively rare; most are squamous cell carcinomas. Vulvar intraepithelial neoplasia (VIN) is a premalignant condition of the vulva.

History
- Chronic vulvar itching
- Dyspareunia
- Burning, tingling, or soreness in the vulvar region

Physical Examination
- Change in appearance including lesions or areas of redness or white, discolored skin
- Slightly raised skin lesions; some may appear darkened like a mole or freckle

Considerations
- Squamous cell carcinomas of the vulva associated with HPV infections are found more commonly in younger women, whereas those associated with differentiated VIN are typically found in older women.
- Risk factors associated with vulvar cancer include HPV infection, cervical cancer history, smoking, and chronic vulvar skin conditions.

Urethral Caruncle
A benign lesion located at the posterior urethral meatus

History
- May be asymptomatic or might note a bump at the urinary meatus
- May cause dyspareunia, dysuria, or bleeding if irritated

Physical Examination
- Bright-red, vascular lesion located on the posterior lip of the urinary meatus

Consideration
- Commonly found in postmenopausal women and premenarchal girls and suspected to be a result of decreased levels of estrogen

Bartholin Gland Cyst
Bartholin gland cysts develop when the gland becomes blocked, which is a common gynecologic problem, especially in women of reproductive age. An uninfected cyst is typically painless and presents as a palpable, nontender lump or swelling. Bartholin cysts can become infected and cause significant pain. Visible erythema and acute tenderness are suggestive of an inflamed cyst and possible abscess (**Figure 14.12**).

PELVIC SUPPORT ISSUES
Pelvic Organ Prolapse
Pelvic organ prolapse is a condition in which there is failure of the anatomic supportive structures to adequately support the organs of the pelvis. It is a common and most often asymptomatic problem that does not

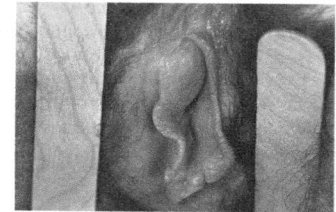

FIGURE 14.12 Infected Bartholin cyst.
Source: Centers for Disease Control and Prevention/Susan Lindsley.

require intervention for most women. Symptoms vary depending on the severity of the defects in the supportive structures. Types of pelvic organ prolapse include the following:

- **Cystocele:** Loss of pelvic support in the anterior vaginal wall causes the bladder to prolapse into the vaginal canal.
- **Rectocele:** Loss of pelvic support in the posterior vaginal wall allows the small bowel and/or rectum to prolapse.
- **Uterine prolapse:** Loss of pelvic support allows the uterus and cervix to prolapse through the vaginal canal; it is often associated with a concurrent cystocele and rectocele.

History
- May be asymptomatic or may have pelvic pressure
- Urinary urgency, feeling of incomplete bladder emptying
- Difficulty with defecation

Physical Examination
- Bulging in the vulvar or vaginal areas
- May have visible tissue at the introitus

Consideration
- Risk factors for development include pregnancy, vaginal delivery and delivery-related injury, family history, obesity, and connective tissue diseases.

GENITAL LESIONS/MASSES: MALIGNANT AND NONMALIGNANT
Cervical Intraepithelial Neoplasia and Cervical Malignancies
Cervical intraepithelial neoplasia (CIN) is a premalignant condition of the squamous epithelial cell of the cervix. Infection with HPV is the most common cause of CIN lesions. There are two common types of CIN: low-grade squamous intraepithelial lesion and high-grade squamous intraepithelial lesion.

History
- History of abnormal Pap testing, HPV infection
- Unusual vaginal bleeding (i.e., after intercourse, between periods, or postmenopause)
- Pelvic pain, dyspareunia

Physical Examination
- Physical examination may be unremarkable.
- Cervix may have erosion, ulcer, or mass.

Consideration
- Several risk factors have been identified in the development of high-grade squamous intraepithelial lesion (HSIL) and cervical cancer, including the subtype of HPV infection, the persistence of the HPV infection, cigarette smoking, and immunosuppressed state.

ADNEXAL MASSES

Adnexal masses have many etiologies, most of which are benign. Appropriate evaluation and monitoring of women with an adnexal mass is important to differentiate between benign, malignant, or emergent causes or conditions. **Figure 14.13** depicts adnexal masses, including ovarian cysts, ectopic pregnancy, ovarian cancer, and uterine fibroids.

Ovarian Cyst

Ovarian cysts are fluid-filled sacs that form in or on a woman's ovaries, most often during ovulation. They are a common ultrasound finding and typically resolve without intervention.

History

- Often asymptomatic; however, can cause acute, unilateral pelvic pain
- Irregular menstrual periods, bloating

Physical Examination

- Ovarian cysts may be palpable during the bimanual physical exam.

Consideration

- More common in premenopausal women

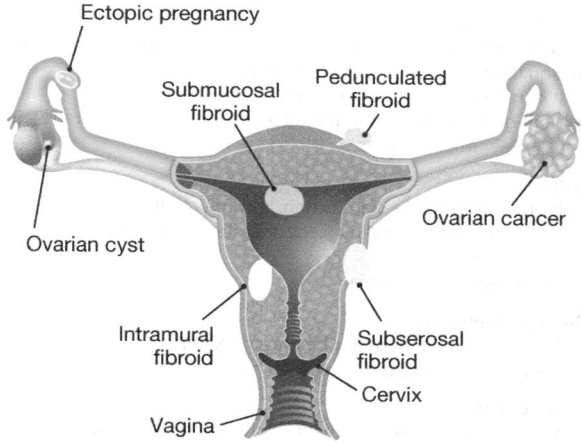

FIGURE 14.13 Adnexal masses, including ovarian cysts, ectopic pregnancy, ovarian cancer, and uterine fibroids.

Ectopic Pregnancy
A potential life-threatening emergency that results from the implantation of a fertilized egg outside of the uterus, most commonly in the fallopian tube

History
- Vaginal bleeding
- Increasing unilateral pelvic pain
- Altered menstrual cycle

Physical Examination
- Positive pregnancy test
- Palpable adnexal mass on bimanual examination
- CMT

Consideration
- Failure to diagnose an ectopic pregnancy in a timely fashion can result in rupture of the fallopian tube, leading to hemorrhage and possible death.

Ovarian Cancer
Ovarian cancer is the second most common gynecologic cancer, most often occurring in women aged 55 to 64 years.

History
- Abdominal distention or bloating
- Early satiety with loss of appetite
- Unexplained pelvic or abdominal pain
- Increased urinary urgency or frequency
- Postcoital bleeding, postmenopausal bleeding
- Unexplained weight loss, fatigue, or change in bowel habits
- Over 50 years of age, with new symptoms of irritable bowel syndrome
- Family history of breast, ovarian, or colon cancer

Physical Examination
- No specific findings
- May palpate mass on pelvic exam, or adnexal fullness

Consideration
- Individuals with suspected ovarian cancer based on presentation should undergo transvaginal ultrasonography to assess ovarian characteristics, and distinguish benign from malignant masses.

Uterine Fibroids
Uterine fibroids are benign growths arising from the smooth muscle (myometrium) of the uterus. They occur in more than half of all women, develop after menarche, and regress post menopause.

History
- Varied symptoms, depending on the size and location of the fibroid
- Can be asymptomatic or cause heavy menstrual bleeding
- Pelvic pain, dyspareunia, bladder dysfunction

Physical Examination
- Lump or mass on abdominal examination
- Enlarged uterus in a nonpregnant woman on bimanual examination
- Irregular contour of the uterus on bimanual examination

Consideration
- Management is individualized; considerations include desire to preserve fertility.

OTHER DISORDERS CAUSING MENSTRUAL IRREGULARITIES

Polycystic Ovarian Syndrome

PCOS is a complex endocrine disorder of unknown etiology. Thought to be genetically linked, it is a common cause of menstrual irregularity and infertility and is associated with insulin resistance.

History
- Presentation variable; can be asymptomatic
- Irregular menstrual cycles
- Infertility
- Weight gain

Physical Examination
- Signs of hyperandrogenism including acne, hirsutism, and acanthosis nigricans
- May have male pattern baldness and thinning hair
- Polycystic ovaries on ultrasound

Consideration
- Women with PCOS are at increased risk for metabolic syndrome, type 2 diabetes, dyslipidemia, and cardiovascular disease.

Endometriosis

Endometriosis is implantation and abnormal growth of endometrial cells outside of the uterus. The endometrial cells induce inflammatory reactions, secrete prostaglandins, and infiltrate tissues and nerves, causing secondary dysmenorrhea, scars, traction, and fibrosis.

History
- Dysmenorrhea, lower abdominal pain, dyspareunia
- May have infertility
- Pain most often cyclic, or intensified during menstrual cycle

Physical Examination
- No specific findings

Consideration
- Visual inspection by laparoscopy is the gold standard for diagnosing endometriosis.

Vasomotor Symptoms
This is a term used to describe the constellation of symptoms commonly referred to as hot flashes or night sweats. Vasomotor symptoms (VMS) are commonly experienced during perimenopause and the menopausal transition as recurrent, transient episodes of flushing accompanied by a sensation of warmth to the upper body and/or face.

History
- Hot flashes, flushing of the face with severe sweating
- Night sweats, sleep disturbances
- May have associated heart palpitations

Physical Examination
- Nonspecific, unless VMS occur during the physical exam

Considerations
- VMS are triggered by caffeine, alcohol, smoking, clothing that is too warm, environmental temperature, stress, eating spicy foods, medications, and co-occurring health conditions.
- VMS have been associated with diminished quality of life for some women.

PHYSICAL EXAMINATION DOCUMENTATION

EXAMPLE OF NORMAL FINDINGS FOR BREAST ASSESSMENT
Breasts symmetric. No retractions, nipple discharge, skin changes, or lesions. No palpable masses, tenderness, or axillary lymphadenopathy.

EXAMPLE OF NORMAL FINDINGS FOR FEMALE GENITALIA EXAM
External genitalia has no lesions or discharge. No inguinal lymphadenopathy. Vulva without lesions, erythema, or discharge. No tenderness to Bartholin or Skene glands. Vagina pink, rugae present, no lesions or discharge. Cervix pink, no lesions or discharge. Nulliparous os. Bimanual exam without pain, no cervical motion tenderness. Uterus normal size, shape, position, and contour. No adnexal tenderness or palpable masses. Anus no hemorrhoids, fissures, or lesions. Rectal wall intact, no masses or tenderness.

REFERENCES

References for this chapter draw from Chapter 21, Evidence-Based Assessment of the Breasts and Axillae, and Chapter 23, Evidence-Based Assessment of the Female Genitourinary System, of the textbook *Evidence-Based Physical Examination: Best Practices for Health and Well-Being Assessment (Second Edition)*. The references may be accessed in the digital version of the handbook at https://connect.springerpub.com/.

15

Evidence-Based Obstetric Assessment

CLINICAL CONSIDERATIONS

- Women should be considered active participants in their care during pregnancy and encouraged to share decision-making with their clinician.
- Recognize that the childbearing year is a time of great growth, stress, and excitement for the entire family unit.
- The clinician should ask about fetal movement, contractions/cramping, vaginal bleeding, and loss of fluid at each visit.
- Collaboration with generalist obstetric providers or perinatologists is key for women with more complicated health histories.
- Many concerns in pregnancy are considered normal. The clinician's job is to determine when these concerns may actually be abnormal and to know how to assess for concerns.
- The initial prenatal visit is an opportunity to provide a wealth of information to patients about their health and pregnancy, as well as an opportunity for the clinician to screen for problems that may arise in later pregnancy.
- The vast majority of women will have a healthy pregnancy.
- Clinicians need to know and understand the red flags from the history and physical examination in order to provide appropriate referrals or emergency care (**Boxes 15.1** and **15.2**).

SUBJECTIVE HISTORY

COMMON REASON FOR SEEKING CARE
- Pregnancy, pregnancy-related concerns

HISTORY OF PRESENT ILLNESS
- Date of the last menstrual period (LMP; unknown, approximate, definite)?
- Date of the last normal menstrual period (if different from LMP)?
- Age at menarche?
- Age at estimated due date (EDD)?

BOX 15.1 Red Flags in Subjective History

- Nausea or vomiting that prohibits intake or causes weight loss
- Dysuria
- Reported decreased or absent fetal movement
- Severe headache
- Use of category D or X medications
- Excessive alcohol use
- Recreational drug use or addiction
- Worsening anxiety or depression
- History of or current domestic or interpersonal violence

BOX 15.2 Red Flags in Objective Exam

- Vaginal bleeding
- Loss of fluid
- Contractions prior to 37 weeks
- Upper right abdominal pain
- Changes in vision
- High blood pressure
- Decreased urine output
- Thrombocytopenia
- Impaired liver function
- Proteinuria
- Seizures
- Symptoms of an ectopic pregnancy (severe, unilateral pelvic pain, dizziness, fainting, or rectal pressure in the first trimester)

- Typical length of cycle (28–30 days most reliable in terms of dating)?
- Is this a planned pregnancy? Was any contraception used at the time of conception?
- Is this a desired pregnancy? If not, discuss pregnancy options, such as continuing pregnancy and keeping the child, continuing pregnancy and adoption, and pregnancy termination.
- See **Box 15.3** for the methods for determining the EDD.

HEALTH HISTORY

Past Medical History

- History of hypertension (HTN) or diabetes mellitus (DM; also relevant polycystic ovarian syndrome [PCOS] or insulin resistance)
- History of asthma or allergic rhinitis
- History of autoimmune disorders, including thyroid disorders

---

BOX 15.3 Methods of Determining Estimated Due Date

- The first day of the LMP may be used if the LMP is certain, the cycles are regular (ideally every 28–30 days), and the LMP was normal for the woman. The accuracy of this can be compromised by several factors: Some women may not know their LMP, some may ovulate later in their cycle than others, and some may have some early pregnancy bleeding that they mistake for a period. Naegele's rule is based on an LMP from a 28-day menstrual cycle. The formula for Naegele's rule is the first day of LMP + 7 days − 3 months = EDD. This is the basis for the calculations performed by most pregnancy wheels and apps. The variation in EDDs obtained by these methods is 1 to 7 days (King et al., 2019).
- If the pregnancy is conceived using ART, such as IUI or IVF, the date of insemination or embryo transfer may be used as the LMP.
- Ultrasound may also be used to confirm an EDD. First-trimester ultrasound (performed before 14 weeks and 0 days) is the most accurate (within 5–7 days). Second-trimester ultrasound is less accurate in terms of dating the pregnancy, with a variance of 7 to 14 days.

ART, artificial reproductive technology; EDD, estimated due date; IUI, intrauterine insemination; IVF, in vitro fertilization; LMP, last menstrual period.

- History of anxiety/depression/postpartum depression or other mental health disorders
- History of varicella (disease or vaccination; if vaccination, how many doses?)
- History of cytomegalovirus (CMV)
- History of clotting disorders or venous thromboembolism (VTE)

Obstetric History (If Relevant)
- GTPAL, that is, **G**ravida (number of pregnancies), **T**erm (number of full-term births 37 weeks 0 days' gestation or later), **P**reterm (number of preterm births 20 weeks 0 days' to 36 weeks 6 days' gestation), **A**bortion (number of elective terminations and/or miscarriages, including births prior to 20 weeks' gestation), **L**iving (number of living children)

- Method of prior births (If vaginal, spontaneous, vacuum, or forceps? If Cesarean section, what kind of incision and what was the indication for Cesarean?)
- Length of labor
- Complications during previous pregnancies and/or births, such as gestational diabetes mellitus (GDM; diet-controlled, controlled with oral medication, controlled with insulin), preexisting DM (type 1 or type 2), essential HTN, gestational HTN, preeclampsia, eclampsia, HELLP (hemolysis, elevated liver enzymes, low platelet count) syndrome, postpartum hemorrhage, shoulder dystocia, retained placenta, third- or fourth-degree perineal laceration, and issues with the child's health
- History of elective termination or miscarriage (Any complications? Weeks of gestation at the time of miscarriage or elective termination? Required medication or dilation and curettage [D&C]?)
- History of miscarriage(s), age of the fetus at the time of miscarriage
- History of preterm labor or birth (20 weeks 0 days–36 weeks 6 days)
- History of fetal/neonatal demise
- History of ectopic pregnancy
- Increased risk of poor outcome in the next pregnancy if poor outcome in previous pregnancy

Gynecologic History
- Last Pap test (with high-risk human papillomavirus [HPV] results if testing performed)
- History of abnormal Pap(s)
- History of sexually transmitted infections (STIs)
- History of loop electrosurgical excision procedure (LEEP) or cone biopsy; if yes, then increased risk for cervical incompetence/preterm labor/preterm birth
- History of gynecologic surgery
- History of endometriosis

Medications
- Prescribed and over-the-counter (OTC) medications or supplements, including dose and frequency (specifically pregnancy category C, D, and X medications)
- Prenatal vitamins

Allergies
- Allergies to medications, or seasonal, environmental, and/or food allergies? If "yes," clarify reactions.

FAMILY HISTORY
- Genetic disorders, including known or suspected genetic disease, multiple malformations, multiple miscarriages, recurrence of the same or similar disorders, intellectual disability, autism spectrum disorders, and consanguinity

- Type 2 DM
- Preeclampsia

SOCIAL HISTORY
- Married/single/divorced/widowed/partnered?
- Is partner involved? If not, who is the support?
- Does partner have any other children?
- Living situation?
- Housing situation?
- Exercise?
- Sleep?
- Dietary restrictions/daily water intake?
- Feels safe at home?
- Tobacco use? If yes, assess readiness to quit.
- Alcohol use?
- Illicit drug use? (Marijuana may or may not be legal depending on state, but still need to counsel on unknown effects during pregnancy.)
- History of substance use disorder?
- Occupational history, such as exposure to workplace hazards (e.g., chemicals/fumes, radiation, chemotherapeutic agents, patients with CMV, small children)?
- Intimate partner violence or history of reproductive or sexual coercion?
  - Identify and document and nonverbal markers of interpersonal violence and/or sexual coercion. These may include bruising, improbable injury, depression, late prenatal care (initiation of care in the second or third trimester), missed prenatal visits, and/or appointments canceled on short notice.

  Note: *Pregnancy is a risk factor for domestic violence beginning or escalating.*

- What kind of diet is followed? Is there a concern for malnutrition (undernutrition or overnutrition)?

REVIEW OF SYSTEMS
- **Constitutional:** Fatigue, weight gain, weight loss, change in appetite
- **Head, eyes, ears, nose, throat:** Visual changes (blurred vision, spots, or floaters), epistaxis, nasal drainage/congestion, bleeding gums, tooth pain
- **Cardiovascular/peripheral vascular:** Heart palpitations, lower extremity swelling, varicosities (lower extremities/vulvar), hemorrhoids
- **Respiratory:** Shortness of breath, wheezing, snoring
- **Breast:** Breast tenderness, breast lumps, nipple discharge, change in breast size

- **Gastrointestinal:** Nausea, vomiting, food aversions, abdominal pain, constipation, diarrhea
- **Genitourinary:** Pelvic pain, vaginal bleeding, vaginal discharge, frequent urination, cramping, contractions, hematuria, dysuria, urinary urgency, urinary incontinence, STI exposure
- **Musculoskeletal:** Muscle cramping, muscle pain, joint pain
- **Skin:** Itching, breast tenderness, breast lumps, nipple discharge
- **Neurologic:** Headache, seizure, dizziness, lightheadedness, syncope
- **Mental health:** Anxiety, depression, irritability, suicidality
- **Endocrine:** Heat or cold intolerance
- **Hematologic:** Easy bruising, excess bleeding
- **Allergic:** Hives, seasonal allergies

PREVENTIVE CARE CONSIDERATIONS

- Up-to-date on cervical cancer screening
- Up-to-date on mammography screening (if applicable)
- Up-to-date on flu vaccine (seasonal, recommended during pregnancy regardless of gestational age), tetanus diphtheria, and pertussis vaccine (recommended between 27 and 36 weeks' gestation during each pregnancy)
- mRNA COVID-19 vaccine (full series, including booster, recommended during pregnancy if not already vaccinated)
- Depression screening
- Intimate partner violence screening
- Tobacco use counseling if patient uses tobacco (advise to stop smoking and provide behavioral interventions for cessation)
- Screening for unhealthy alcohol use (provide brief behavioral counseling interventions to reduce unhealthy alcohol use)
- Pets at home (in particular, patients with cats must be counseled on the risk of toxoplasmosis and precautions; patients who own reptiles must be counseled on the risk of listeriosis and precautions)
- Recent travel of the patient or the partner to areas with Zika virus and timing of the travel; if so, identify mosquito bites and/or Zika virus symptoms
- Current medications/vitamins/supplements (consider safety profile in pregnancy)
- Prepregnancy weight
- Preferred pronouns (he/him, she/her, they/them)
- Preferred name

UNIQUE POPULATION CONSIDERATIONS
Advanced Maternal Age

- Those who will be 35 of age or older at their EDD are considered at advanced maternal age (AMA). There are increased risks with AMA pregnancies, including chromosomal abnormalities, fetal growth restriction, GDM, gestational HTN, preeclampsia, placental insufficiency, preterm birth, and stillbirth.

Trauma-Informed Care

- A gynecologic or obstetric exam, labor, or delivery may trigger posttraumatic stress disorder (PTSD) symptoms from a history of child maltreatment or sexual violence. Similar patterns may be seen in patients who have experienced intimate partner violence or assault as adults. Even without a history of abuse or maltreatment, some people are finding themselves traumatized by their care prenatally, or in labor and delivery.
- Clinicians must educate themselves on trauma-informed care, as well as how best to care for these women during pregnancy without retraumatizing them. Trauma-informed care such as universal screening, clinician comfort with adjusting routine exams and responding to possible reactions of those affected by prior trauma, and the availability of PTSD resources and referrals all play a role in helping to establish a good clinician–patient relationship and contribute to improved perinatal outcomes. For more information on trauma-informed care, refer to Chapter 16, Evidence-Based Assessment of Mental Health Including Substance Use Disorders.

PHYSICAL EXAMINATION

GENERAL SURVEY

- Initial assessment for physiologic stability
- Vital signs including temperature, pulse rate, respiratory rate, and blood pressure (BP)
- Noting whether the patient appears visibly pregnant (fundus above the symphysis pubis)
- Height and weight, with weight recorded at each visit

INSPECTION

- Inspect the breasts and nipples for symmetry. Note any changes to the skin of the breasts, including dimpling, peau d'orange appearance, erythema, or edema. (For more information on breast examinations, please refer to Chapter 14, Evidence-Based Assessment of the Breasts, Female Genitalia, and Reproductive System.)
- A complete visual inspection of the external genitals should be performed, noting any lesions, erythema, edema, or discharge.
- In early pregnancy, Chadwick's sign may be observed during a speculum exam; the cervix appears bluish-purplish in color or cyanotic. Note the presence of any lesions, erythema, edema, discharge, or bleeding inside the vaginal vault or at the cervix.

- The cervical os has a different appearance and feel in nulliparous people versus multiparous people. In nulliparous pregnant persons, the cervical os is pinpoint in size and rounded. In multiparous pregnant persons, the os has the appearance of a slit.

PALPATION

- If >12 weeks' gestation or if dates are unknown, an abdominal exam to assess if the fundus is palpable in the abdomen is useful. See **Figure 15.1** for changes in fundal height.
  - At 12 weeks' gestation, the fundus should be palpable just caudally to the symphysis pubis.
  - At 16 weeks' gestation, the fundus should be palpable midway between the symphysis pubis and the umbilicus.
  - At 20 weeks' gestation, the fundus should be palpable at the umbilicus.

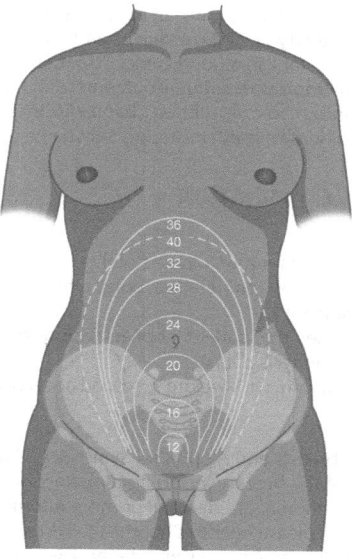

FIGURE 15.1 Changes in fundal height during pregnancy. At 12 weeks' gestation, the fundus of the uterus is palpable just superior to the symphysis pubis. At 16 weeks' gestation, the fundus is palpable midway between the symphysis pubis and the umbilicus. At 20 weeks' gestation, the fundus is in line with the umbilicus. At approximately 28 weeks' gestation, the fundus is palpable midway between the umbilicus and the xyphoid process; the clinician should be able to determine fetal presentation. At 34 weeks' gestation, the fundus is palpable just below the xyphoid process. Sometimes fundal height will decrease at term, as the fetal head engages in the maternal pelvis.

○ As pregnancy progresses past 20 weeks' gestation, the clinician will measure the fundal height at each visit. This is the measurement in centimeters from the top of the symphysis pubis to the fundus (**Figure 15.2**). The measurement approximately correlates with the current number of weeks of gestation. Fundal height measurements alone should not serve as the basis for clinical decision-making or intervention, as ultrasound in the third trimester can be useful in accurately diagnosing abnormalities with fetal growth and amniotic fluid volume.

○ Clinicians will also assess the fetal presentation by utilizing Leopold's maneuvers after approximately 28 weeks' gestation (**Figure 15.3**).

• Gestational age may be estimated by the size of the uterus, either abdominally or with a bimanual exam. In early pregnancy, the clinician may note the Hegar's sign, in which the lower segment of the uterus becomes very soft and compressible in early pregnancy. The clinician may also note the Goodell's sign, which is the softening of the cervix in the first trimester.

• When performing a speculum or bimanual pelvic exam, patient comfort, both physical and emotional, should be considered of utmost importance. Many exams can be done without the need for stirrups; instead, ask the patient to bend at the knee and come down toward the clinician on the exam table. Appropriate draping is important, as well as eye contact with the patient. Some patients may prefer to insert the speculum themselves or view the exam with a handheld mirror. It is helpful to ask the patient if they are ready to be touched before the clinician begins a pelvic exam and to initially touch on the inside of the thigh prior to touching the genitals.

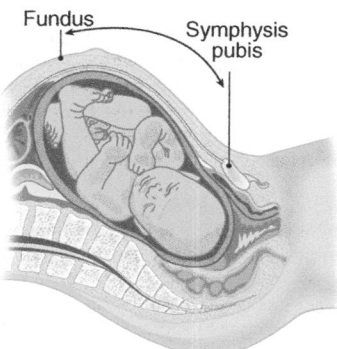

FIGURE 15.2 Measurement of fundal height. Measurement in centimeters from the top of the symphysis pubis to the fundus.

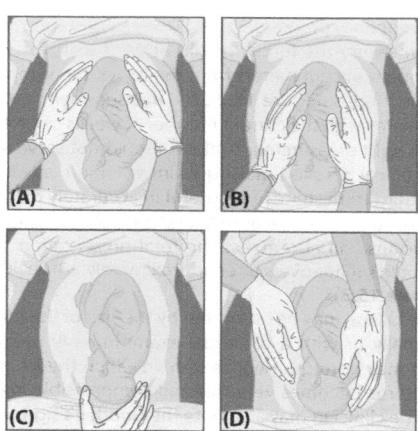

FIGURE 15.3 Performing Leopold's maneuvers. (**A**) Identify the fetal part in the uterine fundus. (**B**) Using the palmar surface of both hands, identify which side of the uterus contains the fetal back and which contains the "small parts" such as the hands and feet. (**C**) Use the thumb and the third finger to identify fetal presenting part. (**D**) Use both hands to outline fetal presenting part.

- In full-term pregnancy or for concerns prior to term, the clinician may need to perform a cervical exam to evaluate for labor/preterm labor. The five main findings from a cervical exam are dilation, effacement, fetal station (**Figure 15.4**), position of the cervix, and consistency of the cervix.

AUSCULTATION

Fetal heart tones are auscultated at each visit, typically with a Doppler. Fetal heart tones can be heard with a Doppler after 10 to 12 weeks' gestation, depending on the strength of the handheld Doppler device. A fetoscope may also be used to auscultate fetal heart tones; however, this requires an experienced clinician and the patient must typically be at least 24 weeks' gestation.

CONSIDERATIONS

- If maternal BP is elevated at the initial prenatal visit, the clinician should attempt to find prepregnancy records to determine if chronic HTN exists.
- Maternal body mass index (BMI) should be calculated at the initial prenatal visit using the prepregnancy weight to guide weight gain recommendations during pregnancy as well as to assess for risk of comorbid conditions (**Table 15.1**).

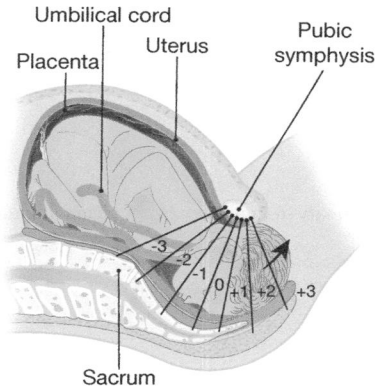

FIGURE 15.4 Fetal station. This is a measurement of the relationship of the presenting part to the ischial spines in the maternal pelvis and signifies the descent of the fetus in the pelvis. Negative numbers (e.g., −2, −1) indicate that the presenting part (typically the bony aspect of the fetal vertex) is above the ischial spines by that many centimeters. The 0 station indicates that the presenting part is in line with the ischial spines. Positive numbers (e.g., +1, +2) indicate that the presenting part is below the ischial spines by that many centimeters. The fetus descends as labor progresses. Most laboring persons will feel a spontaneous urge to push around 0 to +2 cm, particularly without an epidural.

TABLE 15.1 Institute of Medicine Weight Gain Recommendations for Pregnancy

Prepregnancy Weight Category	Body Mass Index[a]	Recommended Range of Total Weight (lb)	Recommended Rates of Weight Gain in the Second and Third Trimesters (Mean Range; lb/wk)[b]
Underweight	<18.5	28–40	1 (1.0–1.3)
Normal weight	18.5–24.9	25–35	1 (0.8–1.0)
Overweight	25–29.9	15–25	0.6 (0.5–0.7)
Obese (includes all classes)	>30	11–20	0.5 (0.4–0.6)

[a]Body mass index is calculated by using the following formula: weight in pounds/height in inches × height in inches × 703.
[b]Calculations assume a 1.1- to 4.4-lb weight gain in the first trimester.

Source: Modified from the Institute of Medicine. (2009). *Weight gain during pregnancy: Reexamining the guidelines.* National Academies Press. © 2009 National Academy of Sciences.

ABNORMAL FINDINGS

ACUTE CYSTITIS (URINARY TRACT INFECTION)
An infection of the lower urinary tract

History
- Dysuria
- Hematuria
- Increased urinary frequency or urgency, incomplete emptying of the bladder
- Flank and/or suprapubic pain
- Uterine contractions/cramping

Physical Examination
- Fever
- Pyuria, positive nitrites, and hematuria on urinalysis

Considerations
- This is not uncommon in pregnant persons due to the effects of progesterone on the motility of the ureters.
- The urinary tract is typically sterile. Urinary tract infections (UTIs) occur when bacteria ascends into the urinary tract. The most common organism causing a UTI is *Escherichia coli*.

ANEMIA IN PREGNANCY
This is a condition in which the blood does not carry enough oxygen to the rest of the body. Iron deficiency is the most common cause of anemia in pregnancy due to increased maternal iron needs, fetal iron needs, and expanded maternal blood volume.

History
- Fatigue, weakness, shortness of breath, headaches
- Leg cramps
- Cold intolerance
- Reported iron-deficient diet
- Pagophagia or pica
- Gastrointestinal (GI) issues affecting iron absorption
- A history of closely spaced pregnancies

Physical Examination
- Pallor
- Tachycardia
- Decreased hemoglobin and ferritin levels

Considerations
- Physiologic anemia is often seen during the second trimester of pregnancy due to increased blood volume.
- Diagnosis and treatment are important as iron deficiency anemia may contribute to preterm birth, intrauterine growth restriction, decrease in maternal blood reserves during birth and increase in need for transfusion after birth, and decreased milk production.

ASYMPTOMATIC BACTERIURIA
The presence of a high level of bacteria in the urine with no patient-reported symptoms

History
- No signs or symptoms consistent with UTI

Physical Examination
- A high level of bacterial growth is found on urine culture ($\geq 10^5$ CFU/mL).
- If bacteriuria is due to group B streptococcus (GBS), treatment threshold is not different; however, the patient should be considered to be GBS-positive during labor and administered intrapartum antibiotic prophylaxis; GBS testing between 36 and 38 weeks' gestation is not indicated in this situation.

Considerations
- This is common in pregnancy and should be treated as these infections have a higher likelihood of ascending to the kidneys.
- Pregnant persons should be universally screened for asymptomatic bacteriuria at their initial prenatal visit.
- Asymptomatic bacteriuria may also cause preterm contractions, so it should be considered when preterm contractions and persistent cramping are complaints.

CONSTIPATION IN PREGNANCY
A condition that causes hard stools; infrequent or hard to pass bowel movements

History
- Reports difficult/painful bowel movements, hard stools, and/or straining with bowel movements
- History of infrequent bowel movements (<3 times week)
- Abdominal pain
- Low-fiber diet
- Decreased fluid intake

- Ignoring the urge to have a bowel movement
- Feeling bloated
- History of laxative or opioid use

Physical Examination
- On abdominal exam, hard, palpable stool in the ascending, descending, and sigmoid segments of the colon
- Hard or impacted stool during a rectal exam

Considerations
- Constipation is a common concern during all trimesters of pregnancy, although it is typically more prevalent during the first trimester. Pregnant people may also experience constipation due to more pressure on the GI tract from the uterus as it grows throughout pregnancy.
- Prenatal vitamins with iron or the addition of an iron supplement during pregnancy can also contribute to constipation.

FIRST-TRIMESTER BLEEDING
Vaginal bleeding during the first trimester, occurring in approximately 20% to 40% of pregnancies

Benign First-Trimester Bleeding
This bleeding would include implantation bleeding, vaginitis, mistaken hematuria or rectal bleeding, or bleeding from a cervical polyp.

History
- Light spotting/vaginal bleeding
- History of recent intercourse

Physical Examination
- Presence of fetal heart tones at 12 weeks' gestation or more with Doppler
- Presence of fetal cardiac activity/fetal movement on ultrasound
- Increasing levels of human chorionic gonadotropin (hCG)

First-Trimester Bleeding That Is Cause for Increased Surveillance or Indicative of Miscarriage
Include blighted ovum, subchorionic hemorrhage (carries increased likelihood of miscarriage), "disappearing" twin gestation, spontaneous abortion (either complete or incomplete), or missed abortion

History
- History of ectopic pregnancy or previous miscarriage
- History of uterine anomaly
- History of adnexal surgery

- History of pelvic inflammatory disease (PID) or endometriosis
- Presence of an intrauterine device (IUD)
- Varying amount of vaginal bleeding, passing tissue and/or large clots from vagina
- Abdominal cramping, back pain
- Lightheadedness

Physical Examination
- Absence of fetal heart tones at 12 weeks' gestation or more with Doppler
- Absence of fetal cardiac activity/fetal movement on ultrasound
- EDD by LMP inconsistent with crown-rump length on ultrasound
- EDD by LMP inconsistent with uterine size on bimanual exam
- Decreasing levels of hCG

Considerations
- 15% to 20% of pregnancies will end in miscarriage and about 80% of those losses will occur in the first trimester.
- It is critical to exclude the possibility of an ectopic pregnancy in any patient with first-trimester bleeding as this can be a life-threatening complication.

GESTATIONAL DIABETES MELLITUS
Diabetes (high blood sugar) that is diagnosed for the first time in pregnancy and usually returns back to normal soon after delivery

History
- Commonly asymptomatic
- May have increased thirst or urination
- Previous history of GDM, prediabetes, or PCOS
- Family history of diabetes
- Lack of physical activity
- Races other than White more susceptible

Physical Examination
- Can be overweight/obese
- Elevated blood sugar during the two-step test

Considerations
- The U.S. Preventive Services Task Force (2016) recommends screening for GDM in all asymptomatic pregnant persons after 24 weeks' gestation. The test is typically performed between 24 and 28 weeks' gestation with an oral glucose challenge.
- Infants born to mothers with GDM have an increased incidence of macrosomia, neonatal hypoglycemia, hyperbilirubinemia, shoulder dystocia, and birth trauma.

HYPERTENSIVE DISORDERS

Chronic or Gestational Hypertension

Chronic hypertension (cHTN) is defined as hypertension diagnosed or present before pregnancy or before 20 weeks of gestation. Additionally, cHTN is hypertension diagnosed for the first time during pregnancy that does not resolve during the postpartum period. *Gestational hypertension* is defined as a systolic BP of ≥140 mmHg or a diastolic BP of ≥90 mmHg on two separate occasions in a pregnant person with previously normal BP. BP readings return to normal in the postpartum period. These measurements must be at least 4 hours apart and after 20 weeks' gestation.

History
- History of kidney disease or DM
- Multiple gestation
- May have no signs or symptoms (other than elevated BP)

Physical Examination
- Elevated BP
- Headache
- Edema
- Nausea/vomiting
- May progress to preeclampsia

Considerations
- Gestational HTN must be distinguished from preeclampsia by the absence of proteinuria or severe features (see next section for the diagnostic criteria for preeclampsia).
- Gestational HTN with a BP in the severe range (a systolic BP of 160 mmHg or greater or a diastolic BP of 110 mmHg or greater) should be diagnosed instead as having preeclampsia with severe features.

Preeclampsia

Preeclampsia is HTN plus proteinuria during pregnancy, with an onset after 20 weeks' gestation. In those with gestational HTN in the absence of proteinuria, preeclampsia may also be diagnosed with the new onset of any severe features (see the following text for list).

History and Physical Examination
- Proteinuria
- Elevated BP
- Severe features

- New-onset headache unresponsive to medication and not accounted for by alternative diagnoses
- New-onset visual disturbances
- Severe persistent right upper quadrant or epigastric pain unresponsive to medication and not accounted for by alternative diagnoses
- Thrombocytopenia (platelet count $<10,000 \times 10^9$/L)
- Renal insufficiency (serum creatinine >1.1 mg/dL or a doubling of the serum creatinine)
- Impaired liver function (doubling of liver transaminases)
- Pulmonary edema

Eclampsia
When preeclampsia is left untreated, it can progress to the serious condition, eclampsia.

History and Physical Examination
- Seizures
- Coma
- Expiry

Consideration
- Up to 50% of pregnant persons with gestational HTN will eventually develop preeclampsia during their pregnancy.

Hyperemesis Gravidarum
Severe symptoms of nausea and vomiting that often require inpatient management in the first and second trimesters

History
- Personal or family history of hyperemesis gravidarum
- Severe nausea
- Having multiples
- Overweight
- Food aversions
- Dizziness/lightheadedness, headaches
- Persistent vomiting ($>3–4$ times daily)

Physical Examination
- Large ketonuria
- Dehydration
- Weight loss (typically at least 5% of prepregnancy weight)
- Abnormalities with electrolytes, thyroid function, and liver function

Considerations
- Nausea and vomiting of pregnancy is modulated by increased hCG and estrogen levels.
- Approximately 50% to 80% of pregnant persons will report nausea and 50% will experience both nausea and vomiting.
- "Normal" pregnancy-related nausea and vomiting should be differentiated from hyperemesis gravidarum. Unfortunately, there is no widely accepted clinical distinction between the two.

Pruritic Urticarial Papules and Plaques of Pregnancy
A benign, self-limiting rash that occurs during pregnancy and most often resolves within 7 to 10 days after delivery

History
- Pruritic rash that typically develops in the third trimester
- History of rapid, excessive weight gain, or multiple gestation
- More likely to occur in first pregnancies

Physical Examination
- Scattered erythematous papules are most often found on the abdomen with a clear area directly around the umbilicus.
- Lesions may spread to the extremities, chest, and back; combine to form plaques. In patients with fair skin, white halos may surround the papules.
- Lesions started in striae.
- There are no lesions in the periumbilical area.
- Typically lesions are not on the face, palms, or soles.

Considerations
- Pruritic urticarial papules and plaques of pregnancy are typically seen in primiparous patients toward the end of pregnancy (mean time of onset is 35 weeks' gestation).
- It is benign, self-limiting, and most often resolves within 7 to 10 days after delivery.
- It occurs in 0.3% to 0.6% of pregnancies and is more common with multiple gestation and male fetuses.

Gestational Thrombocytopenia
Gestational thrombocytopenia is characterized by a platelet count of less than 150×10^9/L. Thrombocytopenia is often asymptomatic and may only be discovered on routine complete blood count (CBC) in pregnancy.

History
- Onset in the mid-second to third trimester
- Often asymptomatic
- No history of bleeding
- No history of thrombocytopenia outside of pregnancy

Physical Examination
- A platelet count of $<150 \times 10^9$/L is typically found on routine screening.
- Thrombocytopenia resolves after pregnancy (within 1–2 months postpartum).

Considerations
- Gestational thrombocytopenia occurs in 5% to 11% of pregnancies.
- A gradual decrease in platelets is expected as pregnancy progresses, but thrombocytopenia may result from both physiologic and pathologic conditions.
- There is no significant maternal or fetal risk with gestational thrombocytopenia, and the diagnosis is one of exclusion. The clinician will want to assess for a history of any bleeding disorders or symptoms associated with platelet disorders, such as petechiae, ecchymosis, epistaxis, gingival bleeding, or a history of menometrorrhagia.

PHYSICAL EXAMINATION DOCUMENTATION

Documentation should include results of inspection, palpation, and auscultation.

EXAMPLE OF NORMAL FINDINGS FROM FIRST PRENATAL VISIT AT 8 WEEKS' GESTATION

Blood pressure 120/80, pulse rate 72 per minute, weight 122 lb

Well-appearing and afebrile. Heart rate and rhythm regular. Lungs clear to auscultation bilaterally. Breasts engorged, no distinct masses or lymphadenopathy palpable. Abdomen soft, nontender, and nondistended. Speculum exam completed without discomfort; no vaginal discharge, erythema, or edema noted. Cervix long, posterior, thick, and closed. Uterine size and shape consistent with 8 weeks' gestation; soft lower uterine segment. No palpable adnexal tenderness. On urinalysis, protein negative. Glucose negative. Labs pending.

EXAMPLE OF NORMAL FINDINGS FROM ROUTINE PRENATAL VISIT (18 WEEKS' GESTATION)

Blood pressure 120/80, pulse rate 72 per minute, weight 130 lb

Well-appearing and afebrile. Weight increased 4 lb from the last visit 4 weeks ago and blood pressure unchanged. No facial or peripheral edema noted. Fundal height 2 cm below the umbilicus. Fetal heart tones 140 beats per minute.

REFERENCES

References for this chapter draw from Chapter 24, Evidence-Based Obstetric Assessment, of the textbook *Evidence-Based Physical Examination: Best Practices for Health and Well-Being Assessment (Second Edition)*. The references may be accessed in the digital version of the handbook at connect.springerpub.com/.

16

Evidence-Based Assessment of Mental Health Including Substance Use Disorders

CLINICAL CONSIDERATIONS

- Normalize discussion of mental health concerns as part of the assessment of health and well-being. Mental status and mental health assessment should be included as part of every health encounter.
- Ask directly about suicidal thoughts, self-harm, and suicide attempts; provide opportunity for individuals to discuss suicidality and mental health concerns openly.
- Be observant for signs and symptoms that suggest a lack of vitality. Lack of energy and/or interest in activities that used to bring enjoyment is the key sign of depression.
- When clinicians assess individuals who are struggling with anxiety, depression, and/or substance use, they should also consider that the patient may have additional physical or mental health disorders.
- Trauma, social isolation, genetic factors, and comorbidities increase the likelihood of brain and nervous system changes that lead to mental health and substance use disorders (SUDs).
- Substance use can be associated with compromised functioning in virtually every system of the body.
- Assessing and engaging effectively with individuals who are unable to control or reduce their use of substances and/or whose use continues despite consequences requires empathy.

COMPREHENSIVE MENTAL HEALTH ASSESSMENT

An assessment of an individual's mental health provides the basis for identifying signs and/or symptoms of any underlying mental health concerns and gives the clinician an understanding of the patient's cognitive, emotional, personality, and psychological functioning. This assessment can be done in the course of an individual's routine history and physical examination in primary care; however, if there are specific mental health concerns or abnormalities found during the evaluation, it is recommended to have a visit specific to these concerns after assuring patient safety. Reviewing the reason for seeking care, history of any recent symptoms or problems, as well as a comprehensive health history provides the clinician with valuable information about mental status and health. Within the mental health assessment, the clinician can identify an individual's strengths and coping and note whether there are concerns that require more in-depth or formal assessment of mental health. The mental health assessment is performed within the context of the patient's age, developmental level, and cultural norms.

An initial visit for a psychiatric concern is described as an initial psychiatric evaluation, comprehensive psychiatric evaluation, psychiatric diagnostic interview, and/or comprehensive mental health assessment. The components and criteria to include are outlined in this chapter, and begin with clarifying the patient's identifying data (name, date of birth, gender, and pronouns), referral source (primary care provider, specialist, or therapist), and reason for the visit.

COMMON REASONS FOR SEEKING CARE

- Depressive symptoms such as sadness, insomnia, guilt or unworthiness, energy loss, change in appetite, anhedonia or loss of interest, psychomotor changes, and suicidality
- Anxiety symptoms such as excessive worry and nervousness
- Substance use concerns, alcohol misuse, and smoking cessation

HISTORY OF PRESENT ILLNESS

- The history of present illness (HPI) questions used to assess mental health concerns can follow the same format for episodic visits, and can be used to determine whether additional screening for mental health disorders is needed. The four examples included (in the text that follows) are intended to show how the HPI assessment can be adapted based on the presenting symptoms for individuals with mental health concerns. Note that the question "Are the symptoms currently interfering with functioning at work (school) and home?" is a key question, as interference with functioning is often one important indicator of a mental health diagnosis.

History of Present Illness Example Incorporating Assessments for Depression and Anxiety

- **Onset:** When did the symptoms start or at what age did you first have these symptoms? Have they been persistent? When are your symptoms better? Worse?
- **Sadness/depressed mood:** Are you feeling sad, helpless, or hopeless? Having trouble concentrating?
- **Insomnia/sleep disturbance:** Are you having difficulty falling asleep? Staying asleep?

- **Guilt or unworthiness:** Are you having feelings of unworthiness?
- **Energy loss or fatigue:** Are you feeling fatigued? Describe your energy level on most days. Has your energy level significantly changed?
- **Changes in appetite:** Has your appetite been decreased? Increased? Has your weight changed? If so, explain.
- **Anhedonia or loss of interest:** Are you finding it difficult to participate in things that you once found enjoyable?
- **Psychomotor changes:** Are you feeling sluggish? Agitated?
- **Suicidality:** Do you have suicidal thoughts? (OR do you think about death or hurting yourself?) Have you ever been suicidal? Have you attempted suicide before? Do you have a plan? Do you have the means to carry out this plan?
- **Severity:** How difficult have these problems made it for you to do your work or take care of things at home, or get along with other people? Are the symptoms currently interfering with functioning at work (school) and home?

History of Present Illness Example for the Individual
Who Currently Smokes Cigarettes
- **Onset:** Time of first cigarette in the morning, waking at night to smoke
- **Location:** Smoking at work, home, in the car, around children
- **Duration:** Age when smoking began, previous attempts to quit
- **Characteristics:** Number of cigarettes smoked each day, most recent cigarette; also noting whether any additional types of nicotine or tobacco are used
- **Associated symptoms:** Cough, wheezing, or respiratory problems; chest pain; fatigue; and/or symptoms associated with smoking cessation attempts
- **Relieving symptoms:** Coping skills, pharmacologic and/or non-pharmacologic methods to quit, previous or current counseling
- **Timing or temporal factors:** Use related to stress or need to relax, concurrent use of substances, personal beliefs about need or desire to quit (i.e., readiness to change)
- **Severity:** How difficult has it been to continue smoking or to quit smoking

History of Present Illness Example for Individual
Who Is Misusing Alcohol
- **Onset:** Time of first drink, amount of drinks per day
- **Location:** Drinking alone, socially, before or associated with driving a motor vehicle
- **Duration:** Occasions of heavy use and binge drinking, average use days per week
- **Characteristics:** Typical amount of alcohol use, type of alcohol use, history of blackouts, most recent use

- **Associated symptoms:** Emotions and beliefs related to use, abstinence; consequences of alcohol use (e.g., unable to attend school or work; effect on relationships; legal issues; health issues, including type 2 diabetes, pancreatitis, cancers, heart disease, dementia, hepatitis, and cirrhosis); recent intoxication, disinhibition, or stupor
- **Relieving symptoms:** Coping skills, support system, pharmacologic and/or nonpharmacologic methods to quit, previous or current counseling or involvement in recovery groups, previous periods of sobriety, and what worked to achieve this
- **Timing or temporal factors:** Use related to stress or need to relax, concurrent use of substances, personal beliefs about need or desire to quit (i.e., readiness to change)
- **Severity:** How difficult has it been to continue drinking or to quit drinking; and if drinking, or problems related to drinking, is interfering with functioning at work (school) and home

History of Present Illness Example Incorporating Screening for Substance Use Disorder

- **Onset:** When did the symptoms start? At what age did you start feeling this way and/or using substances?
- **Location:** Location of any pain or physical symptoms?
- **Duration:** Are the symptoms persistent?
- **Characteristics** (*incorporate a screening tool; CRAFFT Questionnaire (version 2.1) used in this example is appropriate for use in teens and young adults*):

  During the past 12 months, on how many days did you:
  1. Drink more than a few sips of beer, wine, or any drink containing alcohol?
  2. Use any marijuana (weed, cannabis, or hash by smoking, vaping, or in food) or synthetic marijuana (like K2 or spice)
  3. Use anything else to get high (like illegal drugs, prescription or over-the-counter [OTC] medications, or things that you sniff, huff, or vape)?

  If "0" for all questions above, ask CAR question (4) only. Otherwise, ask all six questions that follow and note that two or more YES answers suggest a serious problem and need further assessment:
  4. **C:** Have you ever ridden in a CAR driven by someone (including yourself) who was "high" or had been using alcohol or drugs?
  5. **R:** Do you ever use alcohol or drugs to RELAX, feel better about yourself, or fit in?
  6. **A:** Do you ever use alcohol or drugs while you are by yourself, or ALONE?
  7. **F:** Do you ever FORGET things you did while using alcohol or drugs?

8. **F:** Do your FAMILY or FRIENDS ever tell you that you should cut down on your drinking or drug use?
9. **T:** Have you ever gotten into TROUBLE while you were using alcohol or drugs?

- **Aggravating factors:** What makes your symptoms or use worse?
- **Relieving factors:** When are the symptoms better? What treatment have you tried?
- **Timing:** What actions or activities decrease the symptoms?
- **Severity and scale:** How difficult have these problems made it for you to do your work or take care of things at home or get along with other people? Are the symptoms currently interfering with functioning at work (school) and home?

PSYCHIATRIC REVIEW OF SYSTEMS

- Mental health review of systems (ROS) includes sadness, helplessness, hopelessness, worry, insomnia, hypersomnia, fatigue, and headaches; changes in memory, concentration, or mood, as well as memory loss, mood swings, mania, risk-taking, anxiety, worry, guilt, and shame; and suicidal or homicidal ideation, hallucinations, and delusions.
- Individualize history taking for symptoms of mental health disorders based on reason for seeking care and HPI. Consider use of evidence-based screening tools (**Box 16.1**) for the psychiatric ROS; before screening for experiences of traumatic events, review the tenets of trauma-informed care.

HEALTH HISTORY

Past Psychiatric History

- Onset of first mental health symptoms
- Previous or current diagnosis of anxiety, depression, trauma, or mental health disorders
- Previous or current treatment of mental health concerns
- Hospitalizations, surgeries, ED visits for psychiatric disorders
- Past suicidal ideation (SI), suicide attempts, or self-injury behaviors
- Chronic pain, recent or current acute pain

Substance Use History

- Current and past use of substances, including tobacco, alcohol, marijuana, caffeine, illicit drugs; age of first use, amount used, frequency and route of use; history of misuse
- Previous or current diagnosis of SUD, alcoholism, or addiction
- SUD history of treatment and recovery periods, if applicable

Past Medical History

- Hospitalizations, surgeries, ED visits
- Constitutional changes, including weight loss and fatigue
- Physical disabilities or reduced mobility

BOX 16.1 Evidence-Based Screening Tools

- Evidence-based screening tools are used to identify concerning signs and/or symptoms that may indicate mental health diagnoses. Although these screenings are highly important in helping identify mental health disorders, diagnoses must be confirmed with careful diagnostic evaluation, which goes beyond screening.

Patient Health Questionnaire (PHQ-9 and PHQ-2) Depression Scales
- The nine-item Patient Health Questionnaire (PHQ-9) is a valid and reliable tool for screening and monitoring the severity of depression. Question 9 of the tool screens for the presence and duration of suicidal ideation. The brief two-item Patient Health Questionnaire (PHQ-2) consists of the first two questions of the PHQ-9 and screens for core symptoms of depressive disorder; the following are the two questions:
  ○ Over the past 2 weeks, how often have you been bothered by the following problems?
    1. Little interest or pleasure in doing things
       ♦ Not at all (0)
       ♦ Several days (+1)
       ♦ More than half the days (+2)
       ♦ Nearly every day (+3)
    2. Feeling down, depressed, or hopeless
       ♦ Not at all (0)
       ♦ Several days (+1)
       ♦ More than half the days (+2)
       ♦ Nearly every day (+3)

The total score from the PHQ-2 ranges from 0 to 6. If the score is 3 or greater, depressive disorder is likely.

Generalized Anxiety Disorder Scale (GAD-7 and GAD-2)
- The seven-item Generalized Anxiety Disorder Scale (GAD-7) is a validated screening tool for anxiety that includes a severity scale. The abbreviated two-item Generalized Anxiety Disorder Scale (GAD-2) screening consists of the first two questions of the GAD-7:
  ○ Over the past 2 weeks, how often have you been bothered by the following problems?

(continued)

BOX 16.1 Evidence-Based Screening Tools (*continued*)

1. Feeling nervous, anxious, or on edge
   ♦ Not at all (0)
   ♦ Several days (+1)
   ♦ More than half the days (+2)
   ♦ Nearly every day (+3)
2. Not being able to stop worrying
   ♦ Not at all (0)
   ♦ Several days (+1)
   ♦ More than half the days (+2)
   ♦ Nearly every day (+3) b

The scoring for the GAD-2 is similar to the PHQ-2, ranging from 0 to 6. The recommended cut-point for a positive screening is a score of 3 or greater. The GAD-2 and PHQ-2 can be used together (referred to as the *PHQ-4*) to screen for depression and anxiety.

Single-Question Screenings for Substance Misuse

- Evidence suggests that single-screening questions can be effective tools to identify substance misuse. Note that screening negatively for the misuse of one substance does not negate the need to screen for misuse of other substances. A response of one or more is considered a positive screen.
   ○ **Single-question screen to identify illicit substance use:** "How many times in the past year have you used an illegal drug or used a prescription medication for nonmedical reasons?" If clarification of "nonmedical reasons" is needed, provide the explanation, for instance, "because of the experience or feeling it caused."
   ○ **Single-question screening for alcohol misuse:** "How many times in the past year have you had x or more drinks in a day?" where x is five for men and four for women.

- Motor vehicle accidents
- Chronic physical illness/comorbidities, including seizures, loss of consciousness, traumatic brain injury
- Recent or past infectious disease
- Prescribed or OTC medications or supplements, including dose and frequency
- Allergies to medications, or seasonal, environmental, and/or food allergies, including reactions

FAMILY HISTORY

- Anxiety, depression, bipolar disorder, schizophrenia, psychosis
- Other mental health disorders including learning disabilities (e.g., attention deficit hyperactivity disorder [ADHD])
- Neurologic disorders, seizure disorders
- SUD, alcoholism or addiction
- Deaths by suicide or suicide attempts (trajectory; impact on family)
- Other chronic diseases impacted by smoking, alcohol use, or substance misuse

SOCIAL HISTORY

- Home situation and relationships
  - Married/single/divorced/widowed/partnered?
  - Who lives in the home? Is partner supportive?
  - Substance use in the home?
  - Is housing/home/neighborhood safe? Involved in community activities?
  - Social support system? Close friends? Pets?
- Safety (including work or school environment)
  - Trauma history, including adverse childhood events (ACEs), bereavement, grief, isolation
  - Risk or current victim of violence
  - Stress, anxiety, burnout related to workplace culture, school or work expectations
  - Financial or career concerns
  - Legal problems, justice involvement, history of driving under the influence
  - Access to guns, weapons

Risk Assessment

- A particularly sensitive part of the mental health assessment is risk assessment for danger to self, danger to others, and danger from others.
- To determine **danger to self**, it is imperative to conduct a suicide risk assessment. Screen for suicidal ideation, plan, and means. Use a valid suicide risk screening tool such as the PHQ-9, or Ask Suicide-Screening Questions. Assess history of self-injurious behavior and past attempts. Note that the period just following psychiatric hospital discharge is an extremely high-risk time for patients. Ask directly about current ideation and clarify the plan, including how the patient plans to die by suicide. Ask about the means or ability to carry out their plan, including access to guns or substances. Asking about the use and availability of substances is a critical question when assessing suicide risk, danger to self, or danger to others. Ask whether the individual has ever overdosed, nearly overdosed, or has concerns about or has considered overdose with medications or alcohol.

- Homicidal ideation is risk of **danger to others**. If the patient acknowledges a desire to harm someone else, it is necessary to ask about their plan, intent, available means, and specific target. If they identify someone specifically and have a plan, the intended victim and law enforcement must be informed.
- Screen for safety or **danger from others**, including trauma and ACEs. Determine current and/or previous experiences of violence, abuse, and neglect. Note that younger and older populations are particularly vulnerable to being in danger from others.

Red Flags in Risk Assessment
- Those who have mental health and/or SUDs are at increased risk for dying by suicide; additional risk factors include male gender; increasing age; being single, widowed, or divorced; family history of suicide; and prior suicide attempt. Individuals considering suicide may give verbal and/or nonverbal cues that should always be taken seriously. It is important to note warning signs and directly assess suicidality. Red flags are listed in **Box 16.2**.
- Individuals exhibiting these symptoms should not be left alone; remove any dangerous objects or drugs that could be used in a suicide attempt and seek immediate help. The U.S. National Suicide Prevention Lifeline can be reached 24 hours a day at 9-8-8 or 1-800-273-TALK (8255). The nonprofit Crisis Text Line offers free text counseling; to reach the text line, text "Listen" to 741-741.

BOX 16.2 Red Flags in Subjective History That Indicate Risk of Suicidality (Suicidal Ideation, Plan, and/or Attempts)

- Threatening to hurt or kill themselves
- Seeking access to pills, weapons, or other means
- Talking or writing about death, dying, or suicide
- Feelings or statements of hopelessness
- Rage, anger, seeking revenge; feeling trapped
- Increased alcohol or other drug use
- Withdrawal from others
- Anxiety and agitation
- Sleep problems; insomnia or hypersomnia
- Dramatic mood changes
- Sudden and/or drastic change in behavior
- Feelings or statements that reflect not having a reason to live

MEDICAL REVIEW OF SYSTEMS

- **Neurologic:** Weakness, numbness, loss of consciousness, black-outs, headaches, falls, dizziness, idiopathic seizures, confusion
- **Integumentary:** Dryness, itching, bruising, rashes, lesions, burns, sweating
- **Head, eyes, ears, nose, throat:** Sensory deficits, congestion, sinus pain, sore throat
- **Lymphatic:** Bruising, bleeding, lymphadenopathy
- **Cardiovascular:** Chest pain, shortness of breath, rapid pulse
- **Respiratory:** Dyspnea, wheezing, cough, breathlessness
- **Musculoskeletal:** Injury history, pain, stiffness, or swelling
- **Gastrointestinal/genitourinary:** Weight and/or appetite changes, constipation, diarrhea, abdominal pain, nausea, vomiting, incontinence, poor nutrition

MENTAL STATUS EVALUATION

The mental status evaluation (MSE) is part of the patient's physical examination and can be included in any visit in as much detail as needed. The MSE incorporates observational assessment in seven areas: appearance, behavior, speech, affect (mood, emotion), thought process, thought content, and cognition. The seven MSE components can be remembered by the abbreviation ABSATTC, or the mnemonic **A**ll **B**est **S**tudents **A**re **T**aught **T**o **C**are. MSE observational data components (and descriptors) include the following:

A: Appearance

- General survey (no acute distress)
- Eye contact (direct, good, fair, poor, darting, fleeting, absent)
- Hygiene (neat, clean, malodorous, poor, hygiene, unkempt), appropriateness to situation
- Dress (bizarre, flamboyant, disheveled)
- Body habitus (height, weight, waist circumference, body mass index [BMI]), posture (recumbent, sitting, standing, erect, comfortable); note any limitations or defects

B: Behavior

- Verbal or nonverbal expressions (pain, anxiety, illness, anger, fear, frustration, contentment, or sadness)
- Interactions toward the clinician or others (cooperative, resistant, anxious, defensive, guarded, passive, aggressive, threatening, impulsive, distrustful, evasive, withdrawn)
- Activity level (calm, active, flat, restless); ask about previous/recent/current impulsivity
- Body movements and mobility (coordinated, limited, using assistive devices, and/or abnormal movements, tremor, tics, akathisia, dystonia, tardive dyskinesia); note ambulatory status, mannerisms, and psychomotor agitation or retardation

S: Speech and language
- Amount (minimal, excessive, rambling), latency (halting or pausing)
- Rate (rapid, pressured), rhythm, tone, volume

A: Affect
- The outward expressions of a person's feelings, emotions, or mood
  - Emotional expressions (appropriate, inappropriate, incongruent, manic, blunted, labile, exaggerated, restricted, reactive, flat)
  - Expressions of mood (euthymic, neutral, depressed, guilt, worry, fear, helplessness, or hopelessness; difficulty feeling enjoyment [anhedonia]; elated, euphoric, grandiosity; mood instability; irritability)

T: Thought process
- Flow of thoughts or thought processes may be coherent, incoherent, logical, goal-directed, illogical, poverty of thought, disorganized.

T: Thought content
- Dangerous or unusual ideas, delusions, auditory/visual/tactile/olfactory hallucinations, paranoia, attending to internal stimuli; ALWAYS assess for suicidal and homicidal ideation (See the Risk Assessment section of this chapter for additional assessment considerations)

C: Cognition
- **Orientation to time, person, place, and situation:** Confused, disoriented, delirious; note level of awareness
- **Attention and concentration:** Able to express coherent, organized thoughts, or rapidly shifting from one topic to next; note any concerns with success in work, school, or at home (distracted, poor attention)
- **Judgment:** Assessment of negative patterns of thinking (e.g., all-or-nothing thinking, catastrophizing, overgeneralization, blaming, emotional reasoning, or always being right); irrational fears; overwhelming worry; good, fair, poor (based on recent behavior or exam)
- **Insight:** Good, fair, poor (based on recent behavior or exam)
- **Memory:** Immediate (able to repeat three unrelated words and remember and repeat those words again in 5 minutes); recent, remote (personal past events, general cultural or historical information); concerns about memory loss

ADDITIONAL PHYSICAL EXAMINATION CONSIDERATIONS

- Assess for signs of acute and chronic disease when individuals present with mental health concerns. As noted previously, mental health disorders, including substance use/misuse, are likely to result in development of comorbidities. The following are specific health effects of substances to consider when determining components of the physical exam:

  - Excessive alcohol consumption increases the risk of developing type 2 diabetes, pancreatitis, cancers, cardiomyopathy, dementia, hepatitis, and cirrhosis, in addition to the short-term intoxication, disinhibition, stupor, and potential for coma and death.

  - Tobacco use causes damage to nearly every organ in the body, often leading to lung cancer, heart disease, stroke, emphysema, and chronic bronchitis.

  - Marijuana has not only immediate effects like distorted perception, difficulty problem-solving, and loss of motor coordination, but also has effects with long-term use, including respiratory infections, impaired memory, and exposure to cancer-causing compounds.

  - Opioids not only reduce the perception of pain, but also produce drowsiness, mental confusion, euphoria, nausea, constipation, and respiratory depression. Most overdose deaths from substance use are attributable to opioids.

  - Benzodiazepines are correlated with a high risk of dependency. When combined with other sedatives, opiates or alcohol, the risk of serious side effects increases dramatically, including profound sedation, respiratory depression, coma, and death. Withdrawal from benzodiazepines can precipitate seizures, psychosis, panic attacks, sleep disturbances, and difficulties with memory.

Red Flags in Objective Exam

- Individuals may present with symptoms resulting from ingestion, withdrawal, and/or chronic use of substances, in addition to the symptoms of mental health disorders that are incompletely treated or untreated. Substance use can be associated with compromised function in any or every body system related to the substance used, how the substance was ingested, and/or the high-risk behaviors in which an individual engages.

- **Box 16.3** includes a list of physical signs that may indicate substance misuse, SUD, or addiction. Note that these signs may indicate intoxication, withdrawal, or heavy use. Signs may be related to the type of substance used or method of use. Presence or absence of these signs is not the sole assessment of substance use.

> **BOX 16.3** Red Flags in Objective Exam Indicating Possible Substance Misuse, Substance Use Disorder, or Addiction

- **General survey:** Thin, altered vital signs; unsteady gait
- **Appearance:** Poor personal hygiene; smell of alcohol, tobacco, or drug use
- **Mental status:**
  - Combative, aggressive, or bizarre behavior; may appear fatigued, sedated
  - Impaired cognition, confusion, disorientation
  - Slurred speech
- **Integumentary:** Jaundice, diaphoresis, lesions/rashes, burns, scars, abscesses, very dry skin
- **Head, neck, and lymphatics:** Bruising, bleeding, lymphadenopathy
- **Eyes:** Eye redness or drainage, pupil dilation or constriction
- **Eyes, nose, throat:** Rhinorrhea, deviations or deformities in nasal septum, including perforation, atrophy of the nasal mucosa, epistaxis, pharyngitis
- **Respiratory:** Cough, wheezing, respiratory depression or tachypnea
- **Cardiovascular:** Hypertension, hypotension, tachycardia, edema
- **Gastrointestinal/genitourinary/gynecologic:** Hepatomegaly, splenomegaly, abdominal distention, signs of sexually transmitted infection
- **Neurologic:** Weakness, numbness, loss of consciousness, jitteriness, seizure activity
- **Musculoskeletal:** Pain with movement; neck pain, stiffness, or swelling

- While the clinician completes the history and physical exam, how they communicate with the individual who may be misusing substances is a priority. Clinicians should employ the Screening, Brief Intervention, and Referral to Treatment (SBIRT) framework and avoid implicit bias when completing the assessment of an individual using and/or misusing substances in order to avoid triggering shame, guilt, and resistance to treatment. The use of therapeutic communication strategies, including motivational interviewing, while interacting with the patient is foundational to evidence-based practice and improved patient outcomes.

STRENGTHS, GOALS, AND PREVENTIVE CARE CONSIDERATIONS

Assess strategies to facilitate mental well-being preferred by the patient. Identify strengths, interests, or wellness behaviors that may become part of their treatment goals and plan, including the following:

- Physical activity and exercise
- Typical diet, access to fruits and vegetables
- Adequate sleep and rest
- Alcohol moderation or abstinence
- Family, social, and/or community support, including recovery groups
- Religious beliefs or spiritual practices; holistic practices
- Removal of triggers (sources of stress, caffeine, nicotine)
- Deep breathing
- Movement therapies (yoga, tai chi)
- Meditation, progressive muscle relaxation, mindfulness-based stress reduction
- Bibliotherapy, such as self-help books, workbooks, and psychoeducation
- Counseling, cognitive behavioral therapy

CONSIDERATIONS FOR COMPREHENSIVE MENTAL HEALTH ASSESSMENT

- The environments where people are born, live, learn, work, play, worship, and age affect mental health and wellness outcomes. Individuals experience harmful mental health consequences in response to "everyday discrimination," that is, the microaggressions, disrespect, and recurring indignities faced in society. Hundreds of studies support the correlation between systemic inequities and poorer mental health outcomes. The impact is so significant that the *Diagnostic and Statistical Manual of Mental Disorders, Fifth Edition, Text Revision (DSM-5-TR)* includes a comprehensive review of the impact of racism and discrimination on the diagnosis, signs, and symptoms of mental disorders. The following are two examples that highlight the impact of bias on mental health concerns:
  - In the United States, Black, Hispanic, Native American/Alaska Native, Asian, and Native Hawaiian/Pacific Islander populations have less access to mental health services, are less likely to receive needed care, and are more likely to receive poorer quality care when they obtain care than non-Hispanic White populations.
  - LGBTQIA+ youth experience bullying, social rejection and isolation, diminished peer support, discrimination, verbal abuse, and violence at a disproportionate rate when compared with cisgender, heterosexual peers.

- Chapter 17, Evidence-Based Considerations for Assessment Across the Life Span, in this text reviews history taking appropriate for a child or teen presenting with a mental health or behavioral issue. For adolescents, the Home, Education/Employment, Eating, Activities, Drugs, Sexuality, Suicidal ideation and Safety (HEEADSSS) assessment can be helpful in identifying mental health problems.

MENTAL HEALTH DISORDERS

The mental health disorders listed in this section of the chapter are in alphabetical order, not in order of prevalence. The list is not exhaustive.

ANXIETY AND ANXIETY DISORDERS

These are chronic conditions characterized by excessive and persistent worry, tension, and apprehension, causing difficulty functioning at home, school, work, or social situations. To meet the *DSM-5-TR* criteria for an anxiety disorder, there must be difficulty in functioning owing to the anxiety symptoms at home, school, or social situations. Part of the *DSM-5-TR* criteria for the diagnosis of a generalized anxiety disorder (GAD) are embedded in the GAD-2 and GAD-7 screenings, specifically asking the patient if they feel nervous, anxious, or on edge, and if they have not been able to stop or control the worrying.

History
- Excessive worry, fear, feeling of impending doom
- Inability to concentrate, racing thoughts
- Hypervigilance, restlessness, irritability
- Insomnia
- Fatigue

Physical Examination
- Racing heart rate (with palpitations)
- Sweating, trembling
- May have racing thoughts and restlessness on mental status exam

Considerations
- Types of anxiety disorders include GAD, obsessive-compulsive disorder (OCD), panic disorder, and social phobia or social anxiety disorder. Although posttraumatic stress disorder (PTSD) can be considered an anxiety disorder, the diagnosis is formally classified as a trauma- and stressor-related disorder.
- Comorbidities are common, including depression, ADHD, and SUD.
- Some conditions are misdiagnosed as anxiety (e.g., hyperthyroidism, lead intoxication, migraine headaches, substance misuse, and asthma).

- When screening for excessive worry, nervousness, and anxiousness, clinicians should recognize that this is a good time to ask additionally about the patient's usual coping strategies.

Pediatric Considerations
- Anxiety disorders are the most common mental health disorder in children and teens. Anxiety and fear are normal components of development, but should not be excessive, interfere with functioning, or persist beyond what is appropriate for an individual's developmental stage.
- Children with anxiety disorders often present with somatic symptoms, such as abdominal pain, headaches, or chest pain.

Key History Questions for Children and Adolescents
- Is the anxiety appropriate for the age of the child/teen?
- Do they have symptoms in response to a specific trigger (e.g., social situations)?
- Has the child/teen experienced a traumatic event?
- Is there a history of recent stressful events, including marital transition?
- Does their anxiety or worry interfere with functioning?
- What impact does the anxiety have on their sleep, concentration, appetite, energy, and relationships?
- What medications, prescribed or OTC, are they taking (e.g., antihistamines, antidepressants, stimulants, decongestants, caffeine, steroids, or asthma medications)?
- Is the child or teen using substances to regulate anxiety symptoms?

ATTENTION DEFICIT HYPERACTIVITY DISORDER

Diagnosis of ADHD involves assessment for a constellation of symptoms and is best understood as one of a spectrum of neurologic, developmental, cognitive, and genetic disorders. ADHD is often comorbid with other mental disorders and can present in adulthood. Individuals with ADHD show a persistent pattern of inattention and/or hyperactivity/impulsivity that interferes with function or development. Symptoms occur often (not always) and include the following:

- Inattention
  - Fails to give close attention to details or makes careless mistakes
  - Has trouble holding attention on tasks or playing activities
  - Does not seem to listen when spoken to directly
  - Does not follow through on instructions and fails to finish schoolwork, chores, or duties in the workplace (e.g., loses focus, side-tracked)
  - Has trouble organizing tasks and activities
  - Avoids, dislikes, or is reluctant to do tasks that require mental effort over a long period of time

- Loses things necessary for tasks and activities (e.g., school materials, pencils, books, tools, wallets, keys, paperwork, glasses, cell phones)
- Is easily distracted
- Is forgetful in daily activities
- Hyperactivity and impulsivity
  - Fidgets with or taps hands or feet, or squirms in seat
  - Leaves seat in situations when remaining seated is expected
  - Runs about or climbs in situations where it is not appropriate (adolescents or adults may be limited to feeling restless)
  - Unable to play or take part in leisure activities quietly
  - Is "on the go," acting as if "driven by a motor"
  - Talks excessively
  - Blurts out an answer before a question has been completed
  - Has trouble waiting for their turn
  - Interrupts or intrudes on others (e.g., into conversations or games)
- In addition, the following conditions must be met:
  - Several symptoms present before 12 years of age.
  - Several symptoms present in two or more settings (such as at home, school, or work; with guardians, friends, or relatives; in other activities).
  - Symptoms interfere with, or reduce the quality of, social, school, or work functioning.
  - Symptoms are not better explained by another mental disorder (such as a mood disorder, anxiety disorder, dissociative disorder, or a personality disorder).
- Children, adolescents, and adults can have ADHD that predominantly presents as inattention, or hyperactivity-impulsivity, or both. Because symptoms can change over time, the presentation may change over time as well. ADHD often lasts into adulthood. Symptoms might look different at older ages. For example, in adults, hyperactivity may appear as restlessness.

DEPRESSION AND MOOD DISORDERS

Mood disorders are mental health conditions characterized by disturbances in mood, including elevated mood (mania or hypomania), depressed mood (unipolar depression or major depressive disorder), or cycling between elevated and depressed moods (bipolar depression). Criteria for the diagnosis of depression (mild, moderate, and severe) are embedded in the evidence-based screenings reviewed. The mnemonic SIGECAPS is helpful in remembering the signs and symptoms of depression:

- **Sleep:** Increased (hypersomnia) or decreased (insomnia)
- **Interest:** Decreased, loss of ability to enjoy activities that were once enjoyed
- **Guilt:** Feelings of worthlessness, hopelessness

- **Energy:** Change in energy level, fatigued or restless
- **Concentration:** Difficulty making decisions
- **Appetite:** Changes in appetite, and/or weight increase or decrease
- **Psychomotor activity:** Increased (agitation) or decreased (slowed)
- **Suicidal ideation:** Recurrent thoughts of suicide, plans for committing suicide

If the screening or history is positive for depression, obtain a sense of how long the depressive symptoms have been present. When was the first episode of depression? Menstrual dysphoric disorder (MDD) is present for at least a 2-week period and has to include the presence of either sad mood or anhedonia, in addition to at least four associated symptoms. Persistent depressive disorder is a chronic form of depression and is a consolidated term of the *DSM-IV* chronic major depressive disorder and dysthymic disorder. In adults, symptoms last at least 2 years, and in children and adolescents duration must be at least 1 year. Depression can be related to medical illness, induced by substances including medication, and/or may be related to additional internal or external factors, such as premenstrual dysphoric disorder (PMDD) or with seasonal pattern, which is identified as a specifier according to the *DSM-5-TR*.

Note that the SIGECAPS symptoms listed earlier are nonspecific; that is, they can be associated with other disorders. The PHQ-2 is more specific, and if a person screens positively the PHQ-9 should then be administered. If only the PHQ-2 screening is used, the clinician should also ask about the presence of thoughts about death or dying, as suicidal ideation is *not* one of the two questions on the PHQ-2. It is imperative to conduct a suicide risk assessment.

The term *mood disorder* encompasses unipolar and bipolar depression. Screening for hypomania and mania is key to identifying assessments that may indicate bipolar disorder, which has either manic and depressive states, or manic states alone. Symptoms of hypomania and mania include decreased need for sleep for days to weeks, and persistently elevated, expansive, or irritable mood, along with increased activity or energy, grandiosity, more talkativeness, flights of ideas, distractibility, and involvement in risk-taking behaviors. Key questions include the following:

- Do you have racing thoughts? Those who do can describe those thoughts going so fast that they cannot keep track of them, or like cars on a racetrack.
- Has your speech been so fast that it is hard to follow? Pressured speech and flight of ideas may be correlated with mania.
- Have family or friends commented about your behavior or changes in behavior? If a family member or significant other is available, with the patient's permission, they can provide valuable input into the assessment of a mood disorder.

With bipolar disorder, mania is sometimes not recognized by the person, as insight is limited in this state. Patients with bipolar disorder most often seek help while in the depressed episode. DIGFAST is a mnemonic that can help the clinician remember the symptoms of mania:

- **Distractibility:** Difficulty blocking unimportant distractions
- **Indiscretion:** Excessive involvement in pleasurable activities
- **Grandiosity:** Feelings of invulnerability
- **Flight of ideas:** Racing thoughts, rapid shifting of ideas
- **Activity increase:** Dramatic periods of excitement, enthusiasm
- **Sleep deficit:** Decreased need for sleep
- **Talkativeness:** Pressured speech

Identifying symptoms of mania to differentiate unipolar and bipolar mood disorders significantly informs an individual's treatment plan. Antidepressants prescribed to persons with bipolar disorder can activate mania, often with negative outcomes for that person. Note that bipolar disorder can present first as a depressive disorder. The usual age of onset of serious mental disorders (bipolar disorder, thought disorders, and severe persistent mental health disorders) is generally in late adolescence and young adulthood, but can occur earlier or later.

Pediatric Considerations
Important points to note regarding the assessment of depression in children and teens include the following:

- Young children less than 7 years of age with depression are often misdiagnosed with ADHD as they frequently present with inattention, impulsivity, and hyperactivity.
- Anger is often a presenting symptom in adolescents.
- The mean age of onset for major depressive disorder is 14 years.
- Reoccurrence rate is as high as 60% to 70% and often reoccurs in adulthood; 40% to 70% of affected children/teens have co-morbid mental health conditions, so it is critical to assess for other mental health disorders (e.g., anxiety, substance use, ADHD).

Note that mood disorder symptoms can be nonspecific. Diagnoses that should be ruled out for children, teens, and adults include hypothyroidism, anemia, mononucleosis, eating disorders, substance use or withdrawal, premenstrual syndrome, diabetes, and lead intoxication.

THOUGHT DISORDERS AND SEVERE, PERSISTENT MENTAL ILLNESS

If the clinician has a difficult time following the patient's conversation while completing the history and physical exam, additional assessments may be needed for delusions, hallucinations, or disordered thoughts. These assessments help the clinician identify the red flags associated with severe, persistent mental illnesses, which are disorders defined by their level of severity and disability. The severe persistent mental illness (SPMI) category includes the symptomatology of disordered thought processes that can be associated with severe major depressive disorder, schizoaffective bipolar disorders, schizophrenia, psychoses, and borderline personality disorder. SPMIs are characterized by marked difficulties in self-care, marked restriction in activities of daily living (ADL), frequent deficiencies in concentration, and significant difficulties in maintaining social functioning.

Delirium

Key Assessments

- Fluctuating level of consciousness (i.e., decreased awareness and attention)
- Restless, agitated, combative behavior that may wax and wane; may be withdrawn
- Acutely disoriented; may have hallucinations, bizarre delusions, abnormal behavior

Considerations

- Suspect delirium when a new onset or an acute deterioration in behavior, cognition, or function occurs, especially in older adults or individuals who are depressed.
- In the older adult, delirium is often the presenting symptom of an underlying illness.

Delusions

Key Assessments

- Thoughts not based in reality, for example, "I am the king of this country"
- Usually has some level of paranoia associated
- Associated irritability, anger, especially if delusion is challenged

Considerations

- Symptom of severe, persistent mental illness, such as schizophrenia, delusional disorder, schizoaffective disorder, and schizophreniform disorder
- Can be a symptom of acute or chronic medical or neurologic disorder
- False belief not related to religious, cultural, or educational background
- Strongly held false beliefs; individual absolutely convinced of its truthfulness

Dementia
Key Assessments
- Memory loss, difficulty concentrating, mood changes
- Increasing difficulty with completing familiar tasks
- Confused about time, place; disrupts daily life
- Confusion worse in unfamiliar environments
- Repeated forgetting of recent events, names, faces
- May progress to language and communication problems, personality changes, lack of awareness, mobility issues, incontinence, dysphagia

Considerations
- Types include Alzheimer, vascular, Lewy bodies, and mixed dementia.
- Signs and symptoms vary depending on the type of disease/disorder, usually progressive.

Hallucinations
Key Assessments
- Sensory perception in the absence of real stimulus, caused by physical/mental disorders
- May be auditory, visual, or tactile

Considerations
- Associated with schizophrenia, psychotic disorder, or psychosis
- May be associated with substance use
- Also associated with Parkinson disease, epilepsy, dementia, brain tumor, migraines

TRAUMA- AND STRESSOR-RELATED DISORDERS
Trauma- and stressor-related disorders have many of the same symptoms as anxiety disorders; however, the conditions can be linked to traumatic experiences or significant stress. Diagnostic criteria include the following:

- Exposure to actual or threatened death, serious injury, or sexual violation in either:
  - Directly experiencing the traumatic event
  - Witnessing, in person, the event as it occurred to others
  - Learning that the event occurred to a close family member or close friend
  - Experiencing repeated or extreme exposure to aversive details of the traumatic event (e.g., first responders' on-site experiences, exposure to details of child abuse)
- Presence of the following symptoms:
  - **Intrusive thoughts:** Intrusive memories, flashbacks, recurrent nightmares
  - **Negative mood:** Inability to experience happiness, good emotions
  - **Dissociation:** Altered sense of reality, inability to remember aspects of the trauma

○ **Avoidance symptoms:** Efforts to avoid reminders, triggers of the event (isolation); efforts to avoid memories

○ **Arousal symptoms:** Hypervigilance, sleep disturbance, irritable, angry outbursts, exaggerated startle response, problems with concentration

With trauma- and stressor-related disorders, note that the symptoms are a normal human response to extreme stress and/or trauma. Diagnoses include the following:

- **Adjustment disorders:** These occur within 3 months of the onset of the stressor. Differential diagnoses include adjustment disorders with depressed mood; anxiety; mixed depressed mood and anxiety; disturbance of conduct, which might apply to children/teens who have experienced trauma; and disturbance of emotions and conduct.
- **Acute stress disorder:** Symptoms begin at the time of event and last 3 days to 1 month.
- **PTSD:** Symptoms or disturbances occur after 1 month. There are specific diagnostic criteria for PTSD for ages 6 to adulthood. In children under 6 years, if it is determined at the time of the assessment that the child has experienced trauma or extreme ACEs, it is best to document the examination/assessment and refer to a pediatric trauma specialist. Interestingly, young children respond very quickly to trauma-focused interventions, with much quicker response to treatment than adults.

SUBSTANCE USE DISORDERS

This section includes definitions of terms related to substance use, substance misuse, SUD, addiction, binge drinking, alcoholism, neonatal abstinence syndrome (NAS), and recovery.

MISUSE OF SUBSTANCES

Substance use is defined as the use, even once, of any psychoactive compound or substance. *Substance misuse* is the use of any substance in a manner, situation, amount, or frequency that can cause harm to users or to those around them.

SUBSTANCE USE DISORDER DIAGNOSES

SUD is a medical illness caused by repeated misuse of a substance or substances. SUD is characterized by clinically significant impairments in health, social function, and impaired control over substance use, and is diagnosed by assessment of cognitive, behavioral, and psychological symptoms. SUDs range from mild to severe and from temporary to chronic. SUD typically develops gradually over time, leading to changes in brain chemistry and function. Multiple factors influence whether and how rapidly a person develops an SUD. These factors include the substance itself and the genetic vulnerability of the user. Diagnostic criteria are listed in **Box 16.4**, and withdrawal symptoms that may be associated are listed in **Box 16.5**.

BOX 16.4 Diagnostic Criteria: Substance Use Disorder

Signs and Symptoms Consistent With Substance Use Disorder

- Substance used in larger amounts or over longer periods than intended
- Unsuccessful efforts to cut down or control substance use, despite the desire to do so
- Considerable time spent in activities necessary to obtain and use substance or to recover from the effects of substance use
- Craving or a strong desire to use the substance leading to onset of repeated substance use
- Tolerance resulting in need for increased amounts of the substance to attain the desired effect, or diminished effect with continued use of the same amount of the substance
- Withdrawal symptoms experienced, or the substance used to relieve or avoid withdrawal symptoms
- Recurrent substance use resulting in failure to fulfill major role obligations at work, school, or home
- Continued substance use despite having persistent or recurrent social or interpersonal problems
- Social, occupational, or recreational activities discontinued or reduced as a result of substance use
- Recurrent substance use in hazardous situations or environments
- Continued substance use despite knowledge of having a persistent or recurrent physical or psychological problem that is likely to have been caused or exacerbated by the substance

Note: Mild SUD is defined by two or three signs/symptoms of the 11 listed. Moderate SUD is defined by four to five signs/symptoms. Severe SUD manifests as six or more.

SUD, substance use disorder.

Source: Adapted from the American Psychiatric Association. (2022). *Diagnostic and statistical manual of mental disorders—5th edition—text revision.* https://doi.org/10.1176/appi.books.9780890425787

BOX 16.5 Substance-Specific Withdrawal Symptoms

Alcohol Withdrawal
Two or more of these symptoms:
- Autonomic hyperactivity
- Increased hand tremor
- Insomnia
- Nausea or vomiting
- Transient visual, tactile, or auditory hallucinations
- Psychomotor agitation
- Generalized tonic–clonic seizures

Cannabis Withdrawal
Three or more of these symptoms:
- Irritability, anger, or depression
- Nervousness or anxiety
- Sleep difficulties (e.g., insomnia or disturbing dreams)
- Decreased appetite or weight loss
- Restlessness
- Depressed mood
- Physical symptom that causes significant discomfort (abdominal pain, shakiness/tremors, sweating, fever, chills, or headache)

Opioid Withdrawal
Three or more of these symptoms:
- Moodiness
- Nausea or vomiting
- Muscle aches
- Lacrimation or rhinorrhea
- Yawning
- Pupillary dilation, piloerection, or sweating
- Diarrhea
- Fever
- Insomnia

Stimulant Withdrawal
Two or more of these symptoms:
- Fatigue
- Vivid, unpleasant dreams

(continued)

BOX 16.5 Substance-Specific Withdrawal Symptoms (*continued*)

- Insomnia or hypersomnia
- Increased appetite
- Psychomotor retardation or agitation

Tobacco Withdrawal

Four or more of these symptoms:

- Irritability, frustration, or anger
- Anxiety
- Difficulty concentrating
- Increased appetite or weight gain
- Restlessness
- Depressed mood
- Insomnia
- Decreased heart rate

Source: Adapted from the American Psychiatric Association. (2022). *Diagnostic and statistical manual of mental disorders—5th edition—text revision.* https://doi.org/10.1176/appi.books.9780890425787

Addiction

The most severe form of SUD, addiction, is a chronic brain disease characterized by compulsive or uncontrolled use of one or more substances. This disorder has the potential for relapse (recurrence after a significant time of abstinence), resistance to treatment, and recovery. Alcoholism is the disease of addiction to alcohol, characterized by heavy drinking, dependence, tolerance, and use despite consequences.

Alcohol Use Disorder

- Alcohol use disorder is the mild, moderate, or severe repeated misuse of alcohol. Additional terms are provided for clarity; note that alcoholism is defined by disease progression and consequences, and not by quantity of alcohol consumed, although alcohol misuse is characteristic.
  - **Standard drink:** Based on the 2015 to 2020 Dietary Guidelines for Americans, contains 14 g (0.6 oz) of pure alcohol, which equates to 12 oz of beer (5% alcohol content), 5 oz of wine (12% alcohol content), or 1.5 oz of distilled spirits/liquor (40% alcohol content)
  - **Moderate drinking:** Up to one standard drink per day for women and two drinks per day for men

- ○ **Binge drinking:** Consuming an excessive amount of alcohol on a single occasion; for men, defined as drinking five or more standard drinks; for women, four or more standard drinks
- ○ **Heavy drinking:** For women, consuming eight or more alcoholic beverages per week; for men, consuming 15 or more per week; also defined as binge drinking on 5 days or more in the past month

Opioid Use Disorder
Characterized by the persistent use of opioids despite the adverse consequences of its use

Tobacco Use Disorder
The most common SUD characterized by nicotine dependence and withdrawal symptoms with tobacco cessation attempts

LIFE-SPAN AND FAMILY CONSIDERATIONS

Newborns and Neonatal Abstinence Syndrome
Newborns who are exposed to substances during fetal growth and development can experience short- and long-term sequelae. When an infant is exposed to opiates in utero, the constellation of signs, symptoms, and problems that result is known as *neonatal abstinence syndrome*. The characteristic symptoms of NAS are highly variable and serious and include central nervous system hyperirritability and autonomic nervous system dysfunction. Pregnancy complications associated with opiate use include intrauterine growth restriction, placental abruption, preterm delivery, oligohydramnios, stillbirth, NAS, and maternal death. Opiate use during pregnancy is a major public health crisis and clinicians are cautioned to carefully assess individuals of reproductive age, pregnant persons, newborns, children, and adolescents regarding use and exposure to substances.

Adolescent Considerations
The American Academy of Pediatrics defines *addiction* as a developmental disorder and recommends screening for SUD as a routine part of adolescent care. This position is based on the understanding of neurobiology and the neuroadaptations that result from substance use, which can be more dramatic and happen more quickly during adolescence. Trauma, social isolation, genetic factors, and comorbid physical and mental health disorders increase the likelihood of changes within the brain and nervous system that lead to SUD.

Considerations for the Older Adult
The prevalence rates of SUD are underestimated for older adults. Aging presents risks for harm; biological changes increase the effect of alcohol, medications, and illicit drugs in older adults, causing an increased vulnerability to their effects and interactions. The diagnosis

and treatment of comorbid sleep disorders, cognitive impairment, and chronic illnesses are complicated by concurrent use of alcohol, tobacco, and prescription medications.

Impact on Families
Consequences of substance misuse and SUD are experienced by each member of a family; there are emotional, developmental, social, and/or behavioral effects that can have an impact across time and generations. Clinicians should screen for negative outcomes and provide intervention and support to family members experiencing the effects of substance use. Family environments in which a parent or primary caregiver has an SUD are associated with higher rates of abuse and trauma, poor parenting skills, and poor-quality parent–child interactions, all of which are risk factors for the development of addiction. Assessment should include screening for comorbid developmental delays; mental and physical health disorders; and abuse, neglect, and safety issues. Early intervention in families leads to better outcomes for all family members.

RECOVERY
Although resistance to treatment and relapse are common, individuals with SUD can recover. Recovery is a process of change through which individuals improve their health and wellness, live a self-directed life, and strive to reach their full potential. Being "in recovery" indicates that positive sustained changes have become part of a voluntarily adopted lifestyle. Individuals in recovery have unique and personal stories about their lives before recovery, what happened to motivate their change, and what their lives are like now. Clinicians who want to support continued recovery for individuals with SUD can approach these individuals in a manner similar to anyone with a chronic illness.

- Assess their health in all dimensions of wellness.
- Ask whether they have a safe and secure place to live.
- Support their involvement in ADLs that give them purpose.
- Assess their connections to others, their relationships, and their social networks.
- Ask about sponsorship and sobriety.
- Recognize that positive clinician feedback can be a significant part of breaking the cycle of shame, guilt, stigma, and secrecy.

HISTORY AND PHYSICAL EXAMINATION DOCUMENTATION

Physical exam components are individualized based on subjective history and patient presentation and minimally include observation/inspection to assess mental status.

EXAMPLE OF NORMAL PHYSICAL EXAM FINDINGS

Affect pleasant. Dressed appropriately for the weather and situation. Well-groomed. No repetitive or unusual postures or movements. Judgment intact. Thoughts coherent; able to articulate health history with clarity. Remote and recent memories intact. The two-item Patient Health Questionnaire (PHQ-2) screening for depression and the two item Generalized Anxiety Disorder Scale (GAD-2) screening for anxiety negative, with a total score of 2 on each. Single-question screenings for substance use negative.

EXAMPLE CHARTING NOTE FOR AN ADULT WITH SYMPTOMS OF DEPRESSION

Patient Information
- Name: Mrs. Smith
- Age: 70
- Gender: Female
- Vital signs: Temperature 97.6, heart rate 68 per minute, respiratory rate 12 per minute, blood pressure 118/76, body mass index 25

Chief Concern
The patient presents with symptoms of depression.

History of Present Illness
Mrs. Smith, a 70-year-old woman, presents with a chief concern of persistent feelings of sadness, loss of interest in activities, decreased energy, and changes in appetite and sleep patterns. She reports that these symptoms have been present for the past 6 months since the death of her husband. She states that she has been feeling lonely and isolated since then as she lives alone. Mrs. Smith acknowledges that she has been struggling to cope with her husband's passing and the significant life changes that have resulted from it.

Past Medical and Psychiatric Health History
- No history of surgeries; no history of hospitalizations except for childbirth (G3P3AB0)
- Has hyperlipidemia well-controlled on rosuvastatin 20 mg daily
- History of COVID-19 in 2023 with subsequent heart palpitations, well-controlled on metoprolol 25 mg daily
- No prior history of psychiatric illnesses or depression

Family History
- No significant family history of psychiatric illnesses reported; three uncles with alcohol use disorder
- Two siblings alive and well
- Paternal history of heart disease and hypertension (father died of heart failure at age 70); mother died of "old age"

Social History

Mrs. Smith has lived alone in her own home since the death of her husband 6 months ago. She has three grown adult children, all of whom are married. One of her children lives in the area, providing some support. Mrs. Smith reports limited social interactions and a decreased sense of purpose since her husband's death. She describes feeling a lack of emotional support due to her living situation. She denies financial concerns; she is a retired university educator. She is able to drive to clinician visits, and independently shop, cook, and attend church services. She states she has been sober for more than 40 years and chooses not to drink, related to extended family history of alcoholism. She was never a smoker. She has no guns in the home. She denies suicidal ideation (current or past).

Medical and Psychiatric Review of Systems
- **General:** Reports decreased energy and motivation; no weight loss
- **Psychiatric:** Reports feelings of sadness, loss of interest, and changes in appetite and sleep patterns; does have persistent episodes of crying; denies suicidal ideation/homicidal ideation
- **Neurologic:** Denies dizziness, loss of consciousness, and changes in memory
- **Cardiovascular, respiratory, gastrointestinal, and musculoskeletal systems:** Without change

Physical Exam/Mental Status Evaluation
- General appearance fatigued; alert and oriented; clearly articulates history, although quiet and teary at times; thought processes and content coherent
- Mucosa pink; respirations easy; ambulation easy without assistive devices
- PHQ-2 score of 4 and GAD-2 score of 2

Assessment

Mrs. Smith is exhibiting symptoms consistent with depression. The recent loss of her husband and the subsequent feelings of loneliness and isolation are contributing factors. Differential diagnoses include major depressive disorder, grief, anxiety, and social isolation.

REFERENCES

References for this chapter draw from Chapter 25, Evidence-Based Assessment of Mental Health, Chapter 26, Evidence-Based Assessment of Substance Use Disorder, Chapter 27, Evidence-Based Assessment and Screening for Traumatic Experiences: Abuse, Neglect, and Intimate Partner Violence, and Chapter 4, Evidence-Based, Culturally Sensitive, Therapeutic Communication, in *Evidence-Based Physical Examination: Best Practices for Health and Well-Being Assessment (Second Edition)*. The references may be accessed in the digital version of the handbook at https://connect.springerpub.com/.

Evidence-Based Considerations for Assessment Across the Life Span

CLINICAL CONSIDERATIONS

- Children, teens, and older adults have unique health and wellness needs. Evidence-based history and physical examination requires integrating knowledge of the uniqueness of populations across the life span for accurate assessment of individuals. *Note that this chapter first reviews pediatric and adolescent considerations for assessment, then reviews considerations for older adults. There are also pediatric and older adult considerations in every systems chapter of this handbook.*
- Accurate assessment of children requires evaluation of their growth and development over time. While individuals grow and develop at different rates, failure to grow or reach developmental milestones can be evidence of previous illness, early signs of disease, or threats to wellness. A developmental approach to the history taking and physical exam of children and teens allows for effective anticipatory guidance.
- Adolescence is characterized by accelerating growth, physiologic changes of puberty, and developmental changes in the brain that allow for rapid cognitive development.
- Changes in an older adult's functional assessment can be an indication of mental or physical decline. Identifying functional decline early can allow for implementation of interventions to maximize a person's independence and safety. The use of evidence-based, age-appropriate screenings to assess medication use, independence in activities of daily living (ADLs), fall risks, hearing impairment, and home safety should be used for older adult populations.

SUBJECTIVE HISTORY FOR PEDIATRIC AND ADOLESCENT ASSESSMENT

PEDIATRIC CONSIDERATIONS

Caregivers as Historians

- The main difference between collecting the health history for infants and children compared with adults is that the caregiver becomes the primary historian. As children mature developmentally, they become more able to participate in providing their health history. Therefore, the clinician must be prepared to adjust the approach to history taking accordingly.

- The caregiver's interpretation of the child's signs and symptoms may be inaccurate. For example, a caregiver may report that the child has a "tummy ache" because the child abruptly refuses to eat. However, the child may actually be refusing to eat because of painful lesions in the posterior oropharynx that accompany common viral infections. The clinician may need to rephrase questions to elicit the most accurate clinical data. For example, instead of "How long has your child had leg pain?" the clinician might ask "When did you first notice them limping?" It is also helpful to begin with open-ended questions—for example, "Can you tell me about your child's rash?"—and follow up with more specific and objective questions if needed—"Has your child been scratching the rash?"
- The more severe the symptoms of illness and injury, the more likely there may be interruptions in appetite, sleep, elimination, and activity. To elicit valuable clinical insight into the severity of a child's condition, ask "How is your child eating/sleeping/peeing/pooping?" and "Are they playing like they usually do?" The ill child who is not eating or drinking is at increased risk for dehydration or may be experiencing pain from their illness. Changes in elimination patterns can also alert the clinician to specific disease processes (urinary tract infection, constipation, dehydration, diabetes mellitus), which further guide the focused history and physical assessment.
- If a child is presenting with a mental health or behavioral issue, consider using a screening tool along with the history for a more comprehensive assessment.
- Assess birth history as a component of past medical history, especially for children under 2 years of age, including prenatal care, labor/delivery complications, type of delivery, newborn hospital stay, and newborn screening results.

Children as Historians

- A child over the age of 4 to 5 can usually provide some of their own health history. It is essential to ask questions in an age-appropriate manner according to the developmental age and level of understanding. The clinician should pay close attention to nonverbal cues of comprehension and adjust the questions and terminology as needed. It is important to avoid the use of medical jargon.
- For example, the terms "pain" or "discomfort" may be unfamiliar to a child, whereas "ouchies," "boo-boos," or "where it hurts" may be more relatable. Instead of "Do you have painful bowel movements?" ask "Does it hurt when you poop?" Instead of "Is the pain persistent or does it come and go?" ask "Does it hurt all the time

or just sometimes?" Instead of "Do you have a history of abdominal pain?" ask "Has your belly hurt like this before?" Instead of "Have you had any nausea or vomiting?" ask "Have you felt like throwing up?"

ADOLESCENT CONSIDERATIONS

Confidentiality and Support for Developing Autonomy

- Adolescence is the transition from childhood to adulthood. As such, it is important to gather history from both the caregiver and the adolescent when possible. While caregivers can offer a valuable perspective regarding the adolescent's health history, clinicians should also prioritize the opportunity for a one-on-one conversation with the adolescent. The clinician can support the adolescent's development of autonomy and their responsibility for their own health and wellness.

- Adolescents are prone to engage in high-risk behaviors that cause substantial morbidity and mortality, such as substance abuse, reckless driving, and unprotected sex; moreover, many of the health behaviors that contribute to chronic illnesses in adulthood originate in adolescence, such as diet, activity, and tobacco use. Ensuring an opportunity for a private, confidential conversation with the clinician will improve the accuracy and integrity of the history provided by the teen.

- Prior to beginning the health history, the clinician should assure the adolescent that everything that is discussed will be kept confidential except when disclosure is required by law, as is the case when there are concerns of abuse, suicidal or homicidal ideations, or certain sexually transmitted infections that are reportable to the local health department. It is crucial for clinicians to be aware of their federal and state laws regarding adolescent consent and confidentiality as these laws can vary from state to state.

- The clinician should ask questions in a respectful, nonjudgmental manner. If a clinician appears to disapprove or make negative assumptions or seems uncomfortable asking sensitive questions, the adolescent may not be comfortable answering the questions. A nonjudgmental attitude is vital in establishing a rapport with adolescents. Teenagers can detect insincerity and disapproval.

Screening for High-Risk Behaviors

- A point to note when asking about high-risk behaviors (substance misuse, sexual activity) is that if the teen hesitates before answering it may indicate that they are choosing whether to share or not share. To establish a more trusting environment, the clinician may wish to rephrase questions and normalize behaviors. For example, "Some teens your age have tried drinking alcohol or vaping; have you or any of your friends tried these things?" The same approach can be used when talking about potential romantic partners and sexual activity.

- Avoid medical jargon and use terminology that is common and direct. "What do you consider sex?" "What percentage of the time do you use condoms?" "Has anyone made you have sex when you didn't want to?" Establishing a trusting rapport and straightforward dialogue can assist the clinician in obtaining the most accurate health history to care for the adolescent. Clinicians should take a thorough psychosocial history at each adolescent health supervision visit. The HEEADSSS (or HE²ADS³) acronym is used to complete psychosocial assessments (**Box 17.1**).

BOX 17.1 HEEADSSS Assessment Domains

H: Home
Ask about the adolescent's living situation, including family dynamics, relationships with parents and siblings, and any issues related to their home environment.

E: Education and/or Employment
Assess how the teen is functioning at school or in an educational setting, including academic performance, engagement in extracurricular activities, and any employment or vocational plans.

E: Eating and Exercise
Ask about the adolescent's eating habits, including their relationship with food, dietary patterns, and any issues related to disordered eating or body image concerns. Assess physical activity level and exercise routines.

A: Activities
Ask about the teen's engagement in social activities and their relationships with peers. Assess their involvement in sports, clubs, or hobbies, as well as any issues related to social isolation, bullying, or peer pressure.

D: Drugs
Assess use of tobacco, alcohol, illicit drugs, anabolic steroids, or medications not prescribed to the teen. Identify the adolescent's patterns of use, knowledge about substance-related risks, and any difficulties or concerns related to substance abuse, including driving while intoxicated.

(continued)

> **BOX 17.1** HEEADSSS Assessment Domains (*continued*)
>
> **S: Sexuality**
> Assess the adolescent's understanding of sexual behaviors and health, including their knowledge about contraception, sexually transmitted infections, and boundaries/choice. Ask about concerns or issues related to sexual or reproductive health, gender identity, or sexual orientation.
>
> **S: Suicidality**
> Evaluate the adolescent's mental health and emotional well-being, specifically focusing on symptoms of depression, anxiety, self-harm, and suicidal ideation. Identify their coping mechanisms, support systems, and any history of mental health concerns.
>
> **S: Safety**
> Address issues related to safety, including any history of physical, sexual, or emotional abuse. Ask about the adolescent's exposure to violence in their community or through media, as well as their understanding of personal safety precautions.

PHYSICAL EXAM OF CHILDREN AND TEENS

PEDIATRIC CONSIDERATIONS

- Newborns (0–1 month) and young infants (1–6 months) generally prefer to stay warm and secure. The clinician should perform as much of the physical exam as possible prior to removing blankets, clothes, or diapers. By keeping the infant comfortable, the clinician can facilitate an efficient and successful head-to-toe physical exam. In fact, many physical exam elements can be performed while the caregiver is holding the "quiet" infant. In particular, this is an ideal time to auscultate heart and lung sounds. When it is time for the "active" aspects of the exam, the clinician should perform the remainder of the exam with the infant lying supine safely on the exam table. The active aspects of the exam may include the otoscopic ear exam, oropharynx, abdomen, genitalia, and hips. Conversely, the clinician can also seize the opportunity when an infant is already crying to perform an effective exam of the mouth, dentition, and posterior oropharynx.
- For older infants (6–12 months) and young children (1–4 years), the aspects of the physical exam that typically feel most worrisome are the otoscopic ear exam, the oral exam with tongue

depressor, and/or lying down for abdominal palpation or ano-genital exam. Plan to reserve these exam aspects for last. Because children develop motor, language, cognitive, and psychosocial skills through play, learning to transform the physical exam into play for the child can help the clinician increase cooperation.

- The child, whether cooperative or not, must be secured and properly positioned during certain aspects of the physical exam. Safety is paramount. Young children can be safely secured on a caregiver's lap with their head and arms secured to assist the clinician in performing a safe exam of the ears or posterior oral pharynx. **Figure 17.1** demonstrates three positioning holds with the assistance of the caregiver.

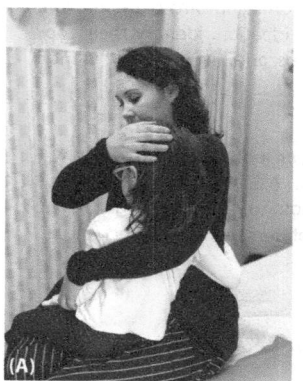
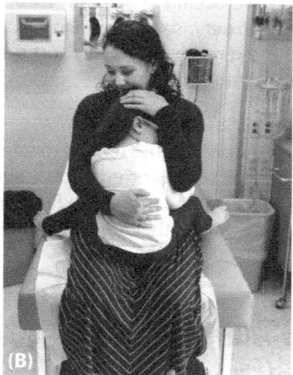
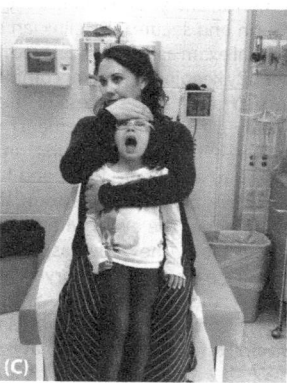

FIGURE 17.1 Positioning holds with a caregiver. **(A)** Sideways. **(B)** Facing the parent. **(C)** Face-front hold for oral exam/throat swab.

Pediatric Vital Signs

Techniques for measurement are discussed in Chapter 2, Evidence-Based General Survey Including Vital Signs, of this text. Normal vital signs by age are listed in **Table 17.1.**

Measurements of Growth

- Infants and children undergo anthropometric assessment at each well-child visit because growth is the primary outcome measure of wellness in children. Deviations in growth trajectories may be indicative of neglect, chronic illness, malnutrition, hormonal conditions, or congenital syndromes. The Centers for Disease Control and Prevention (CDC) recommends using the World Health Organization (WHO) international growth charts for children aged 0 to 23 months and the CDC growth charts for children and adolescents aged 2 to 18 years.
  - Regular assessment should include height/length, weight, head circumference, body mass index (BMI; beginning at age 2), and associated percentiles. Because children are continuously growing, growth measurements are interpreted differently from that of adults. Trends are compared with a reference population of children of the same age and sex and reported as a percentile. These measures should be assessed and documented to allow the clinician to monitor changes over time.

TABLE 17.1 Pediatric Vital Signs

Age	Heart Rate (Beats Per Minute)	Blood Pressure (mmHg)	Respiratory Rate (Breaths Per Minute)
Premature	110–170	SBP 55–75, DBP 35–45	40–70
0–3 months	110–160	SBP 65–85, DBP 45–55	35–55
3–6 months	110–160	SBP 70–90, DBP 50–65	30–45
6–12 months	90–160	SBP 80–100, DBP 55–65	22–38
1–3 years	80–150	SBP 90–105, DBP 55–70	22–30
3–6 years	70–120	SBP 95–110, DBP 60–75	20–24
6–12 years	60–110	SBP 100–120, DBP 60–75	16–22
>12 years	60–100	SBP 110–135, DBP 65–85	12–20

DBP, diastolic blood pressure; SBP, systolic blood pressure.

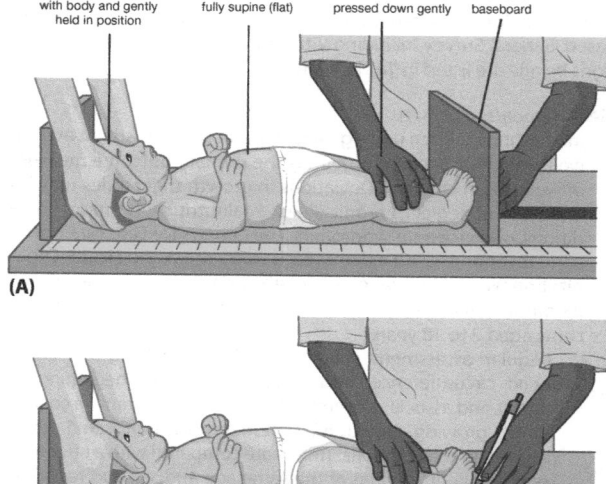

FIGURE 17.2 Obtaining length measurement in an infant.

- Infants and young children under the age of 2 should be measured lying supine with a recumbent infant length board (**Figure 17.2**) and should be weighed nude or in a clean, dry disposable diaper on an accurately calibrated scale (**Figure 17.3**).
- Head circumference should be measured for all children up to the age of 3 with a flexible, non-elastic measuring tape placed just above the brow line anteriorly and over the occipital prominence posteriorly (**Figure 17.4**). It is advisable to measure the head circumference three times in one encounter to ensure the accuracy of the recording.

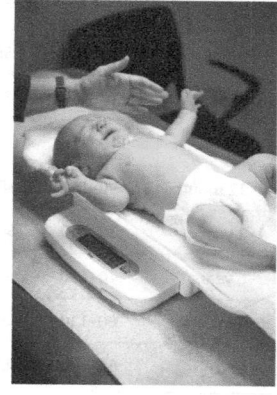

FIGURE 17.3 An infant weighed on a calibrated scale.

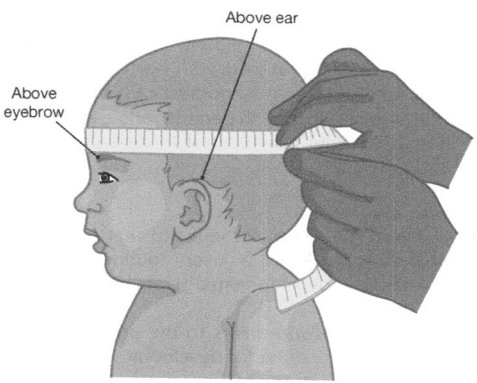

FIGURE 17.4 Measurement of head circumference.

- Length, weight, length-for-weight percentile, and head circumference measurements should be plotted according to age on the WHO growth chart designated for the infant's natal sex.
- Newborns are expected to lose up to 10% of their birth weight in the first few days of life; >10% weight loss should be urgently investigated.
- The normal weight gain for the newborn is 15 to 30 g/day (0.5–1 oz/day). It is normal for breastfed newborns to gain weight on the lower end of the normal range. The newborn should recover birth weight by at least 2 weeks of age. The average infant will double their birth weight by 6 months of age and triple it by 12 months.
- The average length of a newborn is 20 to 21 inches (51 cm). Linear growth velocity averages 2.5 cm/month from birth to 6 months, 1.3 cm/month from 7 to 12 months, and about 7.6 cm/year between 12 months and 10 years of age on average.
- Infants with poor weight gain or growth measurements that trend downward or fall below the third percentile may have failure to thrive and the cause should be investigated. If neglect, organic disease, or severe malnutrition is suspected, the child should be hospitalized for evaluation.
- An upward-trending head circumference may indicate hydrocephalus or other intracranial pathology. A head circumference that stalls in growth may indicate a premature fusion of the sutures/fontanels or a congenital syndrome associated with microcephaly.
- For adolescents and children older than age 2, height, weight, and BMI should be plotted on the CDC growth chart relative to the child's natal sex. Young children and adolescents who can stand steadily without assistance should be weighed with a calibrated

electronic scale or beam balance scale. Height should be measured with a portable or wall-mount stadiometer, with the child standing erect, looking forward, with heels and occiput against the wall. Height and weight should be obtained without shoes. Prior to the accelerated growth period in adolescence, school-age children typically grow an average of 2.5 inches and gain an average of 5 to 7 lb/year.

Developmental Assessment

- Evidence-based guidelines recommend that clinicians perform developmental surveillance at every routine health encounter and a standardized developmental screening at ages 9, 18, and 24 or 30 months.
- *Developmental surveillance* refers to the process of recognizing children who may be at risk for developmental delays. The clinician performs surveillance through physical observation of the child's development and by asking the caregiver whether the child has met age-appropriate developmental milestones.
- *Developmental screening* refers to the use of standardized tools to identify children at risk for delays in the developmental domains of motor (gross and fine), language, cognitive, emotional, and psychosocial.
- All clinicians working with children should be familiar with the early childhood developmental milestones; these are outlined in **Table 17.2.**
- When a child is not developing skills in one or more domains according to expectations, they are exhibiting signs of *developmental delay*.
- Identification of a developmental problem or delay should prompt further diagnostic evaluation and referral for early intervention services (**Box 17.2**).
- *Early intervention* is a collective term describing programs or services (e.g., speech therapy, physical therapy, occupational therapy) that support the development of children aged 0 to 3 years with developmental delays or disabilities. Children aged 0 to 3 years have greater neuroplasticity and therefore higher capacity for improved outcomes the earlier services are established.

ADOLESCENT CONSIDERATIONS

The clinician can implement a typical head-to-toe physical exam sequence and the same techniques used for adults when examining the adolescent. Providing privacy and preserving modesty are paramount. Adolescents often have concerns regarding their developing bodies and they feel self-conscious. It is important to reassure the adolescent when everything is normal.

TABLE 17.2 Developmental Milestones of Early Childhood

Age	Social/Emotional	Language/Communication	Cognitive	Motor
2 months	• Smiles responsively • Seems happy to see caregiver • Calms when spoken to or picked up	• Makes sounds other than crying • Reacts to loud sounds	• Pays attention to faces and follows caregiver's movements with eyes • Looks at a toy for several seconds	• Holds head up when on tummy • Moves both arms and legs
4 months	• Smiles spontaneously at people • Moves or makes sounds to get or keep caregiver's attention	• Cooing (makes sounds like "oohh" and "aahh") • Makes sounds back when talked to • Turns head toward sound of caregiver's voice	• If hungry, opens mouth when seeing breast or bottle • Looks at own hands with interest	• Holds head steady • Brings hands to mouth; uses arm to swing at a toy • Holds toy placed in their hand • Pushes up onto elbows/forearms when on tummy
6 months	• Knows familiar people • Laughs • Likes to look at self in mirror	• Takes turns making sounds with caregiver • Blows "raspberries" • Makes squealing noises	• Puts things in mouth to explore them • Reaches to grab a toy • Closes lips to show they do not want more food	• Rolls from tummy to back • Pushes up with straight arms when on tummy

(continued)

TABLE 17.2 Developmental Milestones of Early Childhood *(continued)*

Age	Social/Emotional	Language/Communication	Cognitive	Motor
9 months	• May have stranger anxiety • Shows several facial expressions, like happy, sad, angry, and surprised • Looks when name is called	• Makes different sounds like "mamamama" and "babababa" • Lifts arms up to be picked up	• Plays peek-a-boo • Develops object permanence (looks for things out of sight) • Bangs things together	• Gets to sitting position independently; sits without support • Uses fingers to "rake" food toward self • Moves things from one hand to the other
1 year	• Plays games such as pat-a-cake	• Waves bye-bye • Understands "no" (pauses or stops when told "no") • Calls a parent "mama," "dada," or another special name	• Puts things in a container, like a block in a cup • Looks for things they see the caregiver hide, like a toy under a blanket	• Pulls up to standing • Cruises (walks while holding on) • Walks holding onto furniture • Drinks from cup without a lid as caregiver holds it • Picks things up between thumb and forefinger (pincer grasp), like small food bits
15 months	• Copies other children when playing • Shows caregiver an object they like • Claps when excited	• Tries to say one or two words besides mama or dada, like "ba" for ball, or "da" for dog • Points to ask for something or to get help	• Tries to use things the right way, like a phone, cup, or book • Stacks at least two small objects, like blocks	• Takes a few steps independently • Uses fingers to feed self

	• Hugs stuffed doll or another toy • Shows affection (hugs, cuddles, kisses)	• Looks at a familiar object when it is named • Follows one-step directions without gestures (like handing over a toy when asked)		
18 months	• Moves away from caregiver but looks to make sure they are close by • Puts hands out to be washed • Looks at pages in book with caregiver • Helps get dressed by pushing arm through sleeve or lifting foot	• Tries to say ≥3 words other than "mama" or "dada"	• Copies caregiver doing chores, like sweeping with a broom • Plays with toys in a simple way, like pushing a toy car	• Walks alone • Drinks from a cup without a lid, may spill sometimes • Tries to use a spoon • Climbs on/off furniture without help • Scribbles
2 years	• Notices when others are hurt or upset, like pausing or looking sad when someone is crying • Looks at caregiver's face to see how they react in new situations	• Says sentences of at least two words, like "more milk" • Points to things in a book when asked • Uses more gestures like blowing a kiss or nodding yes • Points to at least two body parts when asked	• Tries to use switches and knobs • Plays with >1 toy at the same time, like putting toy food on a toy plate • Holds an object in one hand while using the other hand, like holding a container and trying to take the lid off	• Kicks a ball • Runs • Eats with a spoon • Walks (not climbs) up a few stairs, with or without help

(continued)

TABLE 17.2 Developmental Milestones of Early Childhood *(continued)*

Age	Social/Emotional	Language/ Communication	Cognitive	Motor
30 months	• Shows caregiver what they can do by saying, "Look at me!" • Follows simple routines when told, like helping to pick up toys when asked to clean up • Plays next to, and sometimes with, other children	• Says about 50 words • Says ≥2 words together with one action word, like "doggie run" • Names things in a book when pointed to and asked, "What is this?" • Says words like I, me, or we	• Uses things to pretend, like feeding a block to a doll pretending its food • Can identify at least one color • Follows two-step directions, like put the toy down and close the door • Shows problem-solving skills, like using stool to reach something	• Uses hands to twist things, like doorknobs or lids • Takes some clothes off without help • Jumps off the ground with both feet • Turns book pages, one at a time, when read to
3 years	• Calms down within 10 minutes after caregiver leaves, like at childcare drop-off • Notices other children and joins them to play	• Talks in conversation using at least two back-and-forth exchanges • Asks who, what, where, or why questions, "like where is daddy?" • Says first name when prompted • Talks well enough for others to understand most of the time • Says what action is happening in a picture when asked, like eating or playing	• Draws a circle when shown how • Avoids touching hot objects when warned, like a stove	• Strings items together, like large beads • Puts on some clothes independently • Uses a fork • Catches a large ball most of the time

	Social/Emotional	Language/Communication	Cognitive	Movement/Physical
4 years	• Pretends to be something else during play (e.g., superhero or dog) • Asks to play with other children • Comforts others who are hurt or sad, like hugging a crying friend • Avoids danger, like not jumping from tall heights at the playground • Likes to be a "helper" • Changes behavior based on the setting, like a place of worship or playground	• Says sentences with >4 words • Says some words from a song, story, or nursery rhyme • Talks about at least one thing that happened that day, like "I played soccer" • Can answer simple questions, like "What is a coat for?"	• Names a few colors of items • Tells what comes next in a well-known story • Draws a person with ≥3 body parts	• Unbuttons some buttons • Holds crayon or pencil between fingers and thumb (not in a fist)
5 years	• Likes to sing, dance, act, and participate in imaginative play • Follows rules or takes turns when playing games with other children • Does simple chores at home, like matching socks	• Tells a known or made-up story with at least two events • Answers simple questions about a book or story after its read or told to them • Keeps a conversation going with >3 back-and-forth exchanges • Uses or recognizes simple rhymes (e.g., cat-bat)	• Counts to 10 • Names some numbers between 1 and 5 when pointed to • Writes some letters in their name • Uses words about time, like yesterday or tomorrow • Pays attention for 5–10 minutes during activities (screen time does not count)	• Buttons some buttons • Hops on one foot

> **BOX 17.2** Red Flags Indicating Need for Referral and Possible Early Intervention in Children With Developmental Delay
>
> - Any child who fails to move ahead developmentally
> - Any child who begins to deteriorate developmentally
> - Failure to achieve developmental milestones, including:
>   - Inconsistent or lack of response to auditory stimuli
>   - Not sitting with support by 6 months
>   - Unable to sit alone by 9 months
>   - Unable to transfer objects hand to hand by 1 year
>   - Abnormal pincer grasp at 15 months
>   - Unable to walk alone by 18 months
>   - No understandable speech by 18 months
>   - Failure to speak recognizable words by 2 years
>   - Speech predominately unintelligible at 3 years old

Sexual Maturity Rating

Assessment of sexual maturity is important in clinical practice as it confirms expected development, identifies potential alterations, and offers an opportunity for anticipatory guidance. The most commonly used sexual maturity rating (SMR) tool is Tanner staging, which is shown for female pubertal development in **Table 17.3** and male pubertal development in **Table 17.4**. If an adolescent requires a physical examination of the genitalia or a breast exam (for system-specific complaints, or for SMR staging), the use of a chaperone is recommended; however, this should be a shared decision between the clinician and the adolescent. Note that some states have mandatory chaperone laws, so it is important for clinicians to be aware of their respective state laws.

RECOMMENDED SCREENINGS FOR CHILDREN AND TEENS

- Vision and hearing screenings are recommended at routine intervals throughout early childhood and adolescence. Early identification of sensory deficits allows for appropriate early intervention to prevent or minimize the impact of visual/hearing impairments on a child's speech and language, social-emotional, or cognitive and academic development.
- Screening for lead exposure and for iron deficiency anemia are priorities during childhood.
- Routine screening for hypertension, obesity, and dyslipidemia is recommended. Although cardiovascular disease more commonly presents in adulthood, the pathophysiologic processes begin in childhood; therefore, identifiable risk factors that accelerate the disease processes and ultimately increase sequela of the disease can be targeted for screening and prevention.

TABLE 17.3 Female Sexual Maturity Stages

	Breast		Pubic Hair	
Stage 1 Prepubertal	Nipples are small. There is no breast.	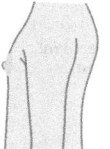	No pubic hair	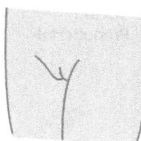
Stage 2 8–15 years	Breast and nipples have just started to grow. The areola has become larger. Breast tissue bud feels firm behind the nipple.	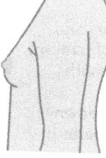	Initial growth of long pubic hairs, which are straight, without curls, and of light colors	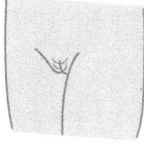
Stage 3 10–15 years	Breast and nipples have grown additionally. The areola has become darker. The breast tissue bud is larger.	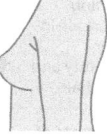	Pubic hair more widespread; hair darker and curls may have appeared	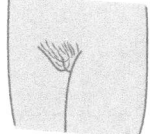
Stage 4 10–17 years	Nipples and areolas are elevated and form an edge toward the breast. The breast has also grown a little larger.	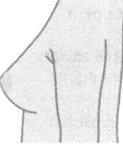	More dense hair growth with curls and dark hair; still not entirely as an adult woman	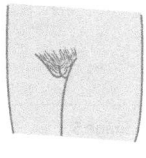
Stage 5 12.5–18 years	Fully developed breast. Nipples are protruding and the edge between areola and breast has disappeared.	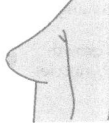	Adult hair growth; dense, curly hair extending toward the inner thighs	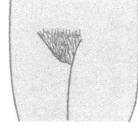

TABLE 17.4 Male Sexual Maturity Stages

Stage	Description	Appearance
Stage 1 Prepubertal	• No secondary sex characteristics • Testicular volume <3 mL (≤2.5 cm in length) • No pubic hair	
Stage 2 9–13 years	• Testes beginning to enlarge (testicular volume ≥3 mL) • Increased texture and pigmentation of scrotum • No change in length/width of penis • Pubic hair long, downy, and variable in pattern	
Stage 3 10–14 years	• Further enlargement of testes • Penile lengthening followed by increase in penile diameter • Increase in quantity and curling of pubic hair	
Stage 4 11–15 years	• Further enlargement of testes and penis • Pubic hair adult-like in quality but not in distribution • Development of axillary and facial hair begins	
Stage 5 12–17 years	• Testes and penis adult in size • Pubic hair adult in quality and distribution • Body hair continuing to grow • Peak of overall growth (height/weight/muscle) velocity	

Source: Illustrations courtesy of J. McHardy; https://commons.wikimedia.org/wiki/File:Tanner_scale-male.png

SUBJECTIVE HISTORY FOR ASSESSMENT OF THE OLDER ADULT

- Older adults often do not have classic symptoms of illness, so it is important for clinicians to complete a thorough health history, which will help detect subtle differences and changes that are often disregarded as "normal aging" or depression.
- It is imperative that the clinician be aware of age-specific differences in disease presentation and red flags for referral or emergency care. (**Box 17.3**)
- Considerations regarding medications include the need for a thorough medication assessment specifically geared at addressing polypharmacy and identifying medications that might be harmful to older adults. The American Geriatrics Society's Beers Criteria* should be considered when the clinician is reviewing the medication list and/or prescribing new medications.
- A thorough medical history for the older adult should also include an assessment of their immunization status. Rather than utilizing chronologic age to determine eligibility for vaccination, clinicians should base recommendations for vaccination on the patient's level of capacity, need for vaccination, and the benefits likely to arise from vaccination.
- Social history should include age-specific considerations, including social support, risk for social isolation, home hazards, financial stability, healthcare and transportation access, nutrition, and experiences of discrimination, isolation, violence, trauma, and/or loss.

OLDER ADULTS AS HISTORIANS

- When obtaining a health history from an older adult, the patient should be addressed and spoken to in the same manner that the

---

BOX 17.3 Red Flags in the History and Physical Exam of the Older Adult

- Unintended weight loss
- History of falls
- Loss of function or disability
- Inability to care for self or complete activities of daily living
- Memory loss that disrupts daily life
- Challenges in planning or solving problems
- Difficulty completing familiar tasks
- Confusion with time or place
- Sudden behavior and/or personality changes
- Signs of elder abuse (physical, sexual, emotional, financial, neglect)

clinician would speak to any other adult. Avoid the use of elder-speak, a style of speech similar to "baby talk," characterized by enhanced intonation, slower rates, and elevated pitch and volume. This can be perceived by the older adult as patronizing, or implying that they are incompetent and lack the cognitive ability to understand their care.

CAREGIVERS AS HISTORIANS

- It is common for caregivers and family members to accompany older adults to their healthcare visits. When possible, the patient should speak for themselves. Some older adults may not want their family member/caregiver present during the visit or the exam portion of the visit. Confidentiality and privacy laws apply when an older adult is competent in their decision-making and has intact cognition. The clinician should ask permission to disclose health information to family members/caregivers and ensure they are in compliance with any federal and state laws.
- In the event that the older adult has significant memory issues or is unable to make informed decisions about their care, it is appropriate to engage the caregiver or family member when needed.

PHYSICAL EXAM OF THE OLDER ADULT

- Vital signs may vary in the older adult due to physiologic changes of aging.
- With advanced age, the body's thermoregulatory measures are less effective. Older adults are less capable of adapting to extreme environmental temperatures, putting them at risk for both hypothermia and heat-related illness. Older adults are also less likely to develop a fever with infection, making body temperature a less reliable indicator of their health status.
- Because the older adult's heart takes longer to recover from activity and stress, if an older adult presents with tachycardia the clinician should review the activities that preceded the assessment to determine whether they are related to the elevated pulse rate. Allow an older adult to rest after a period of activity that may have increased their pulse rate and reassess.
- Older adults are more at risk for hypertension, hypotension, and orthostatic hypotension. Orthostatic blood pressure should be assessed in older adults on blood pressure medications and especially in patients who screen positive for fall risk.
- Assess weight over time. Older adults are at risk for malnutrition due to such things as impaired ability to eat; social isolation; changes in smell, taste, and appetite; dementia; medications; and alcoholism. An older adult losing weight without intention could also mean another condition, such as malignancy or Alzheimer, and they should be closely monitored.

MENTAL HEALTH ASSESSMENT

Refer to Chapter 16, Evidence-Based Assessment of Mental Health Including Substance Use Disorders, for a complete mental health assessment. Note the following variations and considerations for the older adult's mental health exam.

Appearance
- Personal hygiene in the older adult can deteriorate over time due to such things as loss of function, neglect, depression, and dementia.
- Many older adults have kyphosis. This can be due to conditions such as compression fractures, osteoporosis, and degenerative disc disease.

Behavior
- Note the patient's interactions with caregivers, family members, or spouses. Patients with dementia or cognitive impairment may exhibit agitation, apathy, or aggressiveness. They may say inappropriate things or exhibit impulsivity. Depressed older adults may appear flat and speak slowly.
- Observe the patient's body movements and mobility. Older adults often use assistive devices to help improve functional mobility. Ensure their comfort and proper use of these devices.
- Observe for the presence of any abnormal movements or an involuntary tics or tremors which could signify a movement disorder or other underlying condition.

Cognition
- Ask the patient to tell you who they are, the time, and the place. Note any confusion, disorientation, or delirium.
- Observe the older adult's speech pattern and pace. The speech should be coherent and organized in thought and content.
- Test the patient's memory by saying three unrelated words to them, asking them to repeat those words immediately and again in 5 minutes, or have them complete the clock test.
- Complete a depression screening (see the Recommended Screenings for Older Adults section).

TARGETED ASSESSMENTS FOR THE OLDER ADULT

Targeted assessments are important to identify and predict older adults who may be at risk of adverse outcomes. These should include assessment for functional mobility, ADLs, instrumental activities of daily living (IADLs), nutrition, and risk of falls.

Functional Mobility Assessment
- There are many functional mobility assessments. The Timed Up and Go (TUAG) is an example of a functional mobility test that is used to assess a patient's mobility and their risk for falls. Ask the patient to get out of their seat, walk 3 meters across the room,

do a 180° turn, and return to their chair and sit back down. If the patient is able to do this in less than 12 seconds, no further testing is need. If it takes longer than 12 seconds, functional impairment likely exists. This test has been shown to help predict falls, fracture, and mortality.

Activities of Daily Living Assessment

- ADLs are the basic self-care tasks that are considered fundamental in caring for oneself and maintaining independence. Measuring ADLs is an additional way of monitoring a patient's functional status and helps to objectively predict future decline and/or improvement. As a person ages, these gradually take more time to complete.
- A widely used tool to assess ADLs is the Katz Index of Independence in Activities of Daily Living. This tool asks about the ability to independently bathe, dress, toilet, transfer, feed, and have self-control over urination and defecation. It is rated 0 to 6, with a score of 0 indicating that a patient is very dependent and a score of 6 indicating that a patient is very independent.

Instrumental Activities of Daily Living Assessment

- IADLs are another measure of a patient's ability to independently live in the community. These are more complex and are often lost before the basic "activities of daily living." These are essential for independent, safe living and include meal preparation, money management, shopping for groceries and personal items, doing housework, using a telephone, medication management, and having a reliable means of transportation.
- The Lawton–Brody Instrumental Activities of Daily Living Scale is a valid, reliable tool that is scored 0 to 8 for females and 0 to 5 for males. A score of 0 indicates low function and dependence and a score of 5 (for males) or 8 (for females) indicates high functioning and independence.

Nutrition Assessment

- The older adult is at high risk for malnutrition, so nutrition assessments should be part of routine older adult assessments. Nutritional decline often occurs due to preventable factors. Identification and intervention of these underlying factors can make a significant difference in outcomes.
- Asking the older adult about things like dysphagia, problems with dentition or dentures, medication side effects that cause anorexia or nausea, and difficulty handling silverware is important to early identification and intervention.
- There are many valid and reliable nutritional assessment tools available to screen for malnutrition in adults and are typically

used in the nursing home and rehabilitation settings. The Malnutrition Screening Tool (MST) and the Mini Nutritional Assessment* (MNA) are two screening tools that are well known and should be considered if a patient presents with recent weight loss, recent poor intake/appetite, and/or a low BMI. The MST can be found in **Exhibit 17.1**. The MNA can be found at https://www.mna-elderly.com/sites/default/files/2021-10/mna-mini-english.pdf.

Falls Risk Assessment

- Falls are a significant cause of morbidity and loss of independence in the older adult population. Falling once doubles the chances of falling again. Older adults are at higher risk for falls due to a variety of factors including, but not limited to, lower body weakness,

EXHIBIT 17.1 Malnutrition Screening Tool

	Answer	Points
Have you recently lost weight without trying?	No	0
	Unsure	1
If yes, how much weight have you lost? (Answer this question only if *unsure* was marked on the above question.)	2–13 lb	1
	14–23 lb	2
	24–33 lb	3
	34 lb or more	4
	Unsure	2
Have you been eating poorly due to a decreased appetite?	No	0
	Yes	1

Total points

Interpretation of Score for Malnutrition Screening Tool

Risk Category	Total Score
Not at risk	0 or 1
At risk	2+

Source: Reprinted from Ferguson, M., Capra, S., Bauer, J., & Banks, M. (1999). Development of a valid and reliable malnutrition screening tool for adult acute hospital patients. *Nutrition*, *15*, 458–464. https://doi.org/10.1016/S0899-9007(99)00084-2, with permission from Elsevier.

vision problems, home hazards, osteoporosis, difficulties with balance and walking, and vitamin D deficiency.

- The STEADI Algorithm for Fall Risk Screening, Assessment, and Intervention is an evidence-based tool designed to reduce fall risk. It is based on the three-step process of screening, assessing, and intervening where appropriate. This algorithm can be found at www.cdc.gov/steadi/pdf/STEADI-Algorithm-508.pdf.
- There are many other valid and reliable falls risk assessment tools, both for the inpatient setting as well as for the outpatient setting, that can be used with the older adult population.

RECOMMENDED SCREENINGS FOR OLDER ADULTS

- **Hearing, vision, and oral health screenings:** Both hearing and vision decline with aging and can significantly impact quality of life if not identified and corrected. Oral health often declines with age, which puts the older adult at higher risk for dental caries, loose tooth, and periodontal disease. Routine screening and referral to specialists (i.e., optometrists, dentists, and audiologists) are important for maintaining health and function in these areas.
- **Environmental assessment screening:** The goal of completing an environmental assessment is to develop and implement effective strategies to reduce hazards and fall risks and maintain the older adult's ability to function in a safe environment. An assessment can also improve the older adult's accessibility. The Home Safety Checklist assesses 10 domains: housekeeping, floors, bathroom, traffic lanes, lighting, stairways, ladders/step stools, outdoor areas, footwear, and personal precautions. This checklist can be found at https://www.cdc.gov/steadi/pdf/check_for_safety_brochure-a.pdf. Reducing home hazards is an inexpensive intervention to reduce the risk of falls.
- **Depression screening:** Older adults are at an increased risk for depression due to such causes as other serious comorbidities, disability, life changes, and loneliness/social isolation. It can present as grumpiness, irritability, insomnia, attention problems, confusion, or fatigue. The five-item Geriatric Depression Scale is a valid and reliable tool to screen for depression in the older adult. A score of >5 is suggestive of depression and >10 is almost always indicative of depression.

DOCUMENTATION

CHARTING NOTE: WELL-CHILD EXAM

Reason for Seeking Care

A 1-year-old male child (Arris) is here for a routine well-child exam, accompanied by a caregiver (dad).

History of Present Illness
No specific concerns or complaints as reported by dad. Child generally healthy since the last well-child visit at age 9 months. Child "busy, active, and happy" as described by dad. Was breastfed exclusively for the first 6 months of life and currently nurses in the morning and at bedtime.

Medical History
No significant medical history. Vaginal birth. Immunizations up-to-date.

Developmental History
Has been meeting developmental milestones appropriately as reported by caregiver. Can crawl on hands and knees, pull self to standing, cruise around furniture, and walk with one hand held. Speech and language development progressing, says "dada" and three other words. Exhibits nonverbal communication skills, such as waving and pointing. Plays "pat a cake." Feeding skills progressed to self-feeding with table and finger foods. Was very pleased with recent taste of birthday cake as reported by dad.

Review of Systems
- **General:** No fever, weight loss
- **Skin:** No rashes, lesions, or itching
- **Head:** No head injuries
- **Eyes, ears, nose, throat:** No perceived visual difficulties, ear pain, hearing problems; no congestion
- **Respiratory:** No cough, wheezing, or difficulty breathing
- **Gastrointestinal/genitourinary:** Regular pattern of stooling, wet diapers
- **Musculoskeletal:** No limitations in movement
- **Neurologic/psychiatric:** No seizures or recent behavior changes

Physical Examination
- **Temperature:** 37.5°C (temporal scan)
- **Pulse:** 92 per minute with normal rhythm
- **Respiratory rate:** 24 per minute, easy with no retractions
- **Length:** 75th percentile
- **Weight:** 50th percentile
- **Head circumference:** 75th percentile

A 1-year-old male child who is well nourished and hydrated. Awake, alert, and responsive to caregiver. No signs of distress or toxicity. Mucosa pink. Neck supple, no palpable lymphadenopathy. Pupils are equal, round, and reactive to light and accommodation (PERRLA); red reflex intact. Eyes without redness or discharge. Tympanic membranes (TMs) pearly gray with good light reflex bilaterally. No nasal discharge. Oropharynx clear, no visible abnormalities. Breath sounds full, clear and equal bilaterally, respirations easy. Heart rate and rhythm regular, no murmurs or abnormal sounds. Abdomen soft, nontender, and nondistended. No organomegaly or masses palpated. Full range of motion in all extremities on musculoskeletal exam. Motor strength and coordination appropriate for age.

Assessment
Routine well-child exam; healthy 1-year-old meeting developmental milestones

Anticipatory Guidance
- **Diet and nutrition:** Continue to encourage a balanced diet with a variety of fruits, vegetables, and age-appropriate table foods. Offer fluids from a cup.
- **Safety:** Ensure a safe environment for the child, including child-proofing the home, using appropriate car seats, and supervising during play.
- **Oral health:** Begin brushing the child's teeth with a small amount of fluoride toothpaste and schedule the first dental visit.
- **Developmental milestones:** Continue to support the child's development by providing opportunities.

CHARTING NOTE: OLDER ADULT-WELL VISIT
Reason for Seeking Care
A 73-year-old man is here for a routine well visit.

History of Present Illness
Reports feeling well overall. Has recently retired from full-time job. Continues to do activities he has done most of his life. Denies any concerns at this time.

Medical History
Hypertension: Controlled, diagnosed 2009
Hyperlipidemia: Controlled, diagnosed 2009
Benign prostatic hypertrophy: Controlled, diagnosed 2014
Basal cell carcinoma: Removed with clear margins, 2016
Obstructive sleep apnea: Diagnosed 2012, treated with continuous positive airway pressure (CPAP)
Aortic dilation: Mild, sees and monitored by cardiology
Cataract surgery (bilateral): 2016

Medications
Lisinopril 20 mg once daily
Metoprolol succinate 25 mg once daily
Atorvastatin 40 mg once daily
Tamsulosin 0.4 mg once daily
Polyethylene glycol 17 g daily

Family history
Father: Deceased at age 43 due to myocardial infarction
Mother: Deceased at age 76 due to diabetes, pneumonia
Brother: Age 71, rheumatoid arthritis
Brother: Age 69, rheumatoid arthritis
Brother: Age 60, lupus

Social history
Recently retired from engineering business. Lives with his wife of 50+ years. Has three adult daughters and eight grandchildren who he sees regularly. Leads an active lifestyle but has had a sedentary job most of his life. Golfs regularly. Eats a lot of meat and potatoes. Consumes about one fruit/vegetable per day. Denies smoking or recreational drug use. Consumes one to two alcoholic drinks per day. Sexually active with his wife and does not report experiencing any difficulty with sexual drive or intercourse. Sleeps with TV on at night. Has advance directives and living will in order.

Review of Systems
- **General:** No fever, weight loss
- **Skin:** No rashes, lesions, or itching; history of actinic keratosis and basal cell carcinoma (BCC), followed by dermatology
- **Head, eyes, ears, nose, throat:** No perceived visual difficulties, last eye exam 1 year ago, cataracts treated with surgery; denies ear pain or hearing problems; no nasal congestion; last dental cleaning 5 months ago
- **Respiratory:** No cough, wheezing, or difficulty breathing; history of pneumonia; positive exposure to secondhand smoke during childhood, wears CPAP 4 to 5 days a week
- **Gastrointestinal/genitourinary:** Constipation, controlled with polyethylene glycol daily; last colonoscopy 3 years ago; prostate-specific antigen (PSA) checked last year and stable
- **Musculoskeletal:** Occasional aches and pains but nothing chronic or severe; has noted decreased hand strength/grip strength over time
- **Neurologic/psychiatric:** No recent behavior changes; denies difficulty remembering things; denies any falls or feeling unsteady while walking or standing; denies worrying about falling

Physical Examination
- **Temperature:** 37.0°C (oral)
- **Pulse:** 82 per minute with normal rhythm
- **Respiratory rate:** 14 breaths per minute, easy with no retractions
- **Blood pressure:** 130/82 (right), 130/80 (left), sitting
- **Height:** 69 inches
- **Weight:** 180 lb
- **Body mass index (BMI):** 26.6 (up 3 lb from last year)

Alert and oriented × 3. Appears comfortable. Affect and hygiene appropriate. Able to recall three words 5 minutes apart. Neck supple, no palpable lymphadenopathy, no carotid bruits noted bilaterally. Pupils equal, round, and react to light and accommodation (PERRLA). Eyes without redness or discharge. Tympanic membranes (TMs) pearly gray with good light reflex bilaterally. Mild tympanosclerosis noted on left TM at 3 o'clock. Whisper test failed bilateral. No nasal discharge. Oropharynx clear, no visible abnormalities. Dentition intact with tooth 11 missing. No oral caries noted. Breath sounds clear and equal without adventitious breath sounds bilaterally, respirations easy. Heart rate and rhythm regular, no murmurs or abnormal sounds. Abdomen soft, nontender, and nondistended. No visible pulsations, organomegaly, or masses palpated. Full range of motion in all extremities on musculoskeletal exam. Motor strength and coordination appropriate for age. Grip strength 4/5 bilateral.

Timed Up and Go test: 10 seconds
Katz Index score: 6
Lawton–Brody Instrumental Activities of Daily Living Scale score: 5
Nutrition screening: Deferred due to BMI
Geriatric Depression Scale score: 3

Assessment
Routine well visit

Plan
Refer for hearing evaluation.
Recommend 30 minutes of exercise 5 days a week.
Recommend 5+ fruits and vegetables a day.
Wear CPAP nightly.
Continue to follow with cardiology and dermatology.
Arrange environmental assessment screening.

REFERENCES

References for this chapter draw from Chapter 5, Evidence-Based Assessment of Children and Adolescents, Chapter 6, Evidence-Based Assessment of the Older Adult, Chapter 22, Evidence-Based Assessment of the Male Genitalia, Prostate, Rectum, and Anus, and Chapter 23, Evidence-Based Assessment of the Female Genitourinary System, of the textbook *Evidence-Based Physical Examination: Best Practices for Health and Well-Being Assessment (Second Edition)*. The references may be accessed in the digital version of the handbook at https://connect.springerpub.com/.

Index

abdomen and gastrointestinal and urological systems, 260–288
  abdominal aortic aneurysm, 281
  abdominal pain, 275–285
  abdominal palpation, 269
  abdominal percussion technique, 266
  abnormal findings, 274–275
  acute pancreatitis, 276–277
  allergies, 263
  appendicitis, 278
  auscultation, 265–266
    of abdominal aorta, 266
    of renal arteries, 266
  Blumberg's Sign, 272
  celiac disease, 282
  cholecystitis/cholelithiasis, 277
  clinical considerations, 260
  common reasons for seeking care, 260
  constipation, 274–275
  Cullen's sign, 265
  deep palpation, 269
  diarrhea, 275
  differential diagnoses according to localization of pain, 276
  digital rectal examination, 273
  documentation, physical examination, 288
  family history, 263
  gastroesophageal reflux disease/dyspepsia, 283
  gastroparesis, 282
  general survey, 265
  Hackett's grading system for palpable spleen, 270, 271
  health history, 262–263
  heel drop test (Markle test or heel jar test), 273
  hepatitis, 277–278
  history, 274–275
    of present illness, 261–262
  immunizations, 263
  inspection, 265
  irritable bowel syndrome, 283–284
  left lower quadrant pain, 280–281
  left upper quadrant pain, 279–280
  light palpation, 269
  liver palpation, 269–270
  lower urinary tract infection, 285–286
  McBurney's point, 272
  past medical history, 262
  medications, 262
  Murphy's sign, 273–274
  older adults, 274
  palpation, 268–272
  pediatric considerations, 263, 274
  peptic ulcer disease, 284
  percussion, 266–268
  peritonitis, 284–285

abdomen and gastrointestinal and urological systems (*continued*)
periumbilical/epigastric pain, 281–285
physical examination, 261, 264
psoas test, 273
pyelonephritis, 286
regional ileitis/Crohn's Disease, 279
renal colic (urolithiasis, ureterolithiasis), 286–287
review of systems, 264
right lower quadrant pain, 278–279
right upper quadrant pain, 276–278
Rovsing's sign, 273
scratch test, 270
sigmoid diverticulosis/ diverticulitis, 280–281
small bowel obstruction, 285
social history, 263–264
special tests for the abdomen, 272–274
subjective history, 260–264
Traube's space, 267
ulcerative colitis, 281
urinary incontinence, 287–288
urinary system, abnormal findings, 285–288
abdominal aortic aneurysm, 52
abdominal reflex, 207
Achilles reflex, 208
acne, 102–103
actinic keratosis, 103
acute bronchitis, 78–79
acute coronary syndrome, 52–53
acute mild traumatic brain injury (concussion), 140
acute respiratory distress, red flags, 77–78
adnexal masses, 338–340
adults. *See also* older adults
BMI classification, 26
documentation of general survey, example, 33
hypertension, 29
overweight/obesity, 30–31
anal fissures, 305
anaphylactic shock, 30
ankle/foot anatomy, 247–248
anorectal agenesis/imperforate anus, 299
anterior drawer test, 244–245
aorta, coarctation, 56–57
apprehension test, 236
ASCVD risk calculator, 54
assessment across life span, 395–396
activities of daily living assessment, 414
adolescent considerations, 395–396
physical exam, 402, 408
screenings for, 408
caregivers as historians, 412
clinical considerations, 393
developmental milestones of early childhood, 403–407
falls risk assessment, 415–416
female sexual maturity stages, 409–410
functional mobility assessment, 413–414
instrumental activities of daily living assessment, 414
malnutrition screening tool, 415
mental health assessment, 413
nutrition assessment, 414–415
older adult-well visit, charting note, 418–420
older adults
as historians, 411–412
physical exam, 412
recommended screenings, 416

targeted assessments, 413–416
pediatric considerations, 393–395
physical exam, 397–402
screenings for, 408
red flags
developmental delay, 408
in history and physical exam, 411
sexual maturity rating, 408
subjective history, 411
well-child exam, charting note, 416–418
asthma, 79
atherosclerosis, 53–55
atrial septal defect, 55
attention deficit hyperactivity disorder, 378–379
axial traction test, 230
axillae, 121

balanitis and balanoposthitis, 302
Barlow–Ortolani Maneuvers, 249, 250
Bartholin gland cyst, 336
basal cell carcinoma, 104
bed bug bites, 104
Bell's palsy, 213
benign prostatic hyperplasia, 306
blood pressure, 40
body habitus
BMI calculation, 26
height, 25
pediatric, 28
waist and other circumferences, 26–28
weight, 25–26
body mass index
calculation, 26
waist and other circumferences, 26–28
breasts
abnormal findings of the breast and axillae, 324–329
accessory breast tissue, 324
allergies, 312
benign breast mass or lump, 324–325
breast cyst, 324–325
clinical considerations, 309
clinical exam, 314–316
common reasons for seeking care, 310
family history, 313
fibroadenoma, 325
health history, 310–312
past health history, 312
history of present illness, 310
inflammatory breast cancer, 325–326
inspection, 315
invasive ductal carcinomas, 326
invasive lobular carcinomas, 326–327
life-span/special population considerations, 322–323
mastalgia or mastodynia, 327–328
mastitis, 328
medications, 312
nipple discharge, galactorrhea, 328–329
objective exam
red flags in, 323
Paget's disease of the breast, 327
palpation methods, 316
physical examination documentation, 341
quadrants, 315
review of systems, 313–314
sexual history, 312–313
social history, 313
subjective history, 310–314
bronchial breath sounds, 75
bronchiolitis, 79–80
bronchovesicular breath sounds, 75
Brudzinski sign, 211

cachexia, 32
cardiogenic shock, 30
caregivers, as historians,
 393–394, 412
carpal tunnel syndrome, 251
cat scratch disease, 125
cellulitis, 104–105
cervical intraepithelial neoplasia
 and cervical malignancies, 337
cervical spine, 228–229
chest inspection, 40–41
children
 BMI classification, 26
 developmental milestones,
  403–407
 documentation of general
  survey, example, 33–34
 growth and developmental
  assessment, 28
 as historians, 394–395
 overweight/obesity, 30–31
 rashes, 97–101
 recommended screenings
  for, 408
 vital signs, 23–24
chlamydia, 329–330
chronic obstructive pulmonary
 disease, 80
chronic venous insufficiency, 56
compartment syndrome,
 251–252
congestive heart failure, 57–58
contact dermatitis, 105–106
coronary artery disease, 53–55
crackles, 76

De Quervain syndrome, 252
deep vein thrombosis, 58–59
drop arm test, 235–236
drug-induced shock, 30
Dupuytren contracture,
 252–253

ears, nose, and throat, 180–192
 adult ear exam technique.,
  173

air and bone conduction,
 175–176
allergic rhinitis, 185–186
allergies, 171
angioedema, 189–190
aphthous ulcer, 190
audiometry, 176
auditory acuity, 174–175
cholesteatoma, 181–182
clinical considerations, 169
common reasons for seeking
 care, 169
conductive and sensorineural
 hearing loss, 185
documentation physical
 examination, 193
epistaxis, 187–188
eustachian tube dysfunction,
 182
evidence-based assessment,
 169
family history, 172
finger rub test, 175
health history, 170–172
hearing loss, 182
herpangina, 190–191
history, 180, 181, 182
 of present illness, 169–170
immunizations, 172
inspection, 173–174
inspection and palpation of
 the tongue, 179
leukoplakia, 191
lips, 177
malignant otitis externa, 185
medications, 171
mouth, 177
nasal polyp, 188
nasal/oral cancers, 192
nonallergic rhinitis, 186
nose, 185–189
nose and sinuses, 176–177
oral candidiasis, 191–192
oral cavity and posterior
 pharynx, 178
oral examination, 178

otitis media with effusion, 181
otoscope, use of, 177
palpation, 174
  of mouth and jaw, 178–179
paranasal sinuses, 187
pediatric considerations, 172,
  176, 179
physical examination,
  173–179, 180, 185
pneumatic otoscopy, 174
posterior pharynx, 178
review of systems, 172–173
Rinne test, 175–176
septal perforation, 188–189
sinusitis, 186–187
social history, 172
subjective history, 169
  red flags, 173
temporal mandibular
  joint, 179
tinnitus, 185
tongue, 177–178
Weber Screening Test, 175
ectopic pregnancy, 339
eczema (atopic dermatitis), 106
edema, 50
Eichhoff test, 240
elbow, 236, 237
empty can/jobe test, 234–235
endocrine shock, 30
endometriosis, 340–341
environmental exposure
  neurologic system, 197
  respiratory diseases, 69
epidermoid cyst (sebaceous
  cyst), 107
epididymitis, orchitis, and scrotal
  cellulitis, 302
epidural hematoma, 138
epilepsy, 214–215
epispadias and hypospadias, 299
erythema migrans, 107–108
external rotation resistance
  test, 236
eye
  accommodation reflex, 150

acute angle-closure
  glaucoma, 148, 159
allergic conjunctivitis,
  156–157
allergies, 147
bacterial conjunctivitis, 157
cataracts, 156
clinical considerations, 145
common reasons for seeking
  care, 145–146
conjunctivitis, 156–158
corneal abrasion, 158
corneal light reflex, 149
dacryostenosis, 158
diplopia, 159
direct ophthalmoscopy,
  152–153
documentation, physical
  examination, 167
episcleritis, 164–165
extraocular muscles, 151–152
family history, 147
glaucoma, 159–160
Hirschberg test, 149
history of present illness, 146
inspection, 148
macular degeneration, 160
past medical history, 146–147
medications, 147
older adult, 155
open-angle glaucoma,
  159–160
optic neuritis and retrobulbar
  neuritis, 160–161
orbital and periorbital
  cellulitis, 161
pediatric binocular
  assessment, 149
pediatric considerations, 154
physical examination, 148
pingueculum, 161–162
pregnancy considerations,
  155
preventive care
  considerations, 147
pterygium, 162

eye (*continued*)
  pupillary light reflex, 150
  red flags
    in objective exam, 155
    in subjective history, 148
  red reflex, 153
  retinal abnormalities, 162
  retinopathy, 163–164
  review of systems, 147–148
  scleritis, 164–165
  Snellen visual acuity chart,
    153, 154
  social history, 147
  strabismus, 165
  sty (hordeolum), 165–166
  subconjunctival hemorrhage,
    166
  uveitis, 167
  viral conjunctivitis, 157–158
  visual acuity, 153–154
  visual field testing, 150–151

FABER test, 242
facial fractures, 139
female genitalia, and
  reproductive system,
  309–341. *See also* vaginitis/
  vaginosis
  abnormal findings of the
    female genitalia, 329–341
  Bartholin gland cyst, 336
  chlamydia, 329–330
  genital herpes, 332
  genital warts, 331–332
  gonorrhea, 329
  health history, 311
  history, 331
  physical examination,
    314–323
  red flags in subjective history,
    314
  sexually transmitted
    infections, 329–333
  syphilis, 330–331
  trichomoniasis, 330
  urethral caruncle, 336

female sexual maturity stages,
  409–410
Finkelstein test, 240
flexion, abduction, and external
  rotation test, 242, 243
folliculitis, 108

general survey including vital
  signs
  abnormal findings, 28–29
  body habitus, 25–28
  cachexia, 32
  clinical assessment, 11
  common reasons for seeking
    care, 11–12
  documentation of physical
    exam, 33–34
  family history, 14
  history of present illness, 13
  hypertension, 29
  malnutrition, 30
  past medical history, 13
  medications, 13–14
  mental status assessment,
    16–17
  nutritional assessment, 15
  overweight/obesity, 30–31
  pain assessment, 15–16
  pediatric growth and
    developmental
    development, 28
  physical examination, 16
  physiologic stability, 12–13
  prescribed and OTC
    medications, 13
  red flags in emergent
    distress, 12
  review of systems, 14–15
  sarcopenia, 32
  shock, 29–30
  social history, 14
  undernutrition, 30
  vital signs measurement,
    17–25
  weight gain, 31
  weight loss, 31

genetic counseling, 4
genital herpes, 332
genital warts, 331–332
gonorrhea, 329
gout, 253
Gower's sign, 254, 255

hand and wrist bones, 239
Hawkins–Kennedy test, 234
head injury or trauma, 138–140
headache, 137–138
head and neck
  acute, mild traumatic brain
    injury (concussion), 140
  allergies, 131
  auscultation and percussion,
    135
  clinical considerations, 130
  cluster headaches, 138
  common reasons for seeking
    care, 130
  documentation, physical
    examination, 143
  epidural hematoma, 138
  facial fractures, 139
  family history, 132
  head ache, 137–138
  head injury or trauma,
    138–140
  history of present illness,
    130–131
  hyperparathyroidism,
    140–141
  hyperthyroidism, 142
  hypoparathyroidism, 140
  hypothyroidism, 141
  immunizations, 132
  inspection, 133
  past medical history, 131
  medications, 131
  migraine headache, 137
  palpation, 133–135
  parathyroid disorders,
    140–141
  pediatric considerations,
    135–136

pediatric craniofacial
    disorders, 142–143
  red flags
    in objective exam, 136–137
    in subjective history,
      132–133
  review of systems, 132
  secondary headache, risk
    indicators, 133
  skull fractures, 139
  social history, 132
  tension-type headache,
    137–138
  thyroid cancer, 142
  thyroid disorders, 141–142
  traumatic brain injury red
    flags, 137
heart and vascular system
  abdomen, 47
  abdominal aortic aneurysm,
    52
  abnormal findings, 52
  acute coronary syndrome,
    52–53
  allergies, 37
  aorta, coarctation, 56–57
  ASCVD risk calculator, 54
  atherosclerosis, 53–55
  atrial septal defect, 55
  auscultation, 41–42, 47
  blood pressure and vital sign
    assessment, 40
  chest inspection, 40–42
  chronic venous insufficiency,
    56
  clinical consideration, 35
  common reasons for seeking
    care, 35
  congestive heart failure,
    57–58
  coronary artery disease,
    53–55
  deep vein thrombosis, 58–59
  documentation, physical
    examination, 65
  edema, 50

heart and vascular system
(*continued*)
  extremities, 48
  family history, 38
  general survey, 39
  history of present illness,
    35–36
  hypertension, 59
  jugular venous pressure, 46
  past medical history, 36–37
  medications, 37
  mitral valve prolapse, 60–61
  older adults, 50
  palpation, 41, 42–45, 46–47
  pediatric considerations,
    37–38
  pericarditis, 61
  peripheral artery disease,
    61–62
  peripheral vascular
    examination, 45–47
  physical examination, 39
  pulses, grading scale, 50
  Raynaud phenomenon,
    62–63
  red flags in subjective history,
    36, 51
  review of systems, 38–39
  rheumatic heart disease, 63
  seated position examination,
    40–42
  social history, 38
  supine position, 42–47
  tetralogy of Fallot, 63–64
  ventricular septal defect, 64
  Wells' clinical protection
    tool, 59
HEEADSSS assessment domains,
  396–397
heel-to-shin test, 203–204
hernia, 296
herpes zoster (shingles),
  108–109
hip, 241–242
history taking
  chronic care management, 8

common reasons for seeking
  care, 2
episodic visit, 1
family history, 3–4
history of present illness
  (HPI), 2
key consideration, 7
past medical history, 2–3
preventive care
  considerations, 6
process, 1
review of systems, 6–7
social determinants
  of health, 5
social history, 4–5
therapeutic communication, 9
wellness exam, 7–8
human immunodeficiency virus/
  acquired immunodeficiency
  syndrome, 125–126
hydrocele, 300
hyperparathyroidism, 140–141
hypertension, 59
hyperthermia, 28
hypoparathyroidism, 140
hypothermia, 28–29
hypothyroidism, 142
hypovolemic shock, 30

immunizations, 68, 89, 118, 132,
  172, 196, 263
infants, skin, hair, and nails,
  92, 102
inguinal, 123
  hernias, 296

jugular venous pressure, 46

knee, 243

Lachman test, 245
Lasègue's test, 232
lateral epicondylitis (tennis
  elbow), 253
Legg–Calve–Perthes diseases,
  253–254

lifestyle behaviors
   neurologic system, 197
   respiratory disease, 69
lumbar spine, 232
lung cancer, 82
lungs and respiratory system
   acute bronchitis, 78–79
   allergies, 68
   asthma, 79
   auscultation, 74–77
   breathing patterns, 78
   bronchiolitis, 79–80
   chronic obstructive
      pulmonary disease, 80
   clinical consideration, 66
   common reasons for seeking
      care, 66
   cystic fibrosis, 81
   documentation, physical
      examination, 85
   family history, 69
   history of present illness,
      66–67
   immunizations, 68
   influenza, 82
   lung cancer, 82
   past medical history, 67
   medications, 68
   obstructive sleep apnea, 83
   older adult, 77
   palpation, 72–73
   pediatric considerations,
      68, 77
   percussion, 73–74
   peripheral assessment, 71
   pertussis, 83
   physical examination, 71
   pneumonia, 83–84
   pneumothorax, 84
   pulmonary embolus, risk
      indicators, 70–71
   red flags
      in acute respiratory distress,
         77–78
      in objective exam, 77–78
      in subjective history, 70–71

   review of systems, 70
   SARS-CoV-2 (COVID-19),
      80–81
   social history, 69
   subjective history, red flags,
      70–71
   thoracic cage and chest
      movement, 72
   tuberculosis, 84–85
lymphadenitis, 126
lymphangitis, 126–127
lymphatic filariasis, 127
lymphatic system
   axillae, 121
   cat scratch disease, 125
   clinical consideration, 117
   common reasons for seeking
      care, 117
   documentation, physical
      examination, 129
   family history, 118
   head and neck, 120–121
   history of present illness,
      117–118
   human immunodeficiency
      virus/acquired
      immunodeficiency
      syndrome, 125–126
   immunizations, 118
   inguinal, 123
   inspection, 119
   lymphadenitis, 126
   lymphangitis, 126–127
   lymphatic filariasis, 127
   lymphedema, 127–128
   lymphoma, 128
   past medical history, 118
   medications, 118
   mononucleosis (or mono),
      128–129
   older adult, 125
   palpation, 120
   pediatric considerations,
      124
   physical examination,
      119

lymphatic system (*continued*)
  red flags
    in objective physical
      examination, 124
    in subjective history, 119
  review of systems, 119
  social history, 118–119
lymphedema, 127–128
lymphoma, 128

male genital candidiasis,
  302–303
male genitalia, prostate, rectum,
  and anus, 289–308
  abnormal findings, 299–307
  abnormalities, 304–305
  additional assessments
    for specific conditions,
    295–297
  anal fissures, 305
  anorectal agenesis/
    imperforate anus, 299
  assessment for hernia, 296
  balanitis and balanoposthitis,
    302
  benign prostatic hyperplasia,
    306
  clinical considerations, 289
  common reason for seeking
    care, 290
  condyloma, 304
  congenital or developmental
    abnormalities, 299–302
  cremasteric reflex, 295
  digital rectal examination,
    296–297
  documentation, physical
    examination, 307–308
  epididymitis, orchitis, and
    scrotal cellulitis, 302
  epispadias and hypospadias,
    299
  external and internal
    hemorrhoids, 305–306
  health history, 290–293
  history of present illness, 290

hydrocele, 300
infection or inflammatory
  disorders, 302–304
inguinal hernias, 296
inspection, 294–295
male genital candidiasis,
  302–303
manifestations of systemic
  conditions, 304
nonspecific urethritis, 303
older adults, 298
other abnormalities, 304–305
palpation test, 295
pediatric considerations,
  297–298
  digital rectal examination,
    296–297
Peyronie disease, 304
phimosis/paraphimosis, 300
physical examination, 294
prostate cancer, 306
rectal polyps and rectal
  cancer, 307
red flags
  in objective exam,
    298–299
  in subjective history, 294
review of systems, 293–294
sexually transmitted
  infections, 303–304
skin cancer, 304–305
subjective history, 290–294
technique for assessing
  inguinal hernias, 297
testicular torsion, 300–301
testicular tumor/malignancy,
  305
transillumination, 295
undescended testes, 301
varicocele, 301–302
malnutrition, 30
McMurray's test, 246
melanoma, 109
mental health/substance use
  disorders, 363–391
  ABSATTC mnemonic, 17

addiction, 387
adolescent considerations, 388
adult with symptoms of depression, example charting note for, 390–391
  assessment, 391
  chief concern, 390
  family history, 390
  history of present illness, 390
  medical and psychiatric review of systems, 391
  past medical and psychiatric health history, 390
  patient information, 390
  physical exam/mental status evaluation, 391
  social history, 391
alcohol use disorder, 387–388
anxiety and anxiety disorders, 377–378
attention deficit hyperactivity disorder, 378–379
clinical considerations, 363
common reasons for seeking care, 364
comprehensive mental health assessment, 363–377
considerations for the older adult, 388–389
depression and anxiety, 364–365
depression and mood disorders, 379–381
example of normal physical exam findings, 390
family history, 370
generalized anxiety disorder scale, 368–369
health history, 367–369
history of present illness, 364–367
history/physical examination documentation, 389–391
impact on families, 389

life-span and family considerations, 388–389
past medical history, 367–369
medical review of systems, 372
mental health disorders, 377–384
mental status evaluation, 372–373
misusingalcohol, 365–366
newborns and neonatal abstinence syndrome, 388
opioid use disorder, 388
patient health questionnaire, 368
physical examination considerations, 374–375
  objective exam, red flags in, 374–375
past psychiatric history, 367
psychiatric review of systems, 367, 368–369
recovery, 389
single-question screenings for substance use, 369
social history, 370–371
strengths, goals/preventive care considerations, 376
substance use history, 367
tobacco use disorder, 388
trauma and stressor-related disorders, 383–384
mental status evaluation (MSE), 372–373
migraine headache, 137
mitral valve prolapse, 60–61
mononucleosis (or mono), 128–129
muscle strength scale, 226
muscular dystrophy, 254
musculoskeletal system, 222–259
  abnormal findings, 251
  additional pediatric exams, 249
  ankle/foot anatomy, 247–248

musculoskeletal system
(*continued*)
    anterior drawer test, 244–245
    apprehension test, 246–247
    area of snuffbox tenderness,
        239
    carpal tunnel syndrome, 251
    cervical spine, 228–229
    clinical considerations, 222
    common reasons for seeking
        care, 222
    compartment syndrome,
        251–252
    De Quervain syndrome, 252
    dermatomes/myotomes
        of the lower and upper
        extremity, 229, 232
    documentation physical
        examination, 258–259
    hand and wrist bones, 239
    Hawkins–Kennedy test, 234
    head, 226–228
    health history, 223–224
    hip, 241–242
    history, 255
    history of present illness,
        222–223
    knee, 243
    movements, types, 227
    Neer test, 234
    Osgood–Schlatter disease,
        254–255
    osteoarthritis, 255–256
    painful arc test, 235
    palpation, 226
        of spinal processes, 231
    pediatric/adolescent
        considerations, 224
    Phalen test, 240
    physical examination,
        225, 255
    radial head subluxation,
        256–257
    range of motion and special
        tests, 226
    red flags in history and
        physical exam, 225
    review of systems, 225
    rheumatoid arthritis, 257
    rotator cuff tear, 257–258
    scoliosis, 249–250
    shoulder bones, 232–233
    slipped capital femoral
        epiphysis, 258
    social history, 224
    spinal column, 231
    Spurling test, 230
    squeeze test, 248
    Stinchfield test, 242–243
    straight leg raise, 232
    subjective history, 222
    Thomas test, 242
    thoracic/lumbar spine,
        230–232
    Tinel sign, 238
    Trendelenburg test, 243
    valgus stress test, 244
    varus and valgus stress test,
        237
    wrist/hand, 238–239

neurogenic shock, 29
neurologic system, 194–221
    Achilles reflex, 208
    allergies, 196
    Bell's palsy, 213
    biceps and brachioradialis,
        206
    biceps reflex, 207–208
    brachioradialis reflex, 208
    Brudzinski sign, 211
    cerebral palsy, 213–214
    clinical considerations, 194
    common reasons for seeking
        care, 194
    comorbidities or risk factors
        related to neurological
        diseases, 196
    cortical sensory function,
        211–212

corticospinal, basal ganglia, and cerebellar motor pathways, 205
cranial nerve documentation, 221
cranial nerves, 198–203
deep tendon reflexes, 207–208
documentation, physical examination, 221
epilepsy, 214–215
family history, 197
finger abduction, 206
foot/ankle, 206–207
graphesthesia, 211
grip strength, 206
health history, 195–197
hemorrhagic stroke, 215
hip, 206
history and physical exam, 212
history of present illness, 194–195
immunizations, 196
intracranial tumor, 215–216
ischemic stroke, 216–217
joint position sense, 210–211
Kernig sign, 212
knee, 206
past medical history, 195
medications, 196
meningitis, 217
mental status examination, 198
multiple sclerosis, 217–218
muscle strength, 206–207
myasthenia gravis, 218–219
neurological disorders, 197
Parkinson disease, 219
patellar reflex test, 208
pediatric considerations, 196–197
peripheral neuropathy, 220
physical examination, 198–212
primary sensory functions, 210
primitive reflex testing in infancy, 209
pronator drift testing, 205
proprioception and cerebellar function, 203–207
reflexes, 207–209
review of systems, 197–198
sensory function, 209–211
social history, 197
special tests, 211–212
subjective history, 194–195
thumb opposition, 206
trauma, 195
triceps reflex, 208–209
trigeminal neuralgia, 220–221
tuning fork, testing, 210
two-point discrimination test, 211
wrist, 206
neuropathic pain, 15
nociceptive pain, 15
nutritional status, 15

obstetric assessment, 343–361
advanced maternal age, 348–349
allergies, 346
clinical considerations, 343
common reasons for seeking care, 343
family history, 346–347
gynecologic history, 346
health history, 344–346
history of present illness, 343–344
past medical history, 344–345
medications, 346
objective exam red flags, 344
obstetric history, 345–346
obstructive sleep apnea, 83
preventive care considerations, 348

obstetric assessment (*continued*)
  review of systems, 347–348
  social history, 347
  subjective history, 343–349
    red flags, 344
  trauma-informed care, 349
  unique population
    considerations, 348–349
older adult
  activities of daily living
    assessment, 414
  charting note, 418–420
  falls risk assessment, 415–416
  functional mobility
    assessment, 413–414
  heart and vascular system, 50
  as historians, 411–412
  instrumental activities of
    daily living assessment, 414
  lungs and respiratory
    system, 77
  lymphatic system, 125
  malnutrition screening
    tool, 415
  mental health/substance use
    disorders, 363–391
  nutrition assessment,
    414–415
  physical exam, 412
  prostate cancer, 306
  recommended screenings,
    416
  red flags in history and
    physical exam, 411
  skin, hair and nails, 89–90,
    102
  subjective history, 411
  targeted assessments, 413
onychomycosis, 109–110
ovarian cancer, 339
ovarian cysts, 339
overweight/obesity, 30–31

pain
  assessment, 15
  evidence-based tool, 16

types, 15
parathyroid disorders, 140–141
Parkinson disease, 219
pediatric considerations
  anogenital examination,
    297–298
  anxiety disorders, 377–378
  assessment across life span,
    393–395
    physical exam, 397–402
  depression, 379–381
  ear, nose, throat, 172, 176
  gastrointestinal and
    urological systems, 274
  head and neck, 135–136
  hearing problem, 179
  heart and vascular system,
    37–38
  lungs and respiratory
    system, 68
  lymphatic system, 124
  male genitalia, prostate,
    rectum, and anus,
    297–298
  musculoskeletal system, 224
  neurologic system, 196–197
  respiratory disease, 77
  skin, hair, and nails, 89, 92
  vision assessment, 154
peripheral artery disease, 61–62
peripheral assessment, lungs
  and respiratory system, 71
pertussis, 83
pityriasis rosea, 110
pivot shift, 245–246
plantar reflex, 207
pleural rub, 77
pneumonia, 83–84
pneumothorax, 84
polycystic ovarian syndrome
  (PCOS), 340
posterior drawer test, 245
pregnancy, 349–353
  abnormal findings, 354–361
  acute cystitis (urinary tract
    infection), 354

anemia in pregnancy, 354–355
asymptomatic bacteriuria, 355
auscultation, 352
changes in fundal height, 350
chronic or gestational hypertension, 358
constipation, 355–356
eclampsia, 359
fetal station, 353
first-trimester bleeding, 356–357
  benign, 356
general survey, 349
gestational diabetes mellitus, 357
gestational thrombocytopenia, 360–361
hyperemesis gravidarum, 359–360
hypertensive disorders, 358–361
inspection, 349–350
Leopold's maneuvers, 352
measurement of fundal height, 351
miscarriage, 356–357
normal findings from first, 361
palpation, 350–352
physical examination documentation, 361
population considerations, 348–349
preeclampsia, 358–359
pruritic urticarial papules and plaques of pregnancy, 360
weight gain, 353
preterm infants, skin, hair and nails, 92
prostate cancer, 306
psoriasis, 110–111
pulmonary embolus, risk indicators, 70–71
pulses, grading scale, 50

Raynaud phenomenon, heart and vascular system, 62–63
rheumatic heart disease, 63
rheumatoid arthritis, 257
rhonchi, 75
Rinne test, 175–176
rosacea (acne rosacea), 111–112

sarcopenia, 32
SARS-CoV-2 (COVID-19), 80–81
scabies, 112
scoliosis, 249–250
sensory function, 209–211
  monofilament test, 209–210
  testing superficial pain with Wartenberg wheel, 210
  testing vibration with a low-pitched tuning fork, 210
septic shock, 29
sexual maturity rating, 408
shock
  definition, 29
  septic, 29
  types, 29–30
shoulder, 232–233
skin, hair, and nails
  abnormal findings, 102–115
  acne, 102–103
  actinic keratosis, 103
  allergies, 89
  basal cell carcinoma, 104
  bed bug bites, 104
  cellulitis, 104–105
  clinical consideration, 87
  common reasons for seeking care, 87
  contact dermatitis, 105–106
  documentation, physical examination, 115–116
  eczema (atopic dermatitis), 106
  epidermoid cyst (sebaceous cyst), 107
  erythema migrans, 107–108

skin, hair, and nails (*continued*)
  family history, 90
  folliculitis, 108
  herpes zoster (shingles),
    108–109
  history of present illness,
    87–88
  immunizations, 89
  infants, children, and
    adolescents, 92, 102
  inspection, 92
  past medical history, 88–89
  medications, 89
  melanoma, 109
  older adults, 89–90, 102
  onychomycosis, 109–110
  palpation, 92
  pediatric considerations, 89
  physical examination, 91
  pityriasis rosea, 110
  preterm infants, 92
  primary and secondary skin
    lesions, 93–96
  psoriasis, 110–111
  red flags
    in subjective history, 91
  review of system, 90–91
  rosacea (acne rosacea),
    111–112
  scabies, 112
  social history, 90
  specific populations, 102
  squamous cell carcinoma,
    113
  tinea corporis, 113–114
  tinea versicolor, 114
  urticaria (hives), 114–115
  verruca vulgaris (warts), 115
skull fractures, 139
slipped capital femoral
  epiphysis, 258
somatic pain, 15
spinal column, 228
Spurling test, 229, 230
squamous cell carcinoma, 113
squeeze arm test, 230

squeeze test, 248
Stinchfield test, 242–243
straight leg raise (SLR), 232
stridor, 77
substance use disorders,
  384–389
  diagnostic criteria, 385
  misuse of substances, 384
  substance-specific
    withdrawal symptoms,
    386–387
sulcus sign, 236
superficial reflexes, 207
systemic inflammatory response
  syndrome, 29

testicular torsion, 300–301
testicular tumor/malignancy,
  305
tetralogy of Fallot (TOF), 63–64
thessaly test, 246
Thomas test, 242
thoracic/lumbar spine, 230–232
thought disorders and severe
  mental illness, 382–383
  delirium, 382
  delusions, 382
  dementia, 383
  hallucinations, 383
throat, 189–192
  acute pharyngitis, 189
  aphthous ulcer, 190
  strep pharyngitis, 189
thyroid cancer, 142
tinea corporis, 113–114
tinea versicolor, 114
Tinel sign, 238
tobacco use disorder, 5 As
  intervention steps, 69
toxin-induced shock, 30
tracheal breath sounds, 75
transillumination, 295
Traube's space, 267
Trendelenburg test, 243
triceps reflex, 208–209
tuberculosis, 84–85

ulcerative colitis, 281
undernutrition, 30
urinary incontinence, 287–288
urticaria (hives), 114–115
uterine fibroids, 339–340
uterus bimanual exam, 319–321

vaginitis/vaginosis, 333–334
   bacterial vaginosis, 333
   genitourinary syndrome of
     menopause, 334
   vulvar cancers, 335–336
valgus stress test, 244
varicocele, 301–302
varus and valgus stress test, 237
varus stress test, 244
vasomotor symptoms (VMS), 341

ventricular septal defect, 64
verruca vulgaris (warts), 115
vesicular breath sounds, 75
visceral pain, 15
vital signs
   assessment, 40
   blood pressure, 20–22
   pulse rate, 19
   respiratory rate, 19–20
   temperature measurement,
     17–19

weight gain, 31
weight loss, 31
Wells' clinical prediction tool, 59
wheezes, 75
wrist/hand, 238–239